PUBLIC HEALTH IN THE 21ST CENTURY

COVID-19

FROM HEALTH, EDUCATION, ECONOMIC, TO SCIENCE AND TECHNOLOGY IN SOUTH EAST ASIA AND INDIA

PUBLIC HEALTH IN THE 21ST CENTURY

Additional books and e-books in this series can be found
on Nova's website under the Series tab.

PUBLIC HEALTH IN THE 21ST CENTURY

COVID-19

FROM HEALTH, EDUCATION, ECONOMIC, TO SCIENCE AND TECHNOLOGY IN SOUTH EAST ASIA AND INDIA

ASEP BAYU DANI NANDIYANTO
TRYASTUTI IRAWATI BELLINY MANULLANG
RINA MARYANTI
AMIR MACHMUD
A. ANA
AND
ASNUL DAHAR BIN MINGHAT
EDITORS

nova
Medicine & Health
New York

Library of Congress Cataloging-in-Publication Data

Names: Bayu Dani Nandiyanto, Asep, editor.
Title: COVID-19 : from health, education, economic, to science and technology in South East Asia and India / Asep Bayu Dani Nandiyanto, Universitas Pendidikan Indonesia, Bandung, Indonesia [and five others], editors.
Description: New York : Nova Science Publishers, undefined |
Identifiers: LCCN 2020052497 (print) | LCCN 2020052498 (ebook) | ISBN 9781536189032 (hardcover) | ISBN 9781536189926 (adobe pdf)
Subjects: LCSH: COVID-19 (Disease)--Health aspects--Southeast Asia. | COVID-19 (Disease)--Social aspects--Southeast Asia. | COVID-19 (Disease)--Economic aspects--Southeast Asia. | COVID-19 (Disease)--Health aspects--India. | COVID-19 (Disease)--Social aspects--India. | COVID-19 (Disease)--Economic aspects--India.
Classification: LCC RA644.C67 C6834 2021 (print) | LCC RA644.C67 (ebook) | DDC 362.1962/4140959--dc23
LC record available at https://lccn.loc.gov/2020052497
LC ebook record available at https://lccn.loc.gov/2020052498

Published by Nova Science Publishers, Inc. † New York

CONTENTS

PREFACE

This book presents significant results from South East Asia and India in selected areas of health, education, economic, to science and technology during the Corona virus disease 2019 (COVID-19) pandemic outbreak. COVID-19 emerged in December 2019 in China and has been a viral disease as it continues to spread in almost all the countries of the world. It has put us in unprecedented situation and has changed our daily activities. It has also encouraged researchers to scrutinize its effects in our life. Therefore, this new book attempts to share information and scientific evidence and to provide an overview of the topic. This book consists of seven sections, in which each section contains several chapters.

Section one discusses the introduction to COVID-19 and contains one chapter which is written in Chapter 1. In Chapter 1, the authors will give a brief description about the COVID-19 and how it has affected our economic, health, education, science and technology.

Section two explains the general condition of COVID-19. This section consists of five chapters (Chapters 2-6). Chapter 2 deals with a glimpse of the COVID-19 outbreak around the globe. It is based on the review of some literature. The authors will discuss the cause for the coronavirus, the transmission, the epidemiology and the management of COVID-19. Chapter 3 presents COVID-19 pandemic in Indonesia. The author shares the report which describe the epidemiologic and clinical features, as well as the management of COVID-19 patients in Indonesia. Still from Indonesia, in Chapter 4 the authors examine and analyse the challenges Indonesia encountered and how Indonesian combat it. Authors analyse the existing data from current researches on COVID-19 and the reliable mass media. Chapter 5 acknowledges the COVID-19 outbreak in India which has vast population density and how the government have taken multiple major decisions in order to flatten the curve of epidemic outbreak. We also have seen how COVID-19 has affected some countries including in the Philippines as discussed in Chapter 6 where the 'Bayanihan' values among Filipino has also noticed.

In section three, the health state during the COVID-19 is examined. There are two chapters in this section (i.e., Chapters 7 and 8). Chapter 7 does the analysis on the stress of the changes in the life and conditions of patients. The authors paid special attention to the problems of the metaphors of the signals and triggers a psychological transformation. The research aims to analyse the problems of anticipating and minimizing the stress of changes in the life of a person (patient). The authors also discussed the possible treatment to improve immune system as a prevention to COVID-19 since a weak immune response will occur due to fewer nutrients as discussed in Chapter 8.

Section four presents social condition in South East Asia and India, consisting of one chapter (Chapter 9). In Chapter 9, the study of the changes and transformations in human and social life is also examined in order to anticipate and understand events and stresses.

Section five shares research on the education during COVID-19. This section contains eight chapters (Chapters 10-17). In Chapter 10 the authors will analyse the big impact on the education sector in Thailand where the schools and many universities have begun to consider postponing the entrance exam, changing the curriculum, and making the online examination to reduce the risk of student gatherings. Not only the COVID-19 affected education in Thailand, it is also affected the education in Indonesia. As explained in Chapter 11, this chapter scrutinizes how education and information about the COVID-19 virus for students with special needs can be obtained from the family, school, and community. Chapter 12 discusses the science process skills using virtual science laboratory since laboratory experiments have become difficult to conduct in the current COVID-19 pandemic because schools are implementing online learning.

Chapter 13 examines how COVID-19 affects teachers' competencies. It seems that some competencies in the 21st century do not efficient enough to the crisis settings. This crisis teaches a lesson to the educator to rethink the teacher efficiency competences. Chapter 14 describes the perspective of Thai parents on COVID-19 pandemic which affects students learning because the education learning system during the COVID-19 conducted virtually. Chapter 15 reviews the challenges and chances in learning management for Thai students during the COVID-19 outbreak. The challenges and the chances include educational inequality, resource management, readiness and cooperation of parents and family, the adaptation of teachers, and changing behaviours of learners.

In Chapter 16, the authors conduct a research on the role of Malaysian school administrators in facing movement control order during COVID-19. In the era of mobile internet, countries around the world have made various effective attempts at online education, but online education is more of a supplement to school education, and large-scale normal online education lacks cases. In Chapter 17 the authors will analyse the new norms in the world of education from Malaysian school administrator's perspective during pandemic.

Section six scrutinizes the economic condition during COVID-19. There are three chapters (Chapters 18-20) found in this section. In Chapter 18, using the descriptive qualitative method, it discusses the COVID-19 impact on Indonesian economy. Chapter 19 acknowledges the global impact of COVID-19 specifically on the risk and crisis management in the company. The highly uncertain condition makes it difficult for the affected companies' management in decision and policy-making. Chapter 20 examines the consumer purchasing patterns during the pandemic in Indonesia following the adoption of social distancing led to consumer new behaviour in determining purchasing patterns or purchasing decisions.

Lastly, section seven discusses the science and technology and the invention emerges during the COVID-19. There are nine chapters (Chapters 21-29). In the first six chapters (from Chapter 21 to Chapter 26), the authors create devices in solving some of the problems that the society is facing during the pandemic including the application of vending machine as a distribution tool for COVID-19 basic protective assistance (Chapter 21), Health Truck Mobile Community Health Services for the COVID-19 (Chapter 22), Automatic Slit/Window Bod (A Drive Thru System with Physical Distancing) for Delivering Food Assistance (Chapter 23), Mobile Food Truck to Assist People's Food Fulfilment (Chapter 24), Mini Helicopter as Disinfectant Sprayer (Chapter 25), Modification of Public Transportation Car to Prevent the Spread of

COVID-19 (Chapter 26). In the second part of this section, we divided it into three chapters (i.e., Chapter 27, Chapter 28, and Chapter 29). In Chapter 27, the authors examine the Microfluidic Application for COVID-19 Detection Using Polimerase Chain Reaction Method. In Chapter 28, the authors shared the community service the Universitas Pendidikan Indonesia conducted to help local people around the university. Finally, in Chapter 29, authors reviews then Simulation of Multi-Hop Routing Wireless Sensor Network Topology Performance and Its Advantages during COVID-19 Pandemic.

In addition, the present book chapters were supported by World Class University Program and Bangdos in Universitas Pendidikan Indonesia.

Bandung, 30 August 2020

Editors

In: COVID-19 ISBN: 978-1-53618-903-2
Editors: A. B. D. Nandiyanto et al.

Chapter 1

COVID-19 AT A GLANCE: FROM HEALTH, EDUCATION, ECONOMIC, TO SCIENCE AND TECHNOLOGY IN SOUTH EAST ASIA AND INDIA

***Asep Bayu Dani Nandiyanto*[*]*,**
Tryastuti Irawati Belliny Manullang, Rina Maryanti,
Amir Machmud, A. Ana and Asnul Dahar Minghat
Universitas Pendidikan Indonesia, Bandung, Indonesia

ABSTRACT

Corona virus disease 2019 (COVID19) emerged in December 2019 in China and has been a viral disease as it continues to spread in almost all the countries of the world. It has put us in unprecedented situation and has changed our daily activities. It has also forced us to find different ways in conducting our plans. There have been many researches on the COVID-19 conducted around the globe. Among of the many conducted research, we compiled some in this book. The aim of this book, therefore, is to share

---

[*] Corresponding Author's Email: nandiyanto@upi.edu.

information and scientific evidence and to provide an overview of the COVID-19 in South East Asia and India.

Keywords: COVID-19

1. Introduction

On 11 February 2020, World Health Organization (WHO) announced a disease caused by a new coronavirus was a COVID-19, which is the acronym of corona virus disease 2019. This COVID-19 was first identified in Wuhan province, China in December 2019. According to the WHO, viral diseases continue to emerge and represent a serious issue to public health and COVID-19 is one of them because it has claimed hundred thousands of lives worldwide (Anggraeni et al., 2020).

COVID-19 has put us the unprecedented situation where isolation has to be taken to lower the infection. People have to stay indoors and do the activities inside as much as possible. As a result, almost all aspects of our life have been affected from the economy, health, education, information and technology to social condition. At the time, we are working on book chapters, the COVID-19 is still haunting us, while throughout the world, scientists, government, and health authorities are working and making incredible efforts to find the cure for this virus. Others have been working to find ways to adapt to the new life. In Indonesia, in some areas, the government even imposed stricter social restrictions for the so-called "red zones" (Zuhairoh and Rosadi 2020). It also affects the economy which is shown by the potential for shocks in the demand and supply of goods and services (Machmud and Minghat 2020).

There was a significant increase in the number of publications on COVID-19 from 2019 to 2020 (Hamidah, Sriyono and Hudha 2020) such as its effects on vocational education (Ana 2020; Mulyanti, Purnama, and Pawinanto 2020). In the midst of this crisis, the authors of this book have chosen to make use of our time to do our part to contribute to the research world. This book provides us with information from South East Asia and

India during the COVID-19 pandemic outbreak. How the COVID-19 has infected countries like India, Indonesia, Malaysia, Thailand, and The Philippines. This book has given opportunities to researchers from those countries to contribute their research. It represents a collaboration between researchers from different fields and also from different countries. We collected the information and did our researches regarding the COVID-19 effects to the society, education, economy, information, and technology and also provide some insights about COVID-19 from the medical perspectives.

The aim of this book, therefore, is to share information and scientific evidence and to provide an overview of the topic. This book covers general condition of COVID-19, Health State, Social Condition, Education, and Economy during COVID-19 pandemic, as well as Science and Information Technology in Handling COVID-19.

REFERENCES

Ana, A. 2020. "Trends in Expert System Development: A Practicum Content Analysis in Vocational Education for Over Grow Pandemic Learning Problems." *Indonesian Journal of Science & Technology,* vol. 5, no. 2, (March):246-260.

Anggraeni, S., Maulidina, A., Dewi, M. W, Rahmadianti, S., Rizky, Y. P. C., Arinalhaq, Z. F., Usdiyana, D., Nandiyanto, A. B. D., and Al-Obaidi, A. S. M. 2020. "The Deployment of Drones in Sending Drugs and Patient Blood Samples COVID-19." *Indonesian Journal of Science and Technology* vol. 5, no. 2 (March):193-200.

Hamidah, I., Sriyono, and Hudha, M. N. 2020. "A Bibliometric Analysis of COVID-19 Research using VOSviewer." *Indonesian Journal of Science & Technology,* vol. 5, no. 2, (March):209-216.

Machmud, A. and Minghat, A. D. B. 2020. "The Price Dynamics of Hand Sanitizers for COVID-19." *Indonesian Journal of Science & Technology,* vol. 5, no. 2, (March):176-184.

Mulyanti, B., Purnama, W. and Pawinanto, R. E. 2020. "Distance Learning in Vocational High Schools during the COVID-19 Pandemic in West

Java Province, Indonesia." *Indonesian Journal of Science & Technology,* vol. 5, no. 2, (March):271-282.

Zuhairoh, F. and Rosadi, D. 2020. "Real-time Forecasting of the COVID-19 Epidemic using the Richards Model in South Sulawesi, Indonesia." *Indonesian Journal of Science & Technology,* vol. 5, no. 3, (December):456-462.

In: COVID-19
Editors: A. B. D. Nandiyanto et al.
ISBN: 978-1-53618-903-2

Chapter 2

A GLIMPSE OF THE PANDEMIC COVID-19 OUTBREAK AROUND THE GLOBE

Paulami Ghosh[1], Deepanmol Singh[1], Arnab Mondal[2] and Surajit Mondal[3,*]

[1]School of Health Science,
University of Petroleum and Energy Studies, Dehradun, India
[2]CSIR-National Physical Laboratory, New Delhi, India
[3]Research and Development,
University of Petroleum and Energy Studies, Dehradun India

ABSTRACT

A new epidemic emerged as severe acute respiratory syndrome corona virus (SARS-CoV-2) intensely shook the world. The disease is caused by the infection from this deadly virus, known as COVID-19. The number of cases infected by this virus are increasing day by day. Despite all the control measures taken by all healthcare authorities, the number of death toll is not halting. The crown-shaped RNA virus is reported to be transmitted from animal to human and human to human within 14 days of

* Corresponding Author's Email: arnabmondal66@gmail.com.

incubation period. The clinical manifestation of the disease ranges from mild symptoms, including fever, dry cough with sore throat, nasal congestion leading to difficulties in breathing, severe continuous headache, unbearable pain in muscle, as well severe respiratory failure and septic shock. Most of the deaths are observed in old patients or in those with comorbities. Healthcare regulatory authorities including World Health Organization (WHO) and national Center for Drug Control (CDC) are closely monitoring the situation and are continuously giving the necessary guidelines to avoid further transmission of COVID-19.

Keywords: coronaviruses, COVID-19, outbreak, pandemic, SARS-CoV-2

1. Introduction

Combating viral diseases has always been a serious challenge for health authorities throughout the world (Mulyanti, Purnama and Parwinanto 2020). In last two decades, the world has already been threatened by two highly infectious viruses including sever acute respiratory syndrome coronavirus (SARS-CoV), H1N1 influenza and Middle East respiratory syndrome coronavirus (MERS-CoV). The world has not forgotten the damage caused by two of the members of coronavirus family, a novel virus SARS-CoV-2 from the same family has emerged as a biological disaster to mankind.

The second SARS-CoV (known as SARS-CoV-2) infection was first reported in Wuhan, China on 31 December 2019, and the related literature henceforth published can help tracing the origin of the symptomatic individuals back to the early December 2019 (Anggraeni et al., 2020). This virus affects the lower respiratory tract and has some of the symptoms related to pneumonia. Due to unidentifiable etiology of this virus, it was classified as "pneumonia of unknown etiology."

On February 11, 2020, the WHO named the disease as "COVID-19," an acronym of "coronavirus disease 2019" (Razon 2020). The earlier infections caused by SARS-CoV that began in China has caused more than 800 causalities with infection spreading to two dozen states, and MERS-CoV that began in Saudi Arabia was equally threatening.

This new virus has been reported as more contagious and having a higher human to human transmission potential. On February 26, 2020, as the first SARS-CoV-2 positive case was reported in United States without having a travel history to China. SARS-CoV-2 is a member of family of single-stranded RNA viruses (+ssRNA) that can infect multiple animal species, especially mammals (Perlman and Netland 2009). Although mechanism of infection is not completely understood, the illness can range from mild common cold to more serious respiratory depression. Origin of coronavirus is linked to bats, Himalayan palm civet, and dromedary camel. Scientists around the world are working day and night to gather the information on the transmission, virus-host interaction, diagnosis, spectrum of disease, and prevention strategies.

2. Cause for Coronavirus

SARS-CoV-2, like other members of the family, has a crown-like appearance which is due to the presence of spiked glycoproteins on the outer surface. *Coronam* is the Latin term for crown. It is classified under *Coronaviridae* family, *Orthocoronavirinae* sub-family and order *Nidovirales*. Table 1 lists different types of Coronaviruses with their probable hosts (Schoeman and Fielding 2020), (Wang et al., 2020).

HCoV-OC43, and HCoV-HKU1 (betaCoVs of the A lineage); HCoV-229E, and HCoV-NL63 (alphaCoVs) are common human coronaviruses with a viral lineage, and they are potential to infect an individual, causing common cold and self-limiting upper respiratory infections especially in people with a weak immune system (Chan et al., 2013) (Chen, Liu, and Guo 2020). SARS-CoV, SARS-CoV-2, and MERS-CoV are other human betaCoVs with B and C viral lineage have the potential and one of the root causes of severe respiratory and extra-respiratory dysfunctions (Table 1). Multiple reported documents have shown high rates of deaths up to 10-35%. Although SARS-CoV-2 has a lower mortality rate, which is around 2.3%, the reproduction number is higher than SARS-CoV and MERS (Petrosillo et al., 2020).

SARS-CoV-2 is a round or elliptic shaped virus with an approximately 60-140 nm in diameter. It is sensitive to heat and UV rays. It can be made inert with the use of lipid-dissolving solvents, which includes commonly used ethanol, isopropanol, chloroform, and chlorhexidine. It has around 80% genetic similarity with human SARS-CoV, making it named as SARS-CoV-2 (Chan et al., 2020). It has a single stranded RNA containing 29891 nucleotides, which encodes for 9860 amino acids.

Table 1. Types of coronaviruses and their respective hosts

Types	**Species of Coronaviruses**
Type 1 Alpha Coronavirus	Transmissible gastroenteritis coronavirus (TGEV)
	Canine coronavirus (CCoV)
	Porcine respiratory coronavirus (PRCoV)
	Feline coronavirus (FeCoV)
	Porcine epidemic diarrhea coronavirus (PEDV)
	Human coronavirus 229E (HCoV-229E)
	Human coronavirus NL63 (HCoV-NL63)
Type 2 Beta Coronavirus	Bat coronavirus (BCoV)
	Porcine hemagglutinating encephalomyelitis virus (HEV)
	Murine hepatitis virus (MHV)
	Human coronavirus 4408 (HVoV-4408)
	Human coronavirus OC43 (HVoV-OC43)
	Human coronavirus HKU1 (HVoV-HKU1)
	Severe acute respiratory syndrome coronavirus (SARS-CoV)
	Middle Eastern respiratory syndrome coronavirus (MERS-CoV)
Type 3 Gamma Coronavirus	Avian infectious bronchitis virus (IBV)
	Turkey coronavirus (TCoV)
Type 4 Delta Coronavirus	Bulbul coronavirus HKU11
	Thrush coronavirus HKU12
	Munia coronavirus HKU13

3. Transmission of the Disease

The first case of COVID-19 is linked to Seafood Wholesale Market of Wuhan, China. The transmission of virus has been reported to be from the droplets released from the infected person, which is similar to other viruses attacking the respiratory organs such as the rhinovirus and the influenza. The transmission has been thought to be from symptomatic as well as asymptomatic patients. Reports showed that the infection spreads because of close contact with the infected people. The incubation time of this virus is expected to be 3 to 7 days and can go up to 14 days (Li et al., 2020), (Bauch et al., 2005).

4. Epidemiology

WHO (March 03, 10.00 am CET) reported 87,137 confirmed cases in worldwide. Out of which 2977 cases (3.42%) have been found to be deceased. Nearly 92% (79,968 cases) of the total confirmed cases, and 2,873 cases (96.5%) resulted deaths in China. Outside of the People's Republic of China in March 2020, there are approximately 7,169 reported cases, spanning 59 countries which includes the Republic of Korea with 3,736 cases followed by Italy (1,128), international conveyance (Diamond Princess, 705 cases), the Islamic Republic of Iran (593), Japan (239), Singapore (102), France (100), United States of America (62), Germany (57), Kuwait (45), Spain (45), Thailand (42), Bahrain (40), Australia (25), Malaysia (24), United Kingdom (23), Canada (19), United Arab Emirates (19), Switzerland (18), Viet Nam (16), Norway (15), Iraq (13), Sweden (13), Austria (10), Croatia (7), Israel (7), Netherlands (7), Oman (6), Pakistan (4), Azerbaijan (3), Denmark (3), Georgia (3), Greece (3), India (3), Philippines (3), Romania (3). Moreover, two lawsuits were recorded in Brazil, Finland, Lebanon, Mexico, the Russian Federation, and a single event each in Afghanistan, Algeria, Belarus, Belgium, Cambodia, Ecuador, Egypt, Estonia, Ireland, Lithuania, Monaco, Nepal, New Zealand, Nigeria, North Macedonia, Qatar, San Marino, and Sri Lanka.

In India, the death was reported in a 76-year-old male from Karnataka and 68-year-old female from Delhi, and 63-year old man from Maharasthra. All three with co-morbidities (WHO 2020). Data showed correlation of Age and % Case Fatality Rate in China (Table 2) (The Novel Coronavirus Pneumonia Emergency Response Epidemiology Team 2020).

Table 2. Percentage of fatality rates for different age groups

Age (in years)	% Case Fatality Rate
10 to 19	0.2
20 to 29	0.2
30 to 39	0.2
40 to 49	0.4
50 to 59	1.3
60 to 69	3.6
70 to 79	8
80 and above	14.8

Both South Korea and Italy have high number of patients positively diagnosed with COVID-19 but in Italy the percentage fatality rate is higher as 90% of deaths occur in those 70 years old or older. On contrary, in South Korea the percentage fatality rate is significantly low as most of the positively diagnosed population is young (less than 40 years old). The morbidity rates are higher in men as compared to women (Sepkowitz 2020). Although WHO have stated that people irrespective of any certain age-groups can be potentially infected by new corona virus (2019-nCOV), certain population is more vulnerable, which include (WHO 2020):

a. Elderly people over 65 years old
b. Healthcare workers including the doctors, nurses and other staffs
c. People with following medical health conditions:
    1. Asthmatic or people suffering from any kind of chronic lung disease
    2. People with artery blockage conditions and weaker heart
    3. Individuals with high blood glucose levels, otherwise known as diabetic
    4. People with neurological conditions and weaker ability to cough

5. Individuals going through chemotherapy sessions for the treatment of cancer (currently or in recent past)
6. Individuals suffering from chronic kidney disease requiring dialysis
7. Individuals with infections in liver
8. Individuals with lack of spleen
9. Extremely obese individuals with BMI > 40.

d. People who are pregnant* (CDC 2020). Present data shows that there is no transmission of COVID-19 from maternal-fetal (Stower 2020). No maternal morbidity has been observed so far (Mullins et al., 2020).

5. MANAGEMENT OF COVID-19

Although repurposing of several drugs is being done along with the screening of herbal remedies, still health regulatory is continuously advising to take necessary precautions. These preventive steps help to reduce the risk factor, including:

a. Remaining update with the latest information on COVID-19 available on WHO website or nation and local public health agency.
b. Maintaining hygiene is an utmost priority. This includes washing or sanitizing hands after regular interval of time.
c. Maintaining social distancing i.e., at least distance of 1 meter between two persons.
d. Avoiding in touching the face especially eyes, mouth, and nose.
e. Wearing a mask at public places.
f. Practicing good respiratory hygiene by covering the mouth while sneezing or coughing with an elbow.
g. Seeking medical health when symptoms arise. Not following the practice of self-medication.

h. Avoiding spreading false claims which comes without strong justifications.
i. Avoiding public gatherings.

CONCLUSION

It is not the first time that the world has faced an epidemic, but this is certainly one of the most threatening phenomena, at least one in past 100 years. It took few weeks to rise from regional crisis to global threat. To reduce the jeopardy caused by COVID-19, WHO, CDCs, and other organizations are working together to make stringent policies and guidelines to curb the virus transmission.

REFERENCES

Anggraeni, S., Maulidina, A., Dewi, M. W., Rahmadianti, S., Rizky, Y. P. C., Arinalhaq, Z. F., Usdiyana, D., Nandiyanto, A. B. D., and Al-Obaidi, A. S. M. 2020. "The Deployment of Drones in Sending Drugs and Patient Blood Samples COVID-19." *Indonesian Journal of Science and Technology* vol. 5, no. 2 (March):193-200.

Bauch, C. T., Lloyd-Smith, J. O., Coffee, M. P., and Galvani, A. P. 2005. "Dynamically modeling SARS and other newly emerging respiratory illnesses: past, present, and future." *Epidemiology* (Cambridge, Mass.) vol. 16, no. 6 (November): 791-801. doi: https://10.1097/01.ede.0000181633.80269.4c.

Centers for Disease Control and Prevention. 2020. *CDC Worldwide*. https://www.cdc.gov/coronavirus/2019-ncov/specific-groups/high-risk-complications.html.

Chan, J. F., To, K. K., Tse, H., Jin, D. Y., and Yuen, K. Y. 2013. "Interspecies transmission and emergence of novel viruses: lessons from bats and birds." *Trends in microbiology* vol. 21, no 10 (October): 544-55. doi: https://10.1016/j.tim.2013.05.005.

Chan, J. F., Kok, K. H., Zhu, Z., Chu. H., To, K. K., Yuan. S., and Yuen, K. Y. 2020. "Genomic characterization of the 2019 novel human-pathogenic coronavirus isolated from a patient with atypical pneumonia after visiting Wuhan." *Emerging Microbes and Infections* vol. 9, no. 1 (January): 221-236. doi: https://10.1080/22221751.2020.1719902.

Chen, Y., Liu, Q., and Guo, D. 2020. "Emerging coronaviruses: Genome structure, replication, and pathogenesis." *Journal of medical virology* vol. 92, no. 4 (April): 418-423. doi: https://10.1002/jmv.25681.

Li, Q., Guan, X., Wu, P., Wang, X., Zhou, L., Tong, Y., Ren, R., Leung, K., Lau, E., Wong, J. Y., Xing, X., Xiang, N., Wu, Y., Li, C., Chen, Q., Li, D., Liu, T., Zhao, J., Liu, M., Tu, W., Feng, Z. 2020. "Early Transmission Dynamics in Wuhan, China, of Novel Coronavirus-Infected Pneumonia." *The New England journal of medicine* vol. 382, no. 13 (March): 1199-1207. doi: https://10.1056/NEJMoa2001316.

Mullins, E., Evans, D., Viner, R. M., O'Brien, P. and Morris, E. 2020. "Coronavirus in pregnancy and delivery: rapid review." *Ultrasound in Obstetrics & Gynecology.* vol. 55, (March): 586-592. doi: https://10. 1002/uog.22014.

Mulyanti, B., Purnama, W., and Parwinanto, R. E. 2020. "Distance Learning in Vocational High Schools during the COVID-19 Pandemic in West Java Province, Indonesia." *Indonesian Journal of Science and Technology* vol. 5, no. 2 (March):271-282.

Perlman, S., and Netland, J. 2009. "Coronaviruses post-SARS: update on replication and pathogenesis." *Nature Reviews Microbiology* vol. 7, no. 6 (June): 439-50. doi: https://10.1038/nrmicro2147.

Petrosillo, N., Viceconte, G., Ergonul, O., Ippolito, G., and Petersen, E. 2020. "COVID-19, SARS and MERS: are they closely related?" *Clinical Microbiology and Infection* vol. 26. no. 6 (June): 729-734. doi: https://10.1016/j.cmi.2020.03.026.

Razon, B. C. 2020. "COVID 19: Impetus for "Community Spirits" among Filipinos." *Indonesian Journal of Science and Technology* vol. 5, no. 2 (March): 201-208.

Schoeman, D., and Fielding, B. C. 2019."*Coronavirus envelope protein: current knowledge*."

Sepkowitz, K. 2020." Why South Korea has so few Coronavirus deaths while Italy has so many." CNN, March 17, 2020. https://edition.cnn.com/2020/03/16/opinions/south-korea-italy-coronavirus-survivability-sepkowitz/index.html.

Stower, H. 2020. "Lack of maternal-fetal SARS-CoV-2-transmission." *Nature Medicine* vol. 26 (March): 312. https://doi.org/10.1038/s41591-020-0810-y.

The Novel Coronavirus Pneumonia Emergency Response Epidemiology Team. The Epidemiological Characteristics of an Outbreak of 2019 Novel Coronavirus Diseases (COVID-19) - China, 2020 [J]. *China CDC Weekly*, 2020, vol. 2, no. 8 (February): 113-122. doi: https://10.46234/ccdcw2020.032.

Virology Journal, no. 16 (May): 69-90. https://doi.org/10.1186/s12985-019-1182-0.

Wang, L., Wang, Y., Ye. D. and Liu, Q. 2020. "Review of the 2019 novel coronavirus (SARS-CoV-2) based on current evidence." *International Journal Antimicrobe Agents* vol. 5, no. 6 (June):105948. doi: https://10.1016/j.ijantimicag.2020.105948.

World Health Organization. 2020. *WHO Worldwide*. https://www.who.int/emergencies/diseases/novel-coronavirus-2019/advice-for-public/myth-busters.

World Health Organization. 2020. *WHO Worldwide*. https://www.who.int/india/emergencies/india-situation-report.

In: COVID-19 ISBN: 978-1-53618-903-2
Editors: A. B. D. Nandiyanto et al.

Chapter 3

THE COVID-19 PANDEMIC IN INDONESIA

Andika Chandra Putra[*]
Department of Pulmonology and Respiratory Medicine,
Faculty of Medicine, Universitas Indonesia;
National Respiratory Referral Persahabatan Hospital, Indonesia

ABSTRACT

Since the first case of coronavirus disease 2019 (COVID-19) was reported in Wuhan, China, as of 12 June 2020, the total number of confirmed cases of COVID-19 was 7,648,823 cases in 215 countries and regions. In Indonesia, the first confirmed case was reported on 2 March 2020, and since then, the number of cases is rising exponentially on a daily basis. As the largest country in South East Asia, Indonesia is the second-largest number of confirmed cases in South East Asia (36,406 cases) after Singapore (39,850 cases). This situation brings Indonesia like other Asian countries into a catastrophe condition. This report described epidemiologic and clinical features, as well as the management of COVID-19 patients in Indonesia.

Keywords: COVID-19, pandemic, Indonesia

[*] Corresponding Author's Email: andika_cp@staff.ui.ac.id.

1. Introduction

Since 31 December 2019, coronavirus disease or known as COVID-19 was firstly found in Wuhan, China. It has spread all over the world causing the pandemic (Mulyanti, Purnama, and Parwinanto 2020; Anggraeni et al., 2020; Razon 2020). This virus was previously named 2019 novel Coronaviruses or known as 2019-nCoV, but then World Health Organization (WHO) changed its name into COVID-19 on 11 February 2020. COVID-19 is a severe acute respiratory syndrome caused by SARS-CoV2, a new virus that thought of as zoonotic and mutated so that it can infect human (Sun et al., 2020). It has the closest similarity to coronaviruses found in bat, so it is thought to be the primary source. SARS-CoV-2 belongs to betacoronavirus, the same subgenus as Severe Acute Respiratory Syndrome (SARS), and Middle East Respiratory Syndrome (MERS). WHO declared COVID-19 as a Public Health Emergency of International Concern on 30 January 2020, and declared the pandemic on 11 March 2020 (WHO 2020). The first case in Indonesia was on 2 March 2020, and since then, the cases increase exponentially (Indonesia. Kementerian Kesehatan Republik Indonesia 2020).

2. Epidemiology

COVID-19 has a higher rate transmission compared to SARS and MERS. Its basic reproductive number is 2-3, which means one patient can transmit to 2-3 other people. COVID-19 transmission is five times at the early phase. A study in China showed that at an early phase, many patients transmitted a large amount of virus, while the conditions were asymptomatic or mild pneumonia. This caused the virus spread more easily (Wang et al., 2020; Zhou et al. 2020).

COVID-19 is linked to wild animal market in Wuhan, China, pangolins, and snakes. They are linked as the intermediate host. COVID-19 has the closest similarity to coronaviruses found in bat, so it is thought to be the primary source (Sun et al., 2020; Wang et al., 2020; CDC 2020). In China, the majority of patients was men with a median age of 56 years, shown by the fact that patients who need Intensive Care Unit (ICU) were 26% (Zhou et al., 2020). According to other reports in the US, a total patient reaches 5,700 cases, in which 60.30% of them were male and 39.70% were female. Patients with comorbidities are more vulnerable to get COVID-19. The most common comorbidities were hypertension (55.60%), obesity (41.70%), and diabetes (41.70%). Other conditions were cancer (6%), asthma (9%), chronic obstructive disease (5.40%), history of transplant (1%), chronic kidney disease (5%), and others. Patients with no comorbid reach 6.10%, with one comorbid 6.30%, and more than 1 comorbid were 88%. Patients come into emergency with fever (30.70%), shortness of breath (17.30%), and 27.80% of them received oxygenation. Patients who treated in ICU were 14.20%, and 12.20% received invasive mechanical ventilation, and 3.20% receive kidney replacement therapy (WHO 2020).

Until April 2020, WHO reported 3,090,445 positive cases and 217,669 deaths globally. It has spread in all the continents, except Antarctica (WHO 2020). The case for fatality rate among diagnosed cases is about 2-3%, but it varies by countries (Oke and Heneghan 2020). Chinese Center for Disease Control has reported mortality rate of about 3.46%, which is lower than SARS (9.60%) and MERS (34.50%) (Wu, Leung, and Leung 2020). However, the true mortality rate cannot be ascertained because the total positive cases are still unknown. Furthermore, the average incubation day is about 6.40 days but it varies between 0 and 24 days (Wang et al., 2020).

In Indonesia, since the first announced case on 2 March until April 2020, there are 9,771 positive cases and 784 deaths. COVID-19 has been reported in all 34 provinces but it varies depending on demographic and density (Indonesia. Kementerian Kesehatan Republik Indonesia 2020). The highest rate is found in Jakarta (the highest population density), in which mid-May 2020, it has 34.40% of the cases in Indonesia (Indonesia. Dinas Kesehatan DKI Jakarta 2020). Based on the latest data from the COVID-19 task force of the Indonesian government, the susceptible sex was male with a mortality increase in age group ≥ 60 years old. SARS-CoV-2 is also more likely to infect people with chronic comorbidities such as hypertension (55.6%), diabetes (35.2%), cardiovascular disease (20.7%), chronic obstructive pulmonary diseases (COPD) (12.6%) and other respiratory problem (5.6%). Among them, the highest proportion for mortality was COVID-19 with hypertension (14.6%) (Indonesia. Kementerian Kesehatan Republik Indonesia 2020). Among 34 provinces in Indonesia (on 12 June 2020) the capital city of Jakarta and the second-largest city of Surabaya are the higher proportion for COVID-19 patients (Figure 1).

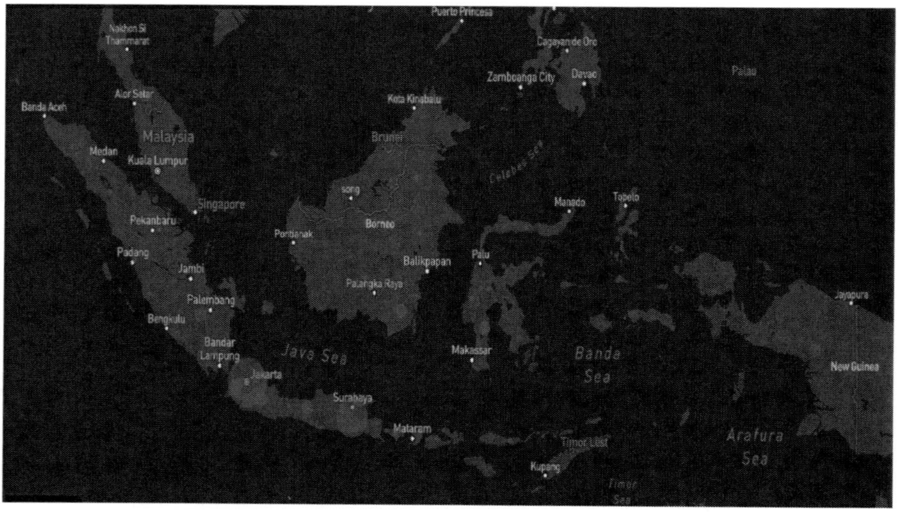

Figure 1. Map of the COVID-19 spread in Indonesia. Size of red circle related with proportion of COVID-19 positive cases. (Source from https://covid19.go.id/peta-sebaran).

3. Clinical Manifestations

The clinical manifestations vary from asymptomatic to severe conditions such as respiratory distress syndrome, septic condition, or multiple organ dysfunction. Chinese Center Disease Control and Prevention (CDC) divided into mild pneumonia, severe, and critical disease. About 1% of positive cases did not have any symptoms. 81% of patients with positive cases are mild or non-pneumonia. Severe disease is defined by respiratory rate $\geq$ 30 times/minutes, oxygen saturation $\leq$ 93%, PaO2/FiO_2, and percentage of oxygen supplied < 300, lung infiltrate in radiograph > 50% in

24 to 48 hours. The severe disease occurred in 14% cases and the critical disease occurred in 5% cases is patient with respiratory failure, septic shock, and/or multiple organ dysfunction syndromes (MODS).

a. *Moderate pneumonia*. Usually patients come with dyspnea and dry cough but without any sign of severe disease
b. *Severe disease*. Patients come with fever and sign of severe dyspnea, saturation < 90%, and respiratory rate > 30x/minutes. But in severe disease, the fever could be absent or slightly increased.
c. *Acute Respiratory Distress Syndrome (ARDS)*. Patients with respiratory failure are divided into (i) Mild (PaO2/FiO_2 between 201-300 mmHg. Patients with no ventilator or non-invasive ventilation by Positive end-expiratory pressure (PEEP) or continuous positive airway pressure (CPAP) $\geq$ 5 cmH_2O; (ii) Moderate (PaO_2/FiO_2 101-200 mmHg), and (iii) Severe (PaO_2/FiO_2 $\leq$ 100 mmHg). Chest radiograph with bilateral opacities not followed by effusions, lung collapses, or lobar also suggested ARDS.
d. *Septic*. Sign of shock includes dyspnea, hypoxemia, hypotension, tachycardia, prolonged capillary refill, hyperthermia or hypothermia, and sign of multi organ dysfunction such as oliguria (decreased kidney function), altered mental status, coagulopathy, hyperbilirubinemia, acidosis, high lactate and others. MODS can be evaluated by sequential organ failure assessment (SOFA) which can predict mortality score on ICU based on clinical and lab data.

MANAGEMENT OF COVID-19 IN INDONESIA

During the COVID-19 pandemic several specialty societies have published treatment guidance and management related to COVID-19, which is divided into two factors: non pharmacology treatment and pharmacology treatment.

Non pharmacology treatment is explained as

1. Patient should use face mask to reduce the aerosol spread to healthcare and place patient in isolation room with negative pressure (Centers for Diseases Control and Prevention 2020).
2. Oxygenation and ventilation (WHO 2020), (National Institutes of Health 2020).
   a. Use oxygen when saturation falls below 90-92% (Alhazzani et al., 2020)
   b. Use nasal cannula 5 lpm or reservoir bag 10-15 lpm with initial target saturation more than 945 (Alhazzani et al., 2020)
   - If the patient is stable, target saturation more than 90% in nonpregnant adults, and 92% in pregnant patients.
   - Saturation target in children is 90% or higher, for children who need urgent resuscitation (apnea or obstructed, distress respiratory syndrome, central cyanosis, shock, seizures, or coma) SpO_2 minimal 94% or higher
   c. High-flow nasal oxygen or non-invasive ventilation has been used to achieve adequate oxygenation (Murthy, Gomersall and Fowler 2020).
   - High flow nasal oxygen is recommended for patients with hypoxemic respiratory failure despite using conventional oxygen therapy. There is evidence that this can reduce the need for intubation and mechanical ventilation (Murthy, Gomersall and Fowler 2020; Huang et.al 2020). However, using this technique can result in higher risk of aerosolization virus and still need emergent intubation if the saturation drops suddenly which can risk providers and put patients in more dangerous condition.
   d. Mechanical ventilation is an option for patient with less saturation who received less invasive measures or patient that cannot maintain breath.
   - Tidal volume settings around 4-8 ml/kg (predicted body weight) and inspiratory pressure < 30 cmH2O.

- Set tidal volume for children 5-8 ml/kg (predicted body weight) for preserved lung compliance and inspiratory pressure < 28 cmH2O.
- PEEP recommended for patient who develop respiratory distress syndrome with higher pressure (>10 cmH2O) better than lower pressure (Alhazzani 2020; Huang et.al 2020).
- Patient with moderate to severe respiratory distress syndrome recommend with prone position in 12-18 hours per day, and for pregnant patient in lateral decubitus.

e. Extracorporeal membrane oxygenation also can be used for severely ill patients if expertise and resources are available (Huang et.al 2020).

3. Fluid therapy
   a. Do not give overhydration because it can precipitate respiratory distress syndrome.
   b. Patient with shock:
      - Crystalloids is recommended (balanced more preferred, example: ringer lactate solution) than colloid fluids such as hydroxyethyl starches, gelatin or albumin for patient critically ill with COVID-19 (Huang et.al 2020).
      - Administer within 15-30 minutes 250-500 ml fluid, with target mean arterial pressure (MAP) 60-65 mmHg for adults' patient.
      - For children administered 10-20 cc/kg bolus within 30 minutes.
      - If there are signs of overhydration or no response then discontinue or reduce the fluid.
      - After initial bolus check the clinical signs (CRT, heart rate, the tactile temperature of extremities, palpable pulse), urinary output (0,5 ml/kg/hour in adult and 1 ml/kg/hour in children), and hemodynamic (MAP > 65 mmHg in adults). If the response is good then titrate continues the fluid (Alhazzani 2020).

Pharmacology treatment is explained in the following. COVID-19 patients are divided into asymptomatic, mild, moderate, and severe pneumonia. They are treated according to their conditions. (Protokol Tatalaksana COVID-19 2020).

1. Asymptomatic
   a. Self-isolation at home for 14 days.
   b. Education for patients (for example: given a leaflet to take home).
   c. Vitamin C 3x500 mg (for 14 days).
   d. Check the temperature twice a day, every morning and night.
   e. Surveillance by medical center officer by phone.
   f. Control in medical center after 14 days surveillance.
2. Mild symptoms
   a. Self-isolation at home for 14 days.
   b. Education for patients (for example: given a leaflet to take home).
   c. Vitamin C 3x500 mg (for 14 days).
   d. Chloroquine 2x 500 mg (for 5 days) or hydroxychloroquine 1x400 mg for 5 days.
   e. Azithromycin 1x 500 mg (for 3 days).
   f. Symptomatic therapy (for example: paracetamol for fever)
   g. Antiviral drug if needed, oseltamivir 2x75 mg or favipiravir 2x .600 mg for 5 days.
   h. Control in medical center after 14 days surveillance.
3. Moderate
   a. Refer to hospital or emergency hospital.
   b. Isolation in hospital for 14 days.
   c. Intravena vitamin C.
   d. Chloroquine 2x 500 mg (for 5 days) or hydroxychloroquine 1x400 mg for 5 days.
   e. Azithromycin 1x 500 mg (for 3 days).
   f. Antiviral drug if needed, oseltamivir 2x 75 mg (for 5 days) or favipiravir loading dose 2x1600 mg for day 1 and then continue with 2x600 mg (day 2-5).

4. Severe
   a. Refer to hospital with facility for COVID-19
   b. Regimen for COVID-19:
      - Chloroquine 2x500 mg (day 1-3) and continue with 2x250 mg (day 4019) or hydroxychloroquine 1x400 mg (day 1-5).
      - Azithromycin 1x500 mg (for 3 days).
      - Antiviral drug: oseltamivir 2x75 mg or favipiravir loading dose 2x1600 mg for day 1 and continue with 2x600 mg (day 2-5).
      - Intravenous drip of vitamin C 200-400 mg in NaCl 0,9% 100 cc.
   a. Supportive therapy (example paracetamol for fever).
   b. Comorbid therapy (if present).
   c. Strictly monitor the patient to prevent respiratory failure.

There are no specific drugs approved for the treatment of COVID-19, but there are some drugs being used under clinical trial and compassionate use protocol based on in vitro study:

1. Remdesivir is antiviral therapy recommended for COVID-19 in severe condition (SpO2 $\leq$ 94% ambient air, need supplemental oxygen, mechanical ventilation, or extracorporeal membrane oxygenation). Although this drug has not been approved by the Food and Drug Administration (FDA). It is issued by the FDA for emergency use as IV remdesivir to treat the severe conditions. According to one placebo-controlled randomized trial, the use of remdesivir is significant in improving recovery time yet does not do any differences for mortality (Gilead 2020). However, remdesivir is not recommended for mild to moderate COVID-19 patients outside the setting of the clinical trial.
2. Chloroquine and hydroxychloroquine have been used in some countries, but the guideline does not recommend high dose chloroquine (2x600 mg for 10 days) because of higher serious effect than the lower dose. It is associated with prolonged QT and risk of arrythmia (Simpson, Kovacs and Stecker 2020). They can be

combined with azithromycin in some protocols, but this also can increase the risk of arrythmia. Infectious Diseases Society of America recommends using this combination only for the clinical trial. NIH guidelines noted when using this combination, patients must be monitored to see the side effects (Clinical Pharmacology 2020).

3. Lopinavir-ritonavir is currently being used to treat HIV. It was used for treating COVID-19 patients but the results are not good.
    a. A study comparing lopinavir-ritonavir with standard treatment shows no difference between improvement time or mortality in 28 days (Cao et al., 2020).
    b. NIH does not recommend using this for treating COVID-19 patients.
4. Immunomodulator is expected to reduce cytokine storm which is estimated to be a factor contributing to respiratory distress syndrome in COVID-19 patients (example: tocilizumab or sarilumab are monoclonal antibodies against interleukin-6).
    a. Convalescent plasma is still uncertain in safety and efficacy for treating COVID-19.
    b. Recently the panel recommends the use of antithrombotic agents to prevent thromboembolic event in COVID-19 patients because COVID-19 has been associated with proinflammation and thrombotic state, increasing fibrin and d-dimers (Han et al., 2020). But the patient who gets antithrombotic drugs should be monitored and evaluated carefully, so this prevention can only be given to inpatients. Outpatients are not allowed to get tested hematology and get prophylaxis except with underlying conditions. This reduces mortality for inpatients with COVID-19.
    c. COVID-19 patients with suspected thromboembolism should get anticoagulant therapy with therapeutic doses like the standard dose for patients without COVID-19Patient with extracorporeal membrane or kidney replacement therapy or thrombosis in

catheters or extracorporeal filters should get anticoagulant therapy like the standard care for patients without COVID-19.

d. Low molecular weight heparin or infraction heparin is preferred for critically ill COVID-19 patients because of their short-lived duration (American Society of Hematology 2020).

5. If the patient falls into septic shock condition, the panel recommends fluid administration first and if the condition persists, adding vasopressin is more recommended (Alhazzani et al., 2020; Murthy, Gomersall and Fowler 2020; Huang et al., 2020).
6. Treatement is started with norepinephrine as the first line. Epinephrine or vasopressin as the second line if norepinephrine is unavailable. The target of mean arterial pressure is 60-65 mmHg.
   a. If the patient is not responding to the usual dose of norepinephrine, adding vasopressin is more recommended than titrating norepinephrine.
   b. If the patient is not responding to norepinephrine and has cardiac dysfunction, adding dobutamine is more recommended than titrating norepinephrine.
   c. Epinephrine is recommended for children and norepinephrine is the second line.

References

American Society of Hematology. *COVID-19 and VTE/Anticoagulation: Frequently Asked Questions.* 2020. https://www.hematology.org/ covid-19/covid-19-and-vte-anticoagulation. Accessed May 22, 2020.

Alhazzani, W., Møller, M. H., Arabi, Y. M., Loeb, M., Gong, M. N., Fan, E., Oczkowski, S., Levy, M. M., Derde, L., Dzierba, A., Du, B., Aboodi, M., Wunsch, H., Cecconi, M., Koh, Y., Chertow, D. S., Maitland, K., Alshamsi, F., Belley-Cote, E., Greco, M., … Rhodes, A. 2020. "Surviving Sepsis Campaign: guidelines on the management of critically ill adults with Coronavirus Disease 2019 (COVID-19)."

Intensive care medicine vol. 46, 5: 854-887. doi:10.1007/s00134-020-06022-5.

Anggraeni, S., Maulidina, A., Dewi, M.W, Rahmadianti, S., Rizky, Y. P. C., Arinalhaq, Z. F., Usdiyana, D., Nandiyanto, A. B. D., and Al-Obaidi, A. S. M. 2020. "The Deployment of Drones in Sending Drugs and Patient Blood Samples COVID-19." *Indonesian Journal of Science and Technology* vol. 5, no. 2:193–200.

Cao, B., Wang, Y., Wen, D., Liu, W., Wang, J., Fan, G., Wang, C. 2020. "A Trial of Lopinavir-Ritonavir in Adults Hospitalized with Severe Covid-19." *The New England Journal of Medicine,* (March). doi: 10.1056/NEJMoa2001282.

Centers for Diseases Control and Prevention. "Coronavirus Disease 2019 (COVID-19): Interim Infection Prevention and Control Recommendations for Patients with Suspected or Confirmed Coronavirus Disease 2019 (COVID-19) in Healthcare Settings." CDC.gov. Updated April 16, 2020. https://www.cdc.gov/coronavirus/2019-ncov/hcp/infection-control-recommendations.html Reviewed April 12, 2020. Accessed May 21st, 2020.

Clinical Pharmacology powered by ClinicalKey. "Azithromycin." *ClinicalKey website*. https://www.clinicalkey.com/#!/content/drug_monograph/6-s2.0-53 Accessed May 21, 2020.

Gilead. *Remdesivir Emergency Use*. 2020. Gilead website. https://www.gilead.com/remdesivir. Accessed May 11, 2020.

Han, H., Yang, L., Liu, R., Liu, F., Wu, K. L., Li, J., Liu, X. H., & Zhu, C. L. 2020. "Prominent changes in blood coagulation of patients with SARS-CoV-2 infection." *Clinical chemistry and laboratory medicine* vol. 58, no. 7: 1116-1120. doi:10.1515/cclm-2020-0188.

Huang, C., Wang, Y., Li, X., Ren, L., Zhao, J., Hu, Y., Cao, B. 2020. "Clinical features of patients infected with 2019 novel coronavirus in Wuhan, China." *The Lancet Articles,* vol. 395, no. 10223: 497-506. https://doi.org/10.1016/S0140-6736(20)30183-5.

Indonesia. Dinas Kesehatan DKI Jakarta. *Data Pemantauan COVID-19 DKI Jakarta* [updated on May 15th 2020]. Accessed https://corona.jakarta.go.id/id/data-pemantauan.

Indonesia. Kementerian Kesehatan Republik Indonesia. 2020. *COVID-19.* Kemkes Worldwide. Updated on April 30 2020. https://infeksiemerging.kemkes.go.id/category/situasi-infeksi-emerging/info-corona-virus/#.XrO8FVOIYzR.

Mulyanti, B., Purnama, W., and Parwinanto, R. E. 2020. "Distance Learning in Vocational High Schools during the COVID-19 Pandemic in West Java Province, Indonesia." *Indonesian Journal of Science and Technology* vol. 5, no. 2:271–282.

Murthy, S., Gomersall, C.D., and Fowler, R.A. 2020. "Care for Critically Ill Patients with COVID". *JAMA.* vol. 323, no.15:1499–1500. doi:10.1001/jama.2020.3633

National Institutes of Health. *COVID-19 Treatment Guidelines: Therapeutic Options for COVID-19 Currently Under Investigation.* NIH Worldwide. Updated April 21, 2020. https://covid19 treatmentguidelines.nih.gov/therapeutic-options-under-investigation/. Accessed May 21st, 2020.

Oke, J., and Heneghan, C. 2020. *Global Covid-19 Case Fatality Rates.* The Centre for Evidence-Based Medicine. Cebm.net. April. https://www.cebm.net/covid-19/global-covid-19-case-fatality-rates/. Accessed April 12, 2020.

Protokol Tatalaksana Covid-19. 2020. *Perhimpunan Dokter Paru Indonesia Worldwide.* April 2020. https://klikpdpi.com/bukupdpi/wp-content/uploads/2020/04/Protokol-Tatalaksana-COVID-19-5OP-FINAL-ok.pdf. [Covid-19 Management Protocol]. April 2020.

Razon, B. C. 2020. "COVID 19: Impetus for "Community Spirits" among Filipinos." *Indonesian Journal of Science and Technology* vol.5, no. 2: 201-208.

Simpson, T.F., Kovacs, R.J and Stecker, E.C. 2020. "Ventricular arrhythmia risk due to hydroxychloroquine-azithromycin treatment for COVID-19." *Cardiology Magazine.* 29 March 2020. https://www. acc.org/latest-in-cardiology/articles/2020/03/27/14/00/ventricular-arrhythmia-risk-due-to-hydroxychloroquine-azithromycin-treatment-for-covid-19.

Sun, J., He, W.-T., Wang, L., Lai, A., Ji, X., Zhai, X., Su, S. 2020. "*COVID-19: Epidemiology, Evolution, and Cross-Disciplinary Perspectives"*

Trends in Molecular Medicine, vol. 25 no. 5 (March): 483-495. doi: 10.1016/j.molmed.2020.02.008.

Wang, Y., Wang, Y., Chen, Y., Qin, Q. 2020." Unique epidemiological and clinical features of the emerging 2019 novel coronavirus pneumonia (COVID-19) implicate special control measures." *Journal of Medical Virology* vol 92, no. 6:568-76. https://doi.org/ 10.1002/jmv.25748.

World Health Organization. "Coronavirus disease (COVID-2019) timeline." *WHO Worldwide.* Updated on April 27 2020. https://www. who.int/news-room/detail/27-04-2020-who-timeline---covid-19. Accessed May 21st, 2020.

World Health Organization. *Coronavirus disease (COVID-2019) situation reports.* [updated on April 30th 2020; cited on May 20st 2020]. Available from: https://www.who.int/docs/default-source/corona viruse/situation-reports/20200430-sitrep-101-covid-19.pdf?sfvrsn =2ba4e093_2. Accessed May 21st, 2020.

World Health Organization, "Clinical Management of Severe Acute Respiratory Infection When Novel Coronavirus (nCoV) Infection Is Suspected: Interim Guidance." *WHO website*. Updated March 13, 2020. https://www.who.int/publications-detail/clinical-management-of-severe-acute-respiratoryinfection-when-novel-coronavirus-(ncov)-infection-is-suspected. Accessed May 21st, 2020.

Wu, J.T., Leung, K., Leung, G.M. 2020. "Nowcasting and forecasting the potential domestic and international spread of the 2019-nCoV outbreak originating in Wuhan, China: a modelling study." *The Lancet* vol.29, no. 395 (February):689-97.

Zhou, F., Yu, T., Du, R., Fan, G., Liu, Y., Liu, Z., Xiang, J., Wang, Y., Song, B., Gu, X., Guan, L., Wei, Y., Li, H., Wu, X., Xu, J., Tu, S., Zhang, Y., Chen, H., and Cao, B. 2020. "Clinical course and risk factors for mortality of adult inpatients with COVID-19 in Wuhan, China: a retrospective cohort study." *Lancet* vol. 395, 10229: 1054-1062. doi:10.1016/S0140-6736(20)30566-3.

In: COVID-19 ISBN: 978-1-53618-903-2
Editors: A. B. D. Nandiyanto et al.

Chapter 4

What We Learn When We Are Facing COVID-19 in Indonesia

Tryastuti Irawati Belliny Manullang**, *Asep Bayu Dani Nandiyanto, Ace Suryadi, Endang Rochyadi and Dingding Haerudin
Universitas Pendidikan Indonesia, Bandung, Jawa Barat, Indonesia

Abstract

As the world is facing a new threat through virus which was found in early December 2019 in Wuhan, China, the changes are happening rapidly. On 2 March 2020, Indonesian government officially announced that the outbreak had finally reached Indonesia. This study conducted to examine and analyze the COVID-19 pandemic outbreak in Indonesia. The main focus of this study was to investigate the challenges Indonesia encountered and how we combat it. Using the existing and evolving information to provide comprehensive picture of the society. The data was taken using the existing data from the current researches on COVID-19 and the reliable mass media. Our research found three major challenges we encountered namely the physical distancing policy, the increasing of the fake news and

* Corresponding Author's Email: manullang@upi.edu.

messages spreading, rising number of unemployment, which eventually bring new changes in our society. The challenges have made us rethinking about our cultural greeting, our news consumption, and its spreading. Also, it made us thinking creatively to change the way we generate our income. On the other hand, it has been a 'blessing in disguise' where the '*gotong royong'* as our cultural heritage has encouraged us to collaborate to help each other, and it has definitely created an opportunity for nature to reclaim itself, and lastly it also lowers the crime rate.

Keywords: COVID-19, education, Indonesia, social humanities

1. INTRODUCTION

In December 2019, when we read the news about the coronavirus disease 2019 (COVID-19) which had emerged in Wuhan province, China, we did not think that the epidemic would cause global shock. The coronavirus is a type of virus that comes from animals. This virus has a very small size and can infect the human body (Maryanti et al. 2020a). The COVID-19 virus is transmitted through droplets, either directly or indirectly. Viruses enter the human body through the nose or mouth. As the death tolls kept increasing, on 30 January 2020, the World Health Organization (WHO) declared it as a Public Health Emergency of International Concern (Anggraeni et al. 2020). The common signs and symptoms of COVID-19 infection include symptoms of acute respiratory disorders such as fever, coughing, and shortness of breath. In severe cases, COVID-19 can cause pneumonia, acute respiratory syndrome, kidney failure, and even death (Tosepu et al. 2020). However, some patients have not shown those symptoms prior to the test. Currently, there has not been any clinical treatments or prevention strategies available for any human coronavirus (Cui, Li and Shi 2019). Even so, there are some simple steps that can be taken in an effort to prevent contracting the COVID-19 virus. We can prevent this virus transmission in several ways by maintaining physical distance (maintaining a minimum distance of 1 meter from other people), using a mask when we leave the house, diligently washing hands with soap, applying hand sanitizer, body booster, be immune to consuming vitamins and a balanced diet, avoid contact with patients, maintain cleanliness, cover mouth and nose when sneezing and coughing, and do not touch nose and mouth before washing hands (Maryanti et al. 2020b).

Elderly patients are having high mortality rates from COVID-19 infection compared to younger patients (Lake 2020). They have weak immune system. Most human coronaviruses are transmitted mainly by the respiratory route or via contact with infected secretions (Chatterjee 2020).

The lock-down in Wuhan has increased the apprehension including the Indonesian citizens who were staying there (Ana 2020). They requested the Indonesian government to evacuate them. As a result, on 30 January 2020, Indonesian government evacuated 238 Indonesian citizens from Wuhan and later quarantined them for 14 days in Natuna Regency, Riau Islands. Two weeks after the quarantine on 15 February 2020, Indonesian Ministry of Health announced to public that all the 238 citizens were all healthy and could continue doing their daily activities (Garnesia 2020).

Prior to that, Indonesian people had been concerned because cases of COVID-19 had been found in other countries. However, Indonesian government had not taken any prevention action although the WHO had announced it as an international concern. On 2 March 2020, Indonesian government officially announced that the outbreak had finally reached Indonesia after two suspected patients were identified. The number of affected people has been rising since the first announcement. On 28 April 2020, Indonesia reported 9,056 laboratories confirmed COVID-19 cases with 765 deaths (WHO 2020). Although the first case had been found in March 2020, the government was reluctant to enforce a complete nationwide lockdown. However, city mayor of Tegal (a city in Central Java) decided to do local lockdown, regardless of resentment that he might receive from the citizens against his decision (Dzulfaroh and Hardiyanto 2020).

The official announcement affected many sectors. School closures started, most of offices decided to apply work-from-home policy, and religious activities were encouraged to be performed at home. No crowds are allowed. Immediately after the declaration, Indonesian risk communication team COVID-19 or also known as *Gugus Tugas Percepatan Penanganan* COVID-19 launched with the goal of communicating relevant information across different target audiences. The objectives of the Task Force on Acceleration of Handling COVID-19 are to improve national resilience in the health sector, to accelerate the handling of COVID-19 through synergy between ministries or institutions and local governments, to enhance anticipation of the escalation developments spread of COVID-19, to develop the synergy of policy making operational, as well as to increase the readiness and proficiency in the prevention, detection and response to COVID-19 (Indonesia. Keppres no.7 tahun 2020).

2. Method

The main focus of this study was to investigate the challenges happening during the COVID-19 pandemic outbreak and how we deal with the challenges. All information was obtained from the news mostly covered by kompas.com; tirto.id; tempo.com; and bbc.indonesia.com. The data was also taken also from the published papers by typing COVID-19 in Indonesia as well as *virus corona di Indonesia* as the key words search. This study is limited; therefore, several considerations should be taken into account when interpreting the findings.

3. Results and Discussion

3.1. Indonesia at Glance

Indonesia has 34 provinces, approximately 16,056 islands spreading over with five main islands namely Sumatra, Java, Kalimantan, Sulawesi, and Papua, and 268 million people (Indonesia. Badan Pusat Statistik 2020). Indonesia has been well-known for its diverse culture, which makes it unique. It is a democratic country and has been independent since 17 August 1945. Indonesia adopts the presidential government system. However, the political and administrative system consists of four levels of government such as the central, the provincial level, the district, the urban municipalities, and the villages (Krishnamohan 2016). Thus, the local government has the right to regulate, allocate, and utilize national resource and intergovernmental fiscal relations between central and local government (Hidayat 2017).

3.2. Challenges during COVID-19 Pandemic Outbreak

The consequences of COVID-19 pandemic outbreak have been affected most of our activities. The situation has been challenging for both government and society. According to us, these three topics are the main challenges that Indonesian encountered besides the economy, health, security, information and technology, and other areas. The three challenges below have been a challenge, however, at the same time enforce us to make a change regardless of our willingness to.

3.3. Physical Distancing

During this COVID-19, local lock down is implemented. We have experienced changes, shifted rapidly after the official announcement. As more information about COVID-19 published on mass media, the more people started to worry because the COVID-19 diseases transfer through droplets (Anggraeni et al. 2020). Maintaining physical distance, improving personal hygiene, including washing hands using soap, and applying hand sanitizers are one of the best preventions that people can take because this virus gives serious threat.

Consequently, people started to panic. Hand sanitizers and masks were two important items that people bought. As a result, the price of these two items rocketed for few weeks after the announcement. Hospitals, clinics and government-mandated community health clinics encountered shortage of Personal Protective Equipment (PPE). This shortage affected the healthcare workers as the frontline because they have to wear PPE in order to prevent the transmission of the virus. However, the shortage has caused a few of the health workers infected.

The physical distancing method has also been affected the way we greet each other. People commonly greet each other in Indonesia by shaking hands. After the COVID-19 case found in Indonesia, it is suggested to avoid this greeting gesture. Shaking hands has been a part of Indonesian culture, however, the virus has forced us to change the greeting into healthier way by clasping hands in front of our chest or simply giving a slight nod.

3.4. Spreading of Fake News and Messages

At the era of social media, misinformation and the spreading of fake news or messages is inevitable. Misinformation and conspiracy theories spread on social media have generated panic and mistrust among the general public, diverted attention away from the outbreak response, and impeded the activities of health-care workers (Cui, Li, and Si 2019). The global pandemic is not only on COVID-19 but also a global epidemic of misinformation—spreading rapidly through social media platforms and other outlets—poses a serious problem for public health (Zarocostas 2020). By 23 March, 2020, there were 44 cases on fake news in Indonesia (Halim and Rastika 2020).

The cases have caused some suspects being charged under the 2016 Electronic Information and Transactions (ITE) Law. The fake news and messages including the death of two volunteers at the Jakarta's makeshift hospital for COVID-19 in the Kemayoran athletes village (Oktaviani 2020), message about prevention of the virus by using UNICEF where one of the statements mentioned that at 26-27°C the coronavirus would die because the viruses cannot live in a hot temperature (Arnani and Wedhaswary 2020).

The spreading of the fake news and messages has made Indonesian police department to conduct round-the-clock cyber patrols, implemented the law enforcement, and continued to educate the public and fight hoaxes with counter-narratives (Antara and Bhwana 2020). It has also made The Indonesian Ulama Council to urge Muslims not to spread hoaxes and false information regarding the disease, as the council had issued a fatwa on declaring such wrongdoing as *haram* (News Desk The Jakarta Post 2020).

3.5. Unemployment Creates New Ways of Generating Revenue

The COVID-19 pandemic has many major consequences not only for one area but also in whole aspects. It has obviously increased the numbers of unemployed citizens as companies were forced to do massive layoffs. The number is predicted to reach 2.9 to 5.2 million unemployed people if the situation is getting worse (Fauzia and Setiawan 2020). In 2019, there were 5.28% of unemployed people in Indonesia which approximately about 7.05 million. In order to prevent the spread of the virus, government is controlling the transmission by lockdowns and travel bans to "flatten the pandemic curve." The lockdown has caused financial challenges and uncertainty. The tourism industry in Bali potentially experience the loss for almost 1 trillion IDR each month because most of the tourists coming are from Australia and China (Gamar and Belarminus 2020). The flight blocking has surely been challenging for the people who work in the tourism industry. Needless to say, the massive layoffs have enforced people to think of new ways to support their families during the pandemic. Due to restrictions, lockdown, and the physical distance policy, many have tried to start their small businesses from home by selling some home-made food and offering the service-based jobs such as courier service and in-home haircut service. Restaurants have changed their services, some have changed their system, where they now open online orders, and some shops have conducted the same approaches by encouraging the staff to sell their products online and to get direct contact with their customers.

The changes had been experienced before. We had online applications where we could order food from restaurants; however, there were some restaurants unwilling to apply the same marketing approaches. The pandemic has obviously changed them.

4. A Silver Lining

Besides the changes aforementioned, there are many other areas that have improved. COVID-19 is a global pandemic and serious threat to human health which halt the economic activities, however it is also considered as a "Blessing in Disguise," where pollution is reducing and nature is reclaiming itself (Muhammad, Long and Salman 2020). Additionally, the criminal cases have been decreased as reported in Papua during March 2020 the cases have been lower to 277% comparing to crime cases in February 2020 (Aditra and Agriesta 2020).

Ultimately, during this pandemic, we also see how the cultural heritage is emerging. In Wonosari, one of the villages in Yogyakarta, the people collaborated to help families that isolated due to the COVID-19. People provided the food supplies for the families. In Bali, the governor worked with local security officers known as *pecalang* to ensure the lockdown is implemented and people maintain the social distancing. Furthermore, as the health care workers are in the shortage of the PPE, this situation emerged solidarity from some citizens including celebrities (CNNIndonesia.com) by organizing the funding to buy more PPE and distribute it to hospitals, clinics, and to government-mandated community health clinics in need.

Conclusion

COVID-19 has affected most of our activities. It has also caused us to encounter unprecedented time and enforced us to start thinking about the 'new normal.' It has caused us to experience new changes at the same time. The challenges have made us rethinking about our cultural greeting, our news consumption and its spreading, as well as also made us thinking creatively to change the way we generate our income. On the other hand, it has been a 'blessing in disguise' where the '*gotong royong*' as our cultural heritage has encouraged us to collaborate to help each other, and it has definitely created an opportunity for nature to reclaim itself, and lastly it lowers the crime rate.

REFERENCES

Aditra, I. P and Agriesta, D. "Angka kriminalitas di papua turun drastis sejak pandemi virus corona." *Kompas.com* 3 April 2020. https://regional.kompas.com/read/2020/04/03/13002291/angka-kriminalitas-di-papua-turun-drastis-sejak-pandemi-virus-corona. [The Crime Rate in Papua has dropped dramatically since the Corona Virus Pandemic]. Kompas.com. 3 April 2020.

Ana, A. 2020. "Trends in expert system development: A practicum content analysis in vocational education for over grow pandemic learning problems." *Indonesian Journal of Science and Technology*, vol. 5, no. 2 (March):246–260.

Anggraeni, S., Maulidina, A., Dewi, M. W, Rahmadianti, S., Rizky, Y. P. C., Arinalhaq, Z. F., Usdiyana, D., Nandiyanto, A. B. D., and Al-Obaidi, A. S. M. 2020. "The deployment of drones in sending drugs and patient blood samples COVID-19." *Indonesian Journal of Science and Technology* vol. 5, no. 2 (March):193–200.

Antara and Bhwana, P. G. "Police tackle 41 cases of hoaxes about COVID-19 spread." *Tempo.com,* 24 March 2020. https://en.tempo.co/ read/1323222/police-tackle-41-cases-of-hoaxes-about-covid-19-spread.

Arnani, M and Wedhaswary, I. D. "[HOAKS] Pesan berantai seputar virus corona mengatasnamakan UNICEF." *Kompas.com*, 13 March 2020. https://www.kompas.com/tren/read/2020/03/13/060300365/-hoaks-pesan-berantai-seputar-virus-corona-mengatasnamakan-unicef?page=2. [[HOAX] A Chain Message Regarding the Corona Virus on behalf of UNICEF]. *Kompas.com*, 13 March 2020.

Chatterjee S. 2020. "Important Steps to Control COVID-19/SARS-CoV-2 Infection." *SN comprehensive clinical medicine*, 1–2. Advance online publication. https://doi.org/10.1007/s42399-020-00271-7.

CNNIndonesia.com. "Ramai-ramai donasi APD dukung tenaga medis lawan corona." *CNNIndonesia.com*, 27 April 2020. https://www.cnnindonesia.com/nasional/20200326155549-20-487176/ramai-ramai-donasi-apd-dukung-tenaga-medis-lawan-corona. [Crowdfunding of PPE Donations to Support Medical Workers against Corona]. *CNNIndonesia.com*, 27 April 2020.

Cui, J., Li, F. and Si, Z. 2019. "Origin and evolution of pathogenic coronaviruses." *Nature reviews. Microbiology* vol. 17,3 (March): 181-192. doi:10.1038/s41579-018-0118-9.

Dzulfaroh, A. N., and Hardiyanto, S. Daftar Wilayah di Indonesia yang terapkan "local lockdown" *Kompas.com*, 29 March 2020. https://www.kompas.com/tren/read/2020/03/29/083900665/daftar-wilayah-di-indonesia-yang-terapkan-local-lockdown-. [List of Regions in Indonesia that Apply "Local Lockdown"] *Kompas.com*, 29 March 2020.

Fauzia, M and Setiawan, S. R. D. "Dampak corona, jumlah pengangguran bisa naik hingga 5,2 Juta Orang." *Kompas.com*, 14 April 2020. https://money.kompas.com/read/2020/04/14/150800726/dampak-corona-jumlah-pengangguran-bisa-naik-hingga-5-2-juta-orang?page=all. [Impact of Corona, the Number of Unemployment Can Increase to 5.2 Million People]. *Kompas.com*, 14 April 2020.

Gamar, R and Belarminus, R. "Akibat Isu Virus Corona, Pariwisata Bali Diperkirakan Merugi Rp 1 Triliun Per Bulan." *Kompas.com*, 13 February 2020. https://regional.kompas.com/read/2020/02/13/17421311/akibat-isu-virus-corona-pariwisata-bali-diperkirakan-merugi-rp-1-triliun-per, *accessed in 11 May, 2020*. [Due to the corona virus issue, Bali tourism is estimated to loss IDR 1 trillion per month]. *Kompas.com*, 13 February 2020.

Garnesia, I. 2020. "Ketika Indonesia Tidak Kebal COVID-19." *Tirto.id*, 26 February 2020. https://tirto.id/ketika-indonesia-tidak-kebal-covid-19-ez18. [When Indonesia is not immune to COVID-19]. *Tirto.id*, 26 February 2020.

Halim, D and Rastika, I. "Bertambah lagi, Total 44 Kasus Hoaks Terkait Virus Corona di Indonesia." *Kompas.com*, 23 March 2020. https://nasional.kompas.com/read/2020/03/23/21275431/bertambah-lagi-total-44-kasus-hoaks-terkait-virus-corona-di-indonesia. [In addition, a total of 44 hoax cases related to the corona virus in Indonesia] *Kompas.com*, 23 March 2020.

Hidayat, R. 2017. "*Political devolution: Lessons from a decentralized mode of government in Indonesia*." SAGE Open, (January). doi:10.1177/2158244016686812.

Indonesia. Badan Pusat Statistik. 2020. *The Statistical Yearbook of Indonesia* 2020, p. 3. http://www.bps.go.id.

Indonesia. Keputusan Presiden Indonesia. 2020. *Decree of President of the Republic Indonesia on Task Force on Acceleration of Handling COVID-19* Number 7. Year 2020. https://peraturan.bpk.go.id/Home/Details/134544/keppres-no-7-tahun-2020.

Krishnamohan, T. 2016. "The local government system in Indonesia and Sri Lanka: A comparative overview." *International Journal in Commerce, IT & Social Sciences- IJCISS* 30, no. 12 (December).

Lake M. A. (2020). "What we know so far: COVID-19 current clinical knowledge and research." *Clinical medicine (London, England)*, *20*(2), 124–127. https://doi.org/10.7861/clinmed.2019-coron.

Maryanti, R., Hufad, A., Sunardi., Nandiyanto, A. B. D., and Al-Obaidi, S. M. 2020a. "Understanding COVID-19 particle contagion through aerosol droplets for students with special needs." *Journal of Engineering Science and Technology* vol.15, no.3:1909-1920.

Maryanti, R, Hufad, A, Sunardi, Nandiyanto, A. B. D, Manullang, T. I. B. 2020b. Understanding Coronavirus (COVID-19) as a Small Particle to Students with Special Needs. *Horizon* vol. 2, no. 1: 121-130.

Muhammad, S, Long, X and Salman, M. 2020. "COVID-19 pandemic and environmental pollution: A blessing in disguise?" *The Science of the total environment* vol. 728 (April): 138820. doi: 10.1016/j.scitotenv.2020.138820.

News Desk. "Police name 30 suspects for allegedly spreading COVID-19 hoaxes. *The Jakarta Post.com*, 20 March 2020." https://www.thejakartapost.com/news/2020/03/20/police-name-30-suspects-for-allegedly-spreading-covid-19-hoaxes.html.

Oktaviani, T. I. Facebook post on death of volunteers at COVID-19 hospital. *The Jakarta Post, 2 April 2020.* https://www.thejakartapost.com/news/2020/04/02/authorities-dismiss-as-hoax-facebook-post-on-death-of-volunteers-at-covid-19-hospital.html.

Tosepu, R., Gunawan, J., Effendy, D., Ahmad, L., Lestari, H., Bahar, H., and Asfian, P. 2020. "Correlation between weather and Covid-19 pandemic in Jakarta, Indonesia." *Science of the Total Environment*. 725 (April): 138436. doi: 10.1016/j.scitotenv.2020.138436.

World Health Organization. 2020. *WHO Worldwide*. https://www.who.int/docs/default-source/coronaviruse/situation-reports/20200428-sitrep-99-covid-19.pdf?sfvrsn=119fc381_2.

Zarocostas, J. "2020. How to fight an infodemic." *World Report*, 395, no. 10225 (February):676. doi: https://doi.org/10.1016/S0140-6736(20)30461-X.

In: COVID-19 ISBN: 978-1-53618-903-2
Editors: A. B. D. Nandiyanto et al.

Chapter 5

COVID-19 OUTBREAK AND THE STEPS TAKEN BY INDIA

***Paulami Ghosh*[1], *Arnab Mondal*[2], *Deepanmol Singh*[1] *and Surajit Mondal*[3]**

[1]School of Health Science, University of Petroleum and Energy Studies, Dehradun, India

[2]CSIR-National Physical Laboratory, New Delhi, India

[3]Research and Development, University of Petroleum and Energy Studies, Dehradun, India

ABSTRACT

The COVID-19 outbreak is now a global pandemic as announced by the World Health Organization. Countries like China and Italy are completely locked down in an attempt to control the situation. Countries like India with vast population density have taken multiple major decisions in order to flatten the curve of epidemic outbreak. Multiple states have announced complete lockdown of major cities and even states. The central government has decided to even halt the passenger trains of Indian Railway services. State government have stopped transport services in their respective states. Some cities even have announced curfews in major areas. Private companies have ordered their employees to work from home.

Major government services like banks, medical shops, and vegetable shops are permitted to be kept open. The citizens are encouraged to socially distance themselves at the stores for purchasing the daily needed products. Thermal scanners are installed at airports, railway stations, and at the entry gates of government institutions. Multiple isolated wards are being made at major hospitals to provide medical facilities to the affected people.

Keywords: COVID-19, India

1. INTRODUCTION

At the beginning of 2020, a new transmission of a virus is found in more than 200 countries in the world started as we experience the Corona Virus Disease 2019 (COVID-19) pandemic outbreak. On 11 February, 2020, the World Health Organization (WHO) named the disease from the corona virus as "COVID-19," an acronym of "coronavirus disease 2019" (Razon 2020). The WHO has officially declared the COVID-19 condition to be a global pandemic and the whole world should pay serious attention to it. Thus, all public activities, including educational institutions with a large number of masses, must be halted to reduce the amount of COVID-19 virus transmission and spread.

The deadly virus had infected the humankind after the consumption of some wild animals/birds which was being sold at the Chinese city of Wuhan (Anggraeni et al. 2020). The infected animal/bird from where the virus originated is yet unknown (WHO 2020). From a small province of Wuhan, China, it is now a global epidemic (WHO 2020), (Hamidah, Sriyono and Hudha 2020).

The World Health Organization (WHO) labelled this outbreak as pandemic (a disease that is spreading in multiple countries around the world at the same time). The appearance of severe acute respiratory syndrome coronavirus 2 (SARS-CoV 2) is also known as novel coronavirus (2019-nCoV) or coronavirus disease 2019 (COVID-19) during the end of 2019 year in the Chinese province of Wuhan is now spreading uncontrollably throughout the world.

Apart from China, European countries like Italy, Spain, and UK are facing huge crisis when it comes to provide proper healthcare and medical facilities to the infected citizens and have lost more lives than China did at the similar stage (Financial Times 2020). The outbreak has taken more than 190 countries into its grip till 22 March 2020 with more than 0.33 million people affected worldwide.

'Quarantine' is one of the most effective strategy to control the outbreak-like situation of epidemics and communicable disease (Wilder-Smith and Freedman 2020). And, 'Social distancing' is a way to reduce contact with the infected to the non-infected individuals. Many countries have failed to contain this deadly virus and now the situation have gone out of control. Developed nations have failed miserably in order to control the outbreak. Scientists and researchers from about 35 leading companies and research institutions are racing hard to come up with vaccines which seem to be a distant dream (Gallagher 2020). Citizens of the countries where the outbreak happed are advised to stay inside and take proper self-care by regularly washing hands with soap and water. The use of sanitizers with more than 50% alcohol content are promoted. People are also advised to use masks and keep social distance from people coughing nearby.

2. Affected Countries

The major countries which have been an epicenter of this COVID-19 pandemic are China where the outbreak happened, followed by European countries like Italy, France, Spain, Switzerland and the UK, the USA and the Asian nations of South Korea and Iran (Figure 1). It is also spreading to other countries of the world spanning over 190 countries and territories, in which there are more than 70 countries with over 100 reported cases as on 23 March 2020. From these 70 countries, San Marino has the highest rate of individuals affected per million people which is 5,158 individuals per million, followed by the countries of Iceland (1,665), Andorra (1,462) and Luxembourg (1,275). On the other hand, India has the lowest rate of affected individuals per million people which is about 0.33 individuals per million.

Other countries on the list in Figure 1 with lowest per million affected people are Vietnam (1), Indonesia, and Mexico at two people per million. Highest deaths due to the COVID-19 outbreak are reported in Italy which is about 5,476 although it has the world's second-best healthcare facilities. China, from where the deadly coronavirus originated, has reported a total death toll of 3,270 individuals, followed by the countries of Spain (1,813) and Iran (1,685) (Table 1).

Indian Council of Medical Research (ICMR), the apex body of India responsible for formulating, coordinating, and promoting the biomedical research has freshly revised its strategies for the containment of the spread of COVID-19 in order to deliver dependable diagnosis to the individuals suspected of being infected by COVID-19. The government has asked the relevant authorities to check every suspected individual who has international travel history within last two weeks; and, as a precautionary measurement, the government has advised the individuals along with their respective families to strictly follow 14-days quarantine.

Furthermore, the government has asked for the COVID-19 test of the individuals suffering from relatable symptoms such as fever, cough, difficulty in breathing, and sore throat. The test should also be done on asymptomatic individuals from day 5 to day 14 if they have come in contact with the infected individuals.

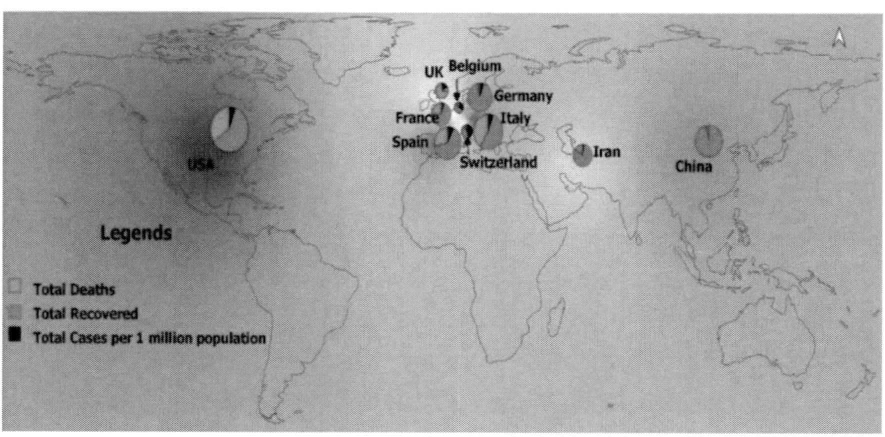

Figure 1. Top 10 countries of coronavirus pandemic outbreak.

Table 1. Top 50 countries of the world to be affected from to outbreak of COVID-19 pandemic

No	Country	Total Cases	Total Deaths	Total Recovered	Cases per 1 M population	Reported 1st case
	World	862,574	42,528	179,127	110.7	Jan-10
1	US	188,592	4,056	7,251	570	Jan-20
2	Italy	105,792	12,428	15,729	1,750	Jan-29
3	Spain	95,923	8,464	19,259	2,052	Jan-30
4	China	81,554	3,312	76,238	57	Jan-10
5	Germany	71,808	775	16,100	857	Jan-26
6	France	52,128	3,523	9,444	799	Jan-23
7	Iran	44,605	2,898	14,656	531	Feb-18
8	UK	25,150	1,789	135	370	Jan-30
9	Switzerland	16,605	433	1,823	1,919	Feb-24
10	Belgium	13,964	828	2,132	1,205	Feb-03
11	Turkey	13,531	214	243	160	Mar-09
12	Netherlands	12,595	1,039	250	735	Feb-26
13	Austria	10,366	146	1,095	1,151	Feb-24
14	South Korea	9,887	165	5,567	193	Jan-19
15	Canada	8,612	101	1,242	228	Jan-24
16	Portugal	7,443	160	43	730	Mar-01
17	Brazil	5,812	202	127	27	Feb-24
18	Israel	5,591	21	226	646	Feb-20
19	Australia	4,862	21	345	191	Jan-24
20	Norway	4,651	39	13	858	Feb-25
21	Sweden	4,435	180	16	439	Jan-30
22	Czechia	3,330	32	45	311	Feb-29
23	Ireland	3,235	71	5	655	Feb-28
24	Malaysia	2,908	45	645	90	Jan-24
25	Denmark	2,860	90	1	494	Feb-26
26	Russia	2,777	24	190	19	Jan-30
27	Chile	2,738	12	156	143	Mar-02
28	Poland	2,347	35	7	62	Mar-03
29	Philippines	2,311	96	50	21	Jan-29
30	Ecuador	2,302	79	58	130	Feb-28
31	Romania	2,245	85	220	117	Feb-25
32	Japan	2,178	57	424	17	Jan-14

Table 1. (Continued)

No	Country	Total Cases	Total Deaths	Total Recovered	Cases per 1 M population	Reported 1st case
33	Luxembourg	2,178	23	80	3,479	Feb-28
34	Pakistan	2,042	26	82	9	Feb-25
35	Thailand	1,771	12	416	25	Jan-12
36	Indonesia	1,677	157	103	6	Mar-01
37	India	1,590	45	148	1	Jan-29
38	Saudi Arabia	1,563	10	165	45	Mar-01
39	Finland	1,418	17	10	256	Jan-28
40	South Africa	1,353	5	50	23	Mar-04
41	Greece	1,314	49	52	126	Feb-25
42	Mexico	1,215	29	35	9	Feb-27
43	Panama	1,181	30	9	274	Mar-09
44	Iceland	1,135	2	198	3,326	Feb-27
45	Dominican Rep.	1,109	51	5	102	Feb-29
46	Peru	1,065	30	394	32	Mar-05
47	Argentina	1,054	27	240	23	Mar-02
48	Singapore	926	3	240	158	Jan-22
49	Colombia	906	16	31	18	Mar-05
50	Serbia	900	23	42	103	Mar-02

Source: https://www.worldometers.info/coronavirus/ (as on 1 April 2020).

3. Indian Scenario and Affected Areas

Below are scenarios that Indian government conducted:

- 'Stay in whichever city you are,' PM Modi urged people; as the number of cases crossed 1700 mark in India (Business Today India 2020).
- Coronavirus cases in India: Several cities across India, including the national capital Delhi and Mumbai were declared to be completely

lockdown as cases of COVID-19 infection continued to surge (Chandrashekhar 2020).

- PM Modi announced a country-wide lockdown for 21 days up to 14 April 2020. For general public (Chandrashekhar 2020). Inter-state travel was completely banned throughout the country and was allowed only with official government documents under special permissions granted by respective state governments (The Hindu Business Line 2020)
- Only the medical staffers and journalists with proper documentation were being permitted to move out during the lockdown (Bloomberg Quint 2020).
- Coronavirus cases in India crossed 1900 on 1 April 2020 with thousands of people testing positive for the infection. Maharashtra and Kerala with 325 and 241 cases respectively were recorded making them worst affecting states of India (India Today Web Desk 2020).
- Followed by the above-mentioned states, southern Indian state of Tamil Nadu had witnessed a rise of 124 corona virus cases, while the national capital Delhi had 123 on-record positive cases.
- Union territories of Jammu and Kashmir, Chandigarh, Ladakh, Andaman and Nicobar Islands and Puducherry were also heavily affected due to the outbreak of the COVID-19 pandemic.

Table 2. Indian states affected from to outbreak of COVID-19 pandemic (as on 1 April 2020)

State/Union Territory	Confirmed	Active	Recovered	Deceased
Maharashtra	325	274	39	12
Kerala	241	215	24	2
Tamil Nadu	124	117	6	1
Delhi	123	115	6	2
Rajasthan	106	103	3	-
Karnataka	105	93	9	3
Uttar Pradesh	104	86	17	1
Telangana	97	77	14	6

Table 2. (Continued)

State/Union Territory	Confirmed	Active	Recovered	Deceased
Andhra Pradesh	87	85	2	-
Madhya Pradesh	86	80	-	6
Gujarat	82	71	5	6
Jammu And Kashmir	55	52	1	2
Punjab	45	40	1	4
Haryana	43	26	17	-
West Bengal	27	18	3	6
Bihar	23	22	-	1
Chandigarh	15	15	-	-
Ladakh	13	10	3	-
Andaman And Nicobar Islands	10	10	-	-
Chhattisgarh	9	7	2	-
Uttarakhand	7	5	2	-
Assam	5	5	-	-
Goa	5	5	-	-
Odisha	4	4	-	-
Himachal Pradesh	3	1	1	1
Puducherry	3	3	-	-
Jharkhand	1	1	-	-
Manipur	1	1	-	-
Mizoram	1	1	-	-
Total	1750	1542	155	53

Source: https://www.covid19india.org/.

4. STEPS TAKEN BY INDIA TO FLATTEN THE CURVE

India with the world's second highest population is now facing a challenge to secure the lives of its citizens from the deadly virus. If the spread of this COVID-19 pandemic spreads like in the US and the European nations, then the country may witness massive loss of human lives as well as severe economic losses. The PM of India has urged people to stay indoors for the restricting the outspread of this disease. For flattening the curve of the reported cases, 21-day country-wide lockdown is announced from 24 March 2020. During the lockdown, the police forces are deployed to ensure public stays inside their houses. The daily necessities and food items are made available to public via home-delivery service. The medical stores are also been ordered to be opened. Indian railways are closed completely to stop people to travel in masses. The railway coaches are being transformed into healthcare bogies to make medical facilities available to distant places in the country. Indian airline companies too are playing a major role in controlling the spread of virus. Indigo has said that it will be operational on only 60% of its routes while Vistara and GoAir have also announced curtailment of their service to help the government in checking the spread of highly infectious COVID-19 (SNS Web 2020). The curfew has been declared basically to break down the chain of spreading the virus between the infected people and others. As a learning from the mistakes of Italy, UK, France, and Iran to prevent the stage 2 to stage 3. If people of India used to go for a minimum quarantine time, in the 3rd and 4th weeks of the crucial time of spreading the virus, India could save its people.

Apart from the central government, respective state governments played their part to control the situation as well. Delhi CM Arvind Kejriwal has ordered the closure of all shops, malls, and other places that are prone to contagion with exceptions given to pharmacies and grocery stores. Delhi CM Arvind Kejriwal announced to even lockdown the national capital to prevent the outbreak of COVID-19 if the situation worsens.

Establishments in the state not to terminate the services of its employees even if they go on leave in view of the COVID-19 outbreak. It also asked these establishments not to deduct the wages of their employees. In his directive, State Labor commissioner Mahendra Kalyankar said that if any worker goes on leave, he should be deemed to be on duty without consequential deduction in wages for this period (The Economic Times 2020). Furthermore, Bihar shutdowns bus services, restaurants, and banquet halls to prevent the spread of COVID-19. However, home-delivery and take-home services of restaurants will remain functional, PTI quoted a health department order (Patna 2020). Odisha lockdowns 40% of the state to knockdown COVID-19, including state capital for a week, 5 districts, and 8 major towns. 70% of the total 3,200 foreign returnees belong to these districts. Airport, railways, bus-stand, and essential services were exempted.

All service providers, including private sector, engaged in COVID-19 relief services, to be declared Emergency Workers: Naveen Patnaik, Chief Minister of Odisha (Mohanty 2020).

The West Bengal government ordered all restaurants, bars, pubs, nightclubs, amusement parks, museums, and zoos to be shut down as a precautionary measure in wake of the COVID-19 pandemic. It aims to prevent all non-essential social gatherings. The strict action would be taken in case of any violation (Deccan Herald 2020). UP government under CM Yogi Adityanath announced to provide financial help to labor (about Rs. 1,000 per month) for meeting their daily requirements due to non-availability of work (India Today Web Desk 2020).

Kerala government under the leadership of CM P. Vijayan announced Rs. 20,000 as a special economic package, for disbursing two-month of advance payment of pension. Those without any welfare pension will be provided Rs. 1,000 each along with free ration for all. Additionally, Rs 500 for health package also being announced (The New Indian Express 2020). Karnataka CM B. S. Yedurappa has stated to release fund of amount 200 crores to fight against the COVID-19 pandemic outbreak. In addition, foreign returning individuals are being stamped to ensure the complete safety of all the residents of Karnataka, and must be quarantine for 15 days (Pinto 2020).

The ministry of health and family welfare have started training for critical care management at 1,000 places through video conference. Health ministry joint secretary Lav Agarwal told reporters that guidelines for coronavirus tests have been revised, directing that asymptomatic direct, and high-risk contacts of confirmed cases should be tested once between day 5 and day 14 of coming in contact with an infected person.

Some initiatives from other institutes for the control of COVID-19 outbreak are:

1. *Teachers to work from home.* Teachers and non-teaching staff of universities, colleges and schools permitted to work from home: Amit Khare, Secretary, Ministry of Human Resource Development (Hindustan Times 2020).

2. *Using of Hand Sanitizer.* In each and every shopping complex are providing sanitizer to each and every customer during the entry to the shopping mall and the exit of the mall. The ministry has also informed to sanitizer maker/provider to provide hand sanitizer under Rs. 100/- for 200 ml (Niyogy 2020).
3. 111 labs to test Covid-19 across the country will be functional from today to test coronavirus (The Economic Times 2020).
4. All restaurants, pubs, bars to remain shut across the country. The restaurants are being allowed to provide home-delivery facilities of food to ensure no citizen goes hungry in the difficult time (Deccan Herald 2020).

CONCLUSION

The government of India was keeping a watch on the situation around the globe and has made efficient strategies to combat this COVID-19 threat, including lockdown whole country, reduce the prices of sanitizers, give fund, increase the testing of sample, disinfect the suspected areas. The statistics showed that the action taken by Indian government has slowed down the spread of COVID-19 infection. Albeit, the number of cases is rising but the rate is not very high as compared to the other countries. The preparedness of India can be shared with other nations as all other nations have been sharing their strategies, experiences, and precautions to reduce the number of positive cases. This COVID-19 pandemic threat faced by the world could be stated as an unpredictable the third world war.

REFERENCES

Anggraeni, S., Maulidina, A., Dewi, M. W., Rahmadianti, S., Rizky, Y. P. C., Arinalhaq, Z. F., Usdiyana, D., Nandiyanto, A. B. D., and Al-Obaidi, A. S. M. 2020. "The Deployment of Drones in Sending Drugs and

Patient Blood Samples COVID-19." *Indonesian Journal of Science and Technology* vol. 5, no. 2 (March):193-200.

Armitage, R and Nellums, L. B. 2020. "Covid-19 and the consequences of isolating the elderly." *The Lancet Public Health Correspondence*, vol. 5, no. 5 (May). https://www.thelancet.com/journals/lanpub/article/PIIS2468-2667(20)30061-X/fulltext.

Bloomberg Quint. "Coronavirus Updates: India Heads for Complete Lockdown as Covid-19 Cases Mount." *Bloombregquint.com.* 22 March 2020. https://www.bloombergquint.com/coronavirus-outbreak/janata-curfew-live-news-updates-coronavirus-covid-19-india-pm-narendra-modi-social-distancing.

Business Today India. 2020. "PM Modi Speech Live Updates: 'Stay where you are,' says PM Modi while declaring complete lockdown in India." *Businesstoday.in.* 24 March 2020. https://www.businesstoday.in/latest/trends/pm-narendra-modi-speech-to-nation-live-updates-coronavirus-in-india-covid-19-outbreak-cases/story/399108.html.

Carlos, W. G., Dela Cruz, C. S., Cao, B., Pasnick, S., and Jamil, S. 2020. "Novel Wuhan (2019-nCoV) Coronavirus." *American Journal of Respiratory and Critical Care Medicine* vol. 201, no. 4 (February): P7-P8. doi:10.1164/rccm.2014P7.

Chandrashekhar, V. "1.3 billion people. A 21-day lockdown. Can India curb the coronavirus?" *sciencemag.com.* 31 March 2020. https://www.sciencemag.org/news/2020/03/13-billionpeople-21-day-lockdown-can-india-curb-coronavirus.

Deccan Herald. "Coronavirus: All restaurants, pubs, bars to remain shut across Bengal till Mar 31." *Deccanherald.com* 21 March 2020. https://www.deccanherald.com/national/east-and-northeast/coronavirus-all-restaurants-pubs-bars-to-remain-shut-across-bengal-till-mar-31-816092.html.

Financial Times. 2020. *Ft.com.* https://www.ft.com/coronavirus-latest.

Gallagher, J. 2020. "Coronavirus vaccine: When will we have one?" *BBC.com.* 21 July 2020. https://www.bbc.com/news/health-51665497.

Hamidah, I., Sriyono, S., and Hudha, M. N. 2020. "A Bibliometric Analysis of COVID-19 Research using VOSviewer." *Indonesian Journal of Science and Technology* vol. 5, no. 2 (March):209-216.

Hindustan Times. "Teachers, non-teaching staff permitted to work from home till March 31, says MHRD." *Hindustantimes.com.* 22 March 2020. https://www.hindustantimes.com/education/teachers-non-teaching-staff-permitted-to-work-from-home-till-march-31-says-mhrd/story-sfUsgS9Yjv3aKpW3T2pzAP.html.

India Today Web Desk. "Covid-29: UP CM Yogi Adityanath says daily wage workers to get Rs 1,000 per month." *Indiatoday.in.* 21 March 2020. https://www.indiatoday.in/india/story/covid-19-coronavirus-uttar-pradesh-yogi-adityanath-1658075-2020-03-21.

India Today Web Desk. "Coronavirus in India: Over 300 new cases take Covid-19 count past 1,900; Delhi total reaches 152." *Indiatoday.in.* 1 April 2020. https://www.indiatoday.in/india/story/coronavirus-india-cases-covid-19-count-news-update-tally-number-1662116-2020-04-01.

Mohanty, M. "A week long lockdown for 40 per cent of Odisha starting tomorrow." *Economictimes.indiatimes.com.* 21 March 2020. https://economictimes.indiatimes.com/news/politics-and-nation/odisha-announces-a-week-long-lockdown-for-40-percent-of-the-state-starting-tomorrow/articleshow/74747444.cms?from=mdr.

Niyogi, S. "Kolkata: Malls adopt steps to create safe zone for customers and staff." *Thetimesofindia.indiatimes.com.* 13 March 2020. https://timesofindia.indiatimes.com/city/kolkata/malls-adopt-steps-to-create-safe-zone-for-customers-and-staff/articleshow/74602013.cms.

Patna. "Coronavirus in India: Bihar shuts down bus services, restaurants, banquet halls till March 31." *Indiatoday.com.* 21 March 2020. indiatoday.in/india/story/coronavirus-india-bihar-shuts-down-bus-services-restaurants-banquet-halls-march-31-1658248-2020-03-21.

Pinto, N. "Coronavirus in Karnataka: CM Yediyurappa announces Rs 200 crore corpus fund to fight Covid-19 outbreak." *Indiatoday.in.* 18 March 2020. https://www.indiatoday.in/india/story/coronavirus-in-karnataka-cm-bs-yediyurappa-covid-19-situation-update-1656984-2020-03-18.

Razon, B. C. 2020. "COVID 19: Impetus for "Community Spirits" among Filipinos." *Indonesian Journal of Science and Technology* vol. 5, no. 2 (March): 201-208.

SNS Web. "Airline to participate in Janta Curfew, curtail operations." *Thestatesman.com.* 21 March 2020. https://www.thestatesman.com/business/airlines-participate-janta-curfew-curtail-operations-1502868339.html.

The Economic Times. "Coronavirus updates: 111 labs across India functional from today for COVID-19 testing, informs govt." *Economictimes.indiatimes.com.* 21 march 2020. https://economictimes.indiatimes.com/news/politics-and-nation/coronavirus-updates-111-labs-across-india-functional-from-today-for-covid-19-testing-informs-govt/videoshow/74750213.cms?from=mdr.

The Economic Times. "Establishments asked not to sack employees in view of Covid-19." *Economictimes.indiatimes.com.* 21 March 2020. https://economictimes.indiatimes.com/news/politics-and-nation/establishments-asked-not-to-sack-employees-in-view-of-covid-19/articleshow/74745984.cms.

The Hindu Business Line. "After curfew, it is lockdown in 75 districts." *Thehindubusinessline.com.* 22 March 2020. https://www.thehindu businessline.com/news/national/coronavirus-states-to-lockdown-75-districts-interstate-travel-restrictions-imposed/article31135152.ece.

The New Indian Express. "Kerala govt announces Rs 20,000 crore special package to tackle coronavirus; highlights. *Newindianexpress.com.* 20 march 2020. https://www.newindianexpress.com/galleries/nation/2020/mar/20/kerala-govt-announces-rs-20000-crore-special-package-to-tackle-coronavirus-highlights-102804.html.

Wilder-Smith, A and Freedman, DO. 2020. "Isolation, Quarantine, Social Distancing and Community Containment: Pivotal Role for Old-Style Public Health Measures in the Novel Coronavirus (2019-Ncov) Outbreak." *Journal of Travel Medicine* 27, no. 2 (March): taaa020. https://doi.org/10.1093/jtm/taaa02.

World Health Organization. 2020. WHO Worldwide. https://www.who.int/health-topics/coronavirus.

World Health Organization. 2020. WHO Worldwide https://www.who.int/emergencies/diseases/novel-coronavirus-2019.

In: COVID-19 ISBN: 978-1-53618-903-2
Editors: A. B. D. Nandiyanto et al. © 2021 Nova Science Publishers, Inc.

Chapter 6

BAYANIHAN VALUES DURING COVID-19

***Brando Cabigas Razon*[1,*]**
***and Tryastuti Irawati Belliny Manullang*[2]**
[1]Sultan Kudarat State University, Tacurong City, Philippines
[2]Departemen Pendidikan Khusus,
Universitas Pendidikan Indonesia, Bandung, Indonesia

ABSTRACT

The Coronavirus Disease in December 2019 (COVID-19) pandemic continued to spread to the whole world. On 12 March 2020, President Rodrigo Duterte announced the month-long lockdown of the entire Metro Manila from 15 March to 14 April 2020. Within this period, vehicles traveling include land, air and sea to and from Metro Manila were suspended, followed by social and religious events involving mass gatherings. Conferences, seminars, and related events were also postponed and people were told to stay home. The government was merely following the usual procedure, such as the implementation of thermal screening at airports to detect arrivals with flu. The COVID 19 was not of great importance for most ordinary people in the Philippines, but the lockdown has both the downsides and the upsides. It has affected the economic,

* Corresponding Author's Email: brandorazon@yahoo.com.

social, and psychological aspects. Needless to say, a tragedy or misfortune to a place or individual may be an advantage for others. Therefore, the economic, social, and ecological aspects have been seen as favorable and beneficial opportunity during this lockdown. We have also learned the value of compassion and empathy during this crisis. This COVID-19 prompted the Philippines to unite to resolve the crisis. '*Bayanihan*' value encourages people to fight the negative and undesirable things in the community and finding the opportunity which can be used and developed.

Keywords: *Bayanihan*, COVID-19 virus, Filipino

1. Introduction

Since December 2019, an increasing number of cases of novel coronavirus (2019-nCoV)-infected pneumonia (NCIP) have been identified in Wuhan (Li et al., 2020). The outbreak of serious acute respiratory syndrome coronavirus (SARS-CoV-2) has now reached pandemic proportions, affecting more than 100 countries in just weeks (Remuzzi and Remuzzi 2020). On 11 February 2020, WHO announced the name for the coronavirus disease as COVID-19. The virus transmitted between humans via respiratory droplets and also with other possibilities that it can be transmitted through direct or indirect contact with mucous membranes in the eyes, mouth, or nose (Li et al., 2020). This shows the reasons why people are aware of COVID-19 since it can attack several organs in the human body. The impact of COVID-19 is a catastrophe because as of 14 April 2020 it has infected no less than 1.9 million people in the world and kills thousands (Corona 24 news 2020).

However, the COVID-19 was not of great importance for most ordinary people in the Philippines. The news about this virus originated from China can be heard in both local and international television networks. It made us recalled the unpleasant experience as we feared the influenza virus (known as H1N1) in 2009. As we heard the news on TV, airports were fitted with a thermal scanner to identify arriving passengers and were instructed to quarantine as detected (Razon 2020). People traveling from countries with H1N1 cases were also advised to do home quarantine to prevent the virus from spreading. It was a monumental experience yet unpleasant. People who took a flight to Osaka, Japan were out on masks uncomfortably as they disembarked. At that period, most ordinary citizens in the Philippines were not affected by the H1N1 pandemic.

Therefore, for Filipinos the coronavirus was just similar to those previously known viruses and was not of big importance. Additionally, most ordinary people including those educated but without scientific inclination do not know what a virus is. Virus is a borderline between living and non-living things, not capable of reproduction but only do this process utilizing the machineries of a living cell. Virus infections are often experienced by most people regardless of status in life such as viruses that cause chickenpox, mumps, sore eyes, and many other illnesses. Some viral infections last for only a short period of time while others serious might last for a longer period and can have a serious impact on the person such as the poliomyelitis virus and many others. International Health organizations such as the World Health Organization (WHO) is making efforts to stop the spread of these viral infections in some ways such as developing vaccines and ensuring the availability of medicines and antiviral agents.

Consequently, countries are working on giving clear and concise information about the symptoms, the transmission, the preventive measures, and the socioeconomical impacts. The continued spread of the virus is the reason why mass media still disseminate awareness through print, television, and other methods to educate people about the best way to wash hands, the proper strategies to sneeze in public and many other acceptable hygiene practices to avoid the widespread. However, cases of confirmed coronavirus positive continued to rise almost exponentially.

Although the outbreak is likely to have started from a zoonotic transmission event associated with a large seafood market which also traded in live wild animals, it soon became clear that efficient transmission from person to person was also happening (Zhou et al., 2020) and consequently the discrimination of the Chinese nationals is also occurring. As an example, in the northern part of the Philippines, before a research conference, the Chinese researcher who supposed to be one of the plenary speakers cancelled the agenda for fear of creating panic to the participants. Another case, when Filipinos encountered Chinese-speaking tourists wearing a mask in the plaza and indeed, they refrain from getting near to them. This was the start where the face masks in the drug stores were out of stock and it was very difficult to find one.

Initially, people did not think this virus would have any significant impacts. However, as the number of people infected by COVID-19 was increasing, at the same time, the fear of getting the virus was also increasing. As a result, some students from the Philippine Science High School in Korondal City commented on the slow action the president took. At that time, airport was still remained open and flights from other countries which considered to increase the spread of the virus were still run. As the death toll was rising, the government became more concerned about the issue of coronavirus. On 12 March 2020, President Rodrigo Duterte announced a month-long lockdown of the entire Metro Manila from 15 March to 14 April 2020. Within this period, vehicles traveling include land, air, and sea to and from Metro Manila were suspended, followed by social and religious events involving mass gathering and also conferences, seminars, and related events were postponed. People were told to stay home. President Rodrigo Duterte announced the effect of the lockdown by on 11 March 2020, night live on ABS CBN (US News 2020).

Regardless of the lockdown, the virus continued to spread rapidly and some Filipinos started to fear the virus since death cases were increasing as it continued to spread. People did not think this virus would have any significant impacts in the Philippines. Due to its simple transmission, the spread of the virus is vast and rapid. Most sick people in the Philippines are those with a travel history outside the country and it spreads to other people in the provinces who also have travel history to the capital city. As the lockdown started, intensive distribution of information and ongoing education to the public was also started. People were given information on the "dos" and "don'ts" while fighting on the COVID-19.

This rapid change is not easy for many people. There were some challenges at the initial stage of the lockdown. There was chaos on the checkpoints, and some people could not stand on the situation. All citizen was encouraged to wear masks, did handwashing as often as possible with soap and water, put on hand sanitizers, and maintained social distancing. The change is inevitable and all Filipinos have been affected. Although the infection is not common among economically challenged people but the effect of the lockdown experience by all citizens regardless of the social status.

Therefore, this study aimed to scrutinize the *Bayanihan* values among Filipino because we believe the values encourage people to fight the negative and undesirable things in the community and finding the opportunity which can be used and developed. As much as the COVID-19 has affected the economic, social, and psychological aspects, however, at the same time we have also learned the values of compassion and empathy during this crisis.

2. Lockdown Effects towards the Local Community

COVID-19 has devastated the income of the people. It affects economic activities, such as disruption in the manufacturing, transport, tourism, and other works sectors, which leads to financial distress among those who are on the status of 'no job no pay.' The lockdown as a way of enforcing group quarantine has clearly resulted in both negative and positive issues for the government and people.

2.1. The Negative Impact

The negative aspects could fall into economic, social, and psychological aspects as commonly observed scenario in our place.

2.1.1. Psychological Effect

As stated earlier that the number of the death toll during the COVID-19 pandemic has infected the mental stated of the people. People are worried that their family might be the victims of this virus. Due to the increasing fear, the panic buying for masks, rubbing alcohols, and hand sanitizers happened. As a result, these items were out of stocks. This can imply that people buy such products to avoid infection or some could hoard supplies, and eventually sell them for higher price.

Additionally, people who are sick or unwell choose not to visit the hospitals for fear of being infected. Although they have different types of sickness, they are reluctant to go for medication. Besides, the fear of running out of food supplies and money during the lockdown has also contributed to their psychological condition. This fear eventually might contribute to depression that people might encounter during this uncertain time.

2.1.2. Economic Effect

COVID-19 has added to the immense economic costs not only for the vulnerable but also for the country as a whole (Mahmud and Minghat 2020). In the Philippines, 50% of the population are poor people (Zoleta 2020). Therefore, it is not easy for the government to solve this issue. The government made a scheme of providing cash amelioration in the amount of Php 5.000 (±100 USD) to this economically challenged family (Colcol 2020). The Department of Social Welfare and Development (DSWD) was assigned to arrange the distribution. A food package consisting of five kilograms of rice, three packages of instant noodles, and three canned sardines were also distributed. Needless to say, that the most affected people are the poor people who only have a budget for one-day consumption and with the lock down, these groups of people cannot go working. They are also still worried about the insufficient supplies during the lockdown. However, few families have started planting easy to grow vegetables in the prevention of the extended and continued lockdown.

2.1.3. Social Effect

As mentioned earlier, vehicles traveling include land, air, and sea to and from Metro Manila were suspended. This has affected the lower-income families the most. So, many people could not go home and could not be with their families during the lockdown. The COVID-19 crisis has a social dimension (Hasanah et al., 2020, Sangsawang 2020). At the beginning, the upper and middle-income classes are specifically affected as they are the ones who have traveled or are acquainted with others who have traveled (National Economic and Development Authority 2020). Government also told people to maintain social distancing and avoid involving mass gathering including social and religious events and also conferences, seminars, and related events were postponed and people were told to stay home. As a result, academia has to reschedule and reconstruct schedules. Socializing outside the house is forbidden and drinking liquor outside the house is also banned. Unfortunately, healthcare front liners have encountered discrimination due to the fear of them carrying the virus.

2.2. The Positive Impact

Undoubtedly, COVID-19 has disrupted our life. However, a tragedy or misfortune to a place or individuals may be an advantage for others. Currently there are plenty of issues that are positive and helpful to many people during the lockdown.

2.2.1. Ecological Aspect

According to the Philippine Department of Environment and Natural Resources, the air pollution in the capital city, Manila, was remarkably reduced since most people stay at home. The burning of fossil fuels is also decreasing as the streets are mostly silent and we do not have both domestic and international flights. Garbage piles are also reducing as most hotels, restaurants, and tourist destinations are closed. Mother Nature is taking its time to recover.

2.2.2. Social Aspect

The social aspect seems not only having a negative impact but also beneficial effects. During this COVID-19 pandemic outbreak, Filipinos have shown the "*Bayanihan*" culture that we have. *Bayanihan* is also called the 'community spirit' where people help out neighbors in order to make the job easier and to ease the burden through collaboration. It is commonly observed during disaster and hardship. Fortunately, it is happening during the COVID-19 pandemic.

Although healthcare workers initially encountered discrimination but realizing the *Bayanihan* value, people stated showing support to them by giving food, water, masks, and other personal protective equipment they need. Some people sing for the healthcare staff and the patients by keeping maintaining the distance, and some send encouragement notes.

Additionally, many families in the Philippines are intact families. The lockdown has given more opportunities for families to devote longer times with their loved ones and do more family bonding activities. This, undoubtedly, has contributed to their immune system as people also promote health practices by taking a balanced diet. People have also learned to affirm their faith and loyalty to God as they show more concern for their fellows. For some Christians, the coronavirus is God's will to make people repent and make them believe that God is still in control above all.

2.2.3. Economic Aspect

As aforementioned that COVID-19 has affected the economic condition adversely (Dirgantari et al. 2020). However, it has also encouraged people to be creative. Due to the lockdown and the social distancing policy, people are not allowed to go out unless they go by motorcycle. Even so, only one person is allowed on the motorcycle. Therefore, people find it difficult to buy their daily needs. But some people came up with the idea of "mobile market." Although the price is higher than the market, but online selling has been more popular. For the seller, they get bigger return than usual and for the buyer it is more practical and less risky than sending one member of the family to go out. In addition, the government-owned employees have been given two months of loan deduction from the Government System Insurance Service in order to help them with their needs during the lockdown.

CONCLUSION

COVID-19 is and has seriously destroyed human lives and disrupted economic development in all nations. It gives pain to the families and relatives of the victims. It challenges all the world leaders to find solutions. However, there are also good things that evolved from this pandemic effect. It can give good results and impact to communities and countries. The lockdown in all parts of the Philippines has brought solidarity between family members and people in the society. In times of crisis, the lesson from the current situation is the importance of compassion and empathy. One of the most significant results of this pandemic is its ability to move the people in the Philippines to reinforce the Filipino importance of *bayanihan* or "community spirits" and to combat this pandemic together as one. The whole world will overcome this crisis, together we heal as one.

REFERENCES

Colcol, E. "Who may receive COVID-29 emergency cash subsidy from gov't? DSWD explains." *MSN.com,* 5 April 2020. (https://www.msn.com/en-ph/news/national/who-may-receive-covid-19-emergency-cash-subsidy-from-govt-dswd-explains/ar-BB12aXae).

Corona 24 News. "Coronavirus in the world - the number infected exceeded 1.9 million people." *Corona24news.com,* 14 April 2020. https://www.corona24.news/c/2020/04/14/coronavirus-in-the-world-the-number-of-infected-exceeded-1-9-million-people.html.

Dirgantari, P. D., Hidayat, Y. M., Mahphoth, M. H., & Nugraheni, R. 2020. "Level of Use and Satisfaction of E-Commerce Customers in Covid-19 Pandemic Period: An Information System Success Model (ISSM) Approach." *Indonesian Journal of Science and Technology*, vol. 5, no. 2 (September): 86-95.

Hasanah, L., Hakim, W. L., Aminudin, A., Sahari, S. K., and Mulyanti, B. 2020. "A Design and performance analysis of a telemetry system for remote monitoring of turbidity of water during the COVID-19 pandemic." *Indonesian Journal of Science and Technology*, vol. 5, no. 2 (September):299-307.

Li, H., Liu, S. M., Yu, X. H., Tang, S. L., Tang, C. K. 2020. "Coronavirus disease 2019 (COVID-19): current status and future perspectives." *International Journal of Antimicrobial Agents,* vol. 55, no. 5 (May). doi: https://10.1016/j.ijantimicag.2020.105951.

Li, Q., Guan, X., Wu, P., Wang, X., Zhou, L., Tong Y. et al., 2020. "Early Transmission dynamics in Wuhan, China, of Novel Coronavirus-Infected pneumonia." The *New England Journal of Medicine* vol. 382 (January):1199-1207.

Machmud, A., and Mighat, A. D. B. 2020. "The Price Dynamics of Hand Sanitizers for COVID-19 in Indonesia: Exponential and Cobweb Forms." *Indonesian Journal of Science & Technology*, vol. 5, no. 2 (September):176-184.

National Economic and Development Authority. "Addressing the Social Economic Impact of the COVID-19 Pandemic." *Neda.gov.* March 2020. http://www.neda.gov.ph/addressing-the-social-economic-of-the-covid-19-pandemic/.

Razon, B. C. 2020. "COVID-19: Impetus for "Community Spirits" Among Filipinos." *Indonesian Journal of Science & Technology,* vol. 5, no. 2 (September): 26-33.

Remuzzi, A., and Remuzzi, G. 2020. "COVID-19 and Italy: What next?" *The Lancet* vol. 395, no. 10231 (March): 1225-1228. https://doi.org/10.1016/S0140-6736(20)30627-9.

Sangsawang, T. 2020. "An Instructional Design for Online Learning in Vocational Education according to a Self-Regulated Learning Framework for Problem Solving during the CoViD-19 Crisis." *Indonesian Journal of Science and Technology*, vol.5, no. 2 (September): 283-298.

US News. Phillipines Duterte Announces Lockdown of Manila to Fight Coronavirus. *US News.com*, 12 March 2020. https://www.usnews.com/news/world/articles/2020-03-12/philippines-duterte-announces-lockdown-of-manila-to-fight-coronavirus.

Visual Capitalist. *COVID-19. "How does it affect you?"* 2020. https://www.visualcapitalist.com/wp-content/uploads/2020/04/covid-19-affects-the-body.html.

Zhou, F, Yu, T., Du, R., Fan, G., Liu, Y., Liu, Z., et al., 2020. "Clinical course and risk factors for mortality of adult inpatients with COVID-19 in Wuhan, China: a retrospective cohort study." *The Lancet*, vol. 395, no. 10229 (March):1054-1062. https://doi.org/10.1016/S0140-6736(20)30566-3.

Zoleta, V. "Understanding Social Sclass in the Phillipines: Which Class Do You Belong to?" *Yahoonews.com*, 16 April 2020. https://sg.news.yahoo.com/understanding-social-class-philippines-class-020037877.html.

In: COVID-19 ISBN: 978-1-53618-903-2
Editors: A. B. D. Nandiyanto et al.

Chapter 7

STRESS OF THE CHANGES IN THE LIFE AND CONDITIONS OF PATIENTS

Mariam R. Arpentieva[1], Asnul Dahar Minghat[2] and Gulzhaina K. Kassymova[3,4,5]

[1]Department at the Development and Education Psychology, Tsiolkovskiy Kaluga State University, Russian Federation
[2]Razak Faculty of Technology and Informatics, Universiti Teknologi Malaysia, University College of Islam Melaka, Malaysia
[3]Institute of Pedagogy and Psychology, Abai Kazakh National Pedagogical University, Kazakhstan
[4]Graduate School, Yogyakarta State University, Indonesia
[5]Institute of Metallurgy and Ore Beneficiation, Satbayev University, Kazakhstan

ABSTRACT

This chapter analyzed the narratives of patients as one of the most productive methods of psychotherapeutic work with adults, particularly work aimed at the development of man, his manhood. The authors paid special attention to the problems of the metaphors of the signals and triggers a psychological transformation. The aim of the study was to analyze the problems of anticipating and minimizing the stress of changes in the life of a person (patient). The research method was theoretically understanding of the problems of anticipating and minimizing the stress of changes in the life of a person (patient). The main results of the study showed the patient overcame estrangement from himself and the world, liminality. A metaphor in a person's life acts as a signal and a trigger for change: its use, one way or another, reveals zones that are subject to changes and stimulates changes themselves. Metaphors manifest themselves in various archetypal structures and in specific metaphors of role models. They allow you to evaluate the direction of the patient's internal movement towards the realization of a particular motivation, intention, support upward and/or slow down downward intentions, as well as comprehend how the patient perceives external changes, how he experiences stress of changes.

Keywords: narrative psychotherapy, markers of change, stress of change, the archetypes, triggers for change

1. Introduction

Stress and change are an integral part of the human life. The stresses of change (a concept introduced by M.R. Arpentieva in 2020) can be smoothed out and transformed by anticipating and understanding them. One approach is to study the precursors of change and transformation by analyzing life scenarios and narratives. This moment is especially relevant in working with people mentally and somatically ill, patients (Arpentieva 2015; Arpentieva and Terentiev 2016; Mindell 1997; Minigalieva 1999).

In working with narratives, special attention should be paid to combining diachronic and synchronous analysis: changing patterns of behavior and the essence of participants' actions at different stages of their life paths, in different worlds and times. Particularly great attention in this context should be given to metaphors - denoting worlds and times, as well as - accomplished or emerging transitions between worlds and times. Metaphors act as bright signals and triggers of change. Each metaphor is a germ or designation of intention, which the heroes follow on their way to themselves, to each other and to God, to happiness and the resolution of the crisis.

The purpose of the study was to analyze the problems of anticipating and minimizing the stress of changes in the life of a person (patient). The research method was a theoretical understanding of the problems of anticipating and minimizing the stress of changes in the life of a person (patient).

2. Results and Discussions

2.1. Transderivational Search and Understanding of Changes

On the way to resolution, the patient overcomes estrangement from himself and the world, liminality. He learns to comprehend changes in himself and the world, recognizing their being and the right to change. Recognizing oneself and other patients in a particular narrative, recognizing themselves and each other as heroes of the narrative, their self-understanding and understanding of other people are processes that can be almost parallel. The condition is semantic resonance: in the process of studying a narrative in the inner world of a person, a search for similar content between the composing narrative and his life world takes place. The fragment of the world' image resonates with a fragment of a fairytale world, a semantic (semantic) resonance arises, due to which it is "unpacked", a new one is updated, productive and more accurate understanding of what is happening (Arpentieva and Terentiev 2016; Bazhov 1993; Hilborn 2004, Meadows 1999. "Transderivational search" - the search for correspondence to the current situation of the patient and fragments of the experience of stress of change, given in the form of a metaphor, story/narrative, script (fabulous or relational).

In order to overcome the non-constructive methods of self-defense associated with this process, to make the structure-schemes and processes-strategies for understanding oneself and the world developed during previous professional and general life experiences, a metaphorical language that integrates the value relationship of a person to himself and the world becomes necessary. As well as ways to translate this relationship into real life - in the process of understanding what is happening and communicating with another person. Metaphors eventually become markers and triggers of change: sometimes nothing acts as strongly as a metaphor applied and/or captured by those who communicate. Moreover, her understanding is the deconstruction of the polylogue of "weak" and "strong" voices (Arpentieva 2015; Packard 2001; Pekar 2010; Ufimstev 2009).

Each of the possible strategies of understanding - based on strong and/or weak signals or voices - acts as a set of ways to understand yourself and another person, the world. Generally speaking, markers and triggers of change can be very intense, explicit, related and declared values and goals of the patient and/or his relationship system. Moreover, they are formed in the form of concepts that have more or less fixed social meanings and personal meanings. They can be weak, hidden, including those associated with implicitly existing, but up to a certain point, not manifested system characteristics. They take shape and arise in dialogue with the therapist and other people in the form of metaphors. Their peculiarity lies in the fact that even minimal changes in the parameters lead to disproportionately significant changes in the behavior of the entire system: these supersensitive zones are usually called "chaos boundaries" (Lewin 2000; Prigozhin and Stengers 1986).

2.2. Between Worlds: Transformations at the Border of Spaces and Times

It is difficult to find "pure chaos" in the surrounding world, and just as it is difficult to find the absolute order. Instead of a limited complex adaptive system surrounded by chaos, the researchers have in front of them an unlimited complex heterogeneous and adaptive environment that looks like an endless "patchwork quilt". There is "relatively pure" chaos as complete uncertainty: the ordering forces here do not act or act differently, including in the direction of increasing chaos. The "boundaries of chaos" can be called the "boundaries of orders": they are located at the junction of the flaps, at the junctions and interactions of the regions of orderliness and homeostatic stability (Beytson 2000; Packard 2001; Prigozhin and Stengers 1986; Ufimtsev 2009). In these junctions there is a conflict and interaction of two (or more) neighboring orders. The "points" of personal or social reality located in them fall under the conflicting influence of two or several homeostatic systems at the same time. This creates a special "tension" in them comparable to the border transition between two hostile countries. One order is contrary, hostile to the other. Where two orders are in contact, tension arises and close mutual attention develops disproportionate sensitivity even to minor events ("provocations"). Here, nonlinear, recursive characteristics appear, which one of the creators of the theory of complex systems Ed pointed out. Lorentz: their ability to be hypersensitive in certain areas, striving for "strange attractors" instead of "logically explainable" (Hilborn 2004; Lorenz 1995; Prigozhin and Stengers 1986). These zones can be called borderline or shimmering, obeying the described the concept of butterfly effect. The butterfly impact denotes the property of some chaotic systems: a slight effect on the system can have large and unpredictable consequences elsewhere and at another time.

The general characteristics of the areas of order are: adaptability; sustainability; the desire for expansion as the development of accessible space; susceptibility to phases of the life cycle, the duration of the phases of which varies depending on the scale and content of the structure (Ufimtsev 2009). Usually it including the phases: the phase of the emergence of "key ideas", the "core", the rapid development and capture of new areas as a result of adaptation to a wide range of conditions (phase of active expansion), a phase of defense against competing structures and a phase of collision with changing external conditions and decay (Ufimtsev 2009).

Common characteristics of "flickering zones" or "areas of collision of orders" are maladaptation, instability/variability, life cycle instability, and the ability to enhance or weaken the expansion of "zones of order". In the border zones or "seams" between the "flaps" of social reality, areas of order are actively clashing, and unique properties of "flickering zones" arise. For example, the "hypersensitivity" of cognitive structures to its periphery, the "sensitivity to problems" of this periphery, and, therefore, the entire "flap" —the concepts, concepts, percentages and (re) constructed by them of social phenomena and objects (Bakurova 2015; Ufimtsev 2009; Van Raj 2012).

Metaphors indicate the presence of "flickering zones'. They, like strict concepts, can denote the same fragments of reality - the same "flickering zones". Moreover, they have different "indicator value", revealing the meaning of the tension of relations between concepts and concepts in the border zone, the "between" zone. The general signs of "indicator value" and the separation of metaphors are as follows: repeated repetition of a metaphor in various circumstances by different people; the metaphor is not repeated literally, but modified with the preservation of meaning; a metaphor is spread socially (Leskov 1981; Ufimtsey 2009).

However, in addition to the artificial metaphors generated by people, there are also natural metaphors created by a stream of socially significant events and pointing to "flickering zones", the existence of which is not yet recognized and which manifest themselves as "strange coincidences". "Irony of fate", "jokers", in practice events that are not connected both in space and in time with each other - synchronisms as manifestations of the collective unconscious: the plots of events are metaphorically identical (Hilborn 2004; Howe and Strauss 1997; Jung 1996; Khlebnikova 2013; Meadows 1999; Van Raj 2012; Zinkevich-Evstigneeva 2013). Through synchrony of apparently unrelated events, the collective unconscious "indicates" the appearance of "flickering zones" of social reality in which significant events occur (Frants 1998; Jung 2003

2.3. Identification of Markers of Change and the Transformation of Reality

At the junction of reality, borderline or "flickering zones" there are points that are most effective and productive from the point of view of understanding the essence of development difficulties and the productive transformation of reality: influences can be produced with more or less purposeful directing of events and facts that have metaphorical significance.

To increase the likelihood and intensity of the desired effect of interventions in these zones, one can resort to methods of increasing their "indicator value". We can resort to repeated use of a language or event metaphor, its variation while preserving the essence, and widespread use of language - artificial or event - natural metaphors in social space. For example, we can resort to "sowing" as repeated use of event and language metaphors along the "target" "flickering zone".

D. Meadows, a student of J. Forrester (Forrester et al. 1977; Meadows 1999; Meadows 1999) examines the limits of the cybernetic approach to the study of complex social systems. J. Forrester already in the 60s of the XX century began to model and study complex social systems ("system dynamics" - the study and prediction of complex systems using computer simulation methods based on cybernetic schematizations). He wrote about the presence of "sensitive points" in these systems, which are the preferred targets for interventions in complex systems. These targets allow you to purposefully change the behavior and condition of large and complex systems with minimal loss of strength and means (Forrester et al. 1977). D. Meadows used the term that is used by system analysts - "leverage points", which can also be translated as "sensitive points" - places in complex systems in which even a small shift can lead to big changes in the whole system. She believed that people often intuitively know where sensitive points are located, but either do not pay attention to it, or try to put pressure on it in a direction that is not productive for the individual or group: errors of intuition arise. Therefore, J. Forrester called these points "counter-intuitive": everyday life and its intuition suggest incorrect movements, leading to a systemic deterioration of the problem (Forrester et al. 1977; Meadows 1999; Meadows 1999; Sangsawang 2020; Hasanah et al. 2020). In terms of the metacognitive approach, we are talking about the fact that the use of everyday heuristics without reflection of the areas of their application often leads to errors (Arpentieva 2015; Arpentieva and Terentiev 2016; Minigalieva 1999).

In the work of D. Harris and St. Zeisler on weak signals as "signs of big changes" (Harris and Zeisler 2002) disclosed one of the approaches to forecasting, based on the representation of social reality as a complex adaptive system in which the so-called weak signals appear and the development of "weak signal amplifiers" to help understand them. The richest source of weak signals is the periphery of culture: 1) interdisciplinary, inter-traditional; 2) kitsch and simulated, pseudo-art and pseudoscience; 3) extra-traditional, cultural, anti-science and anti-art. That is, rejected and forbidden, unusual and rare, devoid of price - worthless and priceless, and also magical, fabulous, which is why narrative therapy has the most significant psychotherapeutic potential among other types of psychotherapy.

According to the theory of "amplification of weak signals", a targeted search for weak signals at the boundary of chaos is the first step in their search. The second step is to understand weak signals, which should not be carried out by methods that understand strong trends: statistics and sorting are unproductive here. An intermediate procedure for understanding them is the "weak signal amplifier" - which helps to filter out weak signals from noise by their ability to cause changes in a complex adaptive system (Ufimtsev 2009.

However, the future makes itself felt not in one weak signal, but in their series distributed in various parts of the "flickering zones". A weak signal, unlike noise, combines (often unusual and incomprehensible) a number of cognitively significant factors that are pointless to "sort through" individually and logically and linearly calculate their potential. Therefore, the "fishing" and the "breadcrumb road" described by E. Mindell are more productive: simply waiting for a "weak signal" without the intention to typologize it and create a space/study of its self-realization space (Mindell 1997). Closest to him is the "integrating impression" regarding the methods and strategies of understanding. All the "crumbs" of the picture are important. They are all transferred from the "background - periphery" to the "center-figure". All of them find their gestalt: where the gestalt is destined to be acquired. In addition, in order to use the weak signal amplifier and other techniques for working with metaphors that serve as indicators (markers) of changes, it is necessary to identify the perspective that helps to search for weak signals. If this is impossible, then you just need to adopt the idea of the need to develop "sensitivity to problems/signals", being in a state of "active listening", including:

1. The irregularities of the "psychological texture", errors and holes (gaps) in a complex system and its manifestations;
2. "Information leaks", blocks - resistances and facades - interaction barriers;
3. Repeating and ignored zones, concepts and concepts;
4. Ordinary and unusual forms and contents of interaction,
5. Discovering both problems and methods of solving problems in the functioning and development of the system.

Instability zones ("flicker zones") are the boundaries of chaos that arise at the junction of stable zones. At these points, control signals come from a number of stable regions and enter into non-linear interactions, "quasi-chaos". It is at these points that the system is very sensitive and variable (Ufimtsev 2009). Areas of sustainability are areas of established and self-sustaining collective representations (values) of oneself and the world, unstable areas are areas of "cognitive flicker", conflict, and the transformation of various meanings. To find weak signals, you need to find significant things/events in the border areas - seams and joints - stable areas that are characterized by unusual and asymmetric, strange coincidences and repetitions.

M. Scheffer et al. also consider the topic of "early warning signals" of critical transitions to models from catastrophe theory: they call the point when the system is between two possible equilibrium states, jumping from one to the other under the action of even minimal influences, a bifurcation point or a phase or critical transition point (Scheffer et al. 2009). In their opinion, there are signs of approaching this point. Decrease in system resistance and its "critical slowdown" - the system is long restored from various fluctuations and perturbations, in contrast to the equilibrium system, which immediately returns to the state of homeostasis and relative isolation).

The critical state of a complex system can be more precisely related to the scale invariance (fractality) of the system structures: when the system structures acquire the property of "scale invariance", they become self-similar, then the system is in a critical/transition state, and the fact that designated self-similarity and there is a "weak signal." A fractal is a typically recursive model, each part of which repeats in its development the development of the entire model as a whole and is reproduced at various scales without major changes. The erosion of the characteristic spatial and temporal relationships in the system and the general drop in energy are common signals of approaching a critical transition (Scheffer et al. 2009; Ufimtsev 2009).

In metaphors, the unity of diachronic and synchronous, dialectics of life, the difficulties of life "grasp" especially easily and harmoniously: a person gains access to understanding the value of his experience - both for himself and for those around him. In psychotherapeutic communication, where the unconscious is almost inevitably involved, the metaphorical language of the narrative is valuable for a number of reasons (Arpentieva 2015; Arpentieva and Terentiev 2016; Bakurova 2015; Zinkevich-Evstegneeva 2012; Zinkevich-Evstegneeva 19980. It is more open to analysis and understanding; it is more powerful in terms of psychotherapeutic intervention, it gives the consciousness the opportunity to relax, and activates the awareness that are ignored by the patient in everyday life, also it reveals "weak signals" or markers of change and it can be used to create change as a trigger.

Metaphors allow us to comprehend the most complex, incomplete or ambivalent aspects of problem relations for a patient and a psychotherapist, including, in the context of the theory of archetypes/archetypal structures, to form on the basis of their analysis more productive in relation to a particular period of a person's life in one or another community, and more conscious role models that underlie the "paradigm" of understanding oneself and the world (Briggs-Myers 1998; Chernyshov 2011; Fromm 2010). In technical terms, this means the use of techniques such as "fishing" and "the road of their breadcrumbs" by E. Mindell (Mindell 1997) "an amplifier of weak signals" or the analysis and transformation of archetypal and role structures of a person's relationship to himself and the world. For these aims we the use of techniques similar to the analysis of projective techniques, including those developed by us to optimize the processing of TAT, "Self-attitude test", "Rules of the three" test and other projective techniques (Arpentieva 2015; Harris and Zeisler St 2002; Mindell 1997; Ufimtsev 2009). In addition, the idea of "weak", intertext signals formed the basis of our tales (Arpentieva and Terentiev 2016; Leskov 1981).

CONCLUSION

A metaphor in a person's life acts as a signal and a trigger for change: its use, one way or another, reveals zones that are subject to changes and stimulates changes themselves. Metaphors manifest themselves in various archetypal structures and in specific metaphors of role models. They allow you to evaluate the direction of the patient's internal movement towards the realization of a particular motivation, intention, support upward and/or slow down downward intentions, as well as comprehend how the patient perceives external changes, how he experiences stress of changes.

REFERENCES

Arpentieva, M. R. (2015). *Vzaimoponimanie kak fenomen mezhlichnostnykh otnosheniy (na materiale psikhologicheskogo konsul'tirovaniya).* Diss. …grand dokt. psikhol. nauk. Moscow: Lomonosov Moscow State University, 1-497. [*Understanding as a phenomenon of interpersonal relationships (based on psychological counseling*). Diss. ...grand doctor of the psychol. Sciences. Moscow: Lomonosov Moscow State University, 1-497.

Arpentieva, M. R. & Terentiev, A. A. (2016). "Skazkoterapiya v razvitii ponimaniya sebya i mira." Kaluga: *KGU Publ.*, 1-792. ["Fairytale therapy in the development of self-understanding and peace"]. Kaluga: KGU Publ., 1-792.

Bakurova, O. N. (2015). "Chuvstvitel'nost' k probleme: psikhologicheskie podkhody k opredeleniyu i izucheniyu ["Sensitivity to the problem: psychological approaches to the definition and study"]. *Vestnik Kaluzhskogo universiteta*, [*Bulletin of the Kaluga University*], *3*, .82-90.

Bazhov, P. P. (1993). *Ural'skie skazy*. Moscow: Zenit, 1-336. [Ural tales]. Moscow: Zenit, 1-336.

Beytson, G. (2000). *Ekologiya razuma*. Moscow: Smysl Publ., 1-476. [Ecology of the mind]. Moscow: Smysl Publ., 1-476.

Briggs-Myers, I., McCaulley, M. H., Quenk, N. L. & Hammer, A. l. L. (1998). *Manual: A Guide to the Development and Use of the Myers-Briggs Type Indicator*. Palo Alto, Calif: Consulting Psychologists Press, 1-420.

Chernyshov, A. V. (2011). *Russkie arkhetipy v brendinge i effektivnost' telereklamy*. Avtoref. diss… kand. sotsiol. Nauk. Nizhniy Novgorod: N. I. Lobachevskiy Novgorod State University Publ., 1-22. [*Russian archetypes in branding and the effectiveness of television advertising*. Abstract. PhD in sociology]. Nizhniy Novgorod: N. I. Lobachevskiy Novgorod State University Publ., 1-22.

Forrester, Dzh., Render, Yu., Medouz, D. & Bekhrens, V. (1977). "Sovremennye problemy kibernetiki: Sb. Statey Znanie. Ser. Matematika i kibernetika". *Knowledge. - Ser. Mathematics and cybernetics*, *1*- 45. ["Modern problems of cybernetics"], *Knowledge. - Ser. Mathematics and cybernetics*, 1-45.

Frants, fon M. L. (1998). "Proritsanie i sinkhroniya. Psikhologiya znachimogo sluchaya." *St. Petersburg: B.S.K. Publ.*, 107. ["Divination and synchrony. Psychology of a significant case"]. *St. Petersburg: B.S.K. Publ.*, 107.

Fromm, E. (2010). *Zabytyy yazyk. Vvedenie v nauku ponimaniya snov, skazok, mifov*. Moscow: AST, 624. [*Forgotten language. Introduction to the science of understanding dreams, fairy tales, myths*]. Moscow: AST, 624.

Hasanah, L., Hakim, W. L., Aminudin, A., Sahari, S. K. & Mulyanti, B. (2020). "A Design and performance analysis of a telemetry system for remote monitoring of turbidity of water during the COVID-19 pandemic." *Indonesian Journal of Science and Technology*, vol. *5*, no. 2, (March), 299–307.

Harris, D. & Zeisler, St. (2002). "Weak signals: Detecting the next big thing." *The Futurist*, vol. *36*, no. 6, 21-29.

Howe, N. & Strauss, W. (1997). "The Fourth Turning." New York: Broadway Books, 1-400.

Jung, K. (1996). *Dusha i mif. Shest' arkhetipov.* Kiev, Kiev Publ., 236. [*Soul and myth. Six archetypes*]. Kiev, Kiev Publ., 236.

Jung, K. G. (2003). *Sinkhroniya*. Moscow: "Refl-buk" Publ, Kiev: Vakler Publ, 1-320. [*Synchrony*]. Moscow: "Refl-buk" Publ, Kiev: Vakler Publ, 1-320.

Jung, K. G., Semyuels, E., Odaynik, V. & Khabbek, Dzh. (1995). *Analiticheskaya psikhologiya: Proshloe i nastoyashchee.* Zelenskiy V. V., Rutkevich A. M. (comp.). Moscow: Martis, 1-320. [*Analytical Psychology: Past and Present*]. Zelenskiy V. V., Rutkevich A. M. (comp.). Moscow: Martis, 1-320.

Khlebnikova, S. A. (2013). "Ispol'zovanie arkhetipov K.-G. Yunga v tselyakh pozitsionirovaniya territorial'nykh brendov." *Fundamental'nye issledovaniya*, 10-11, 184187. [The use of archetypes K.-G. Jung for the positioning of territorial brands]. *Fundamental research*, 10-11, 184187.

Leskov, N. S. (1981). "Levsha Sobranie sochineniy." In 5 volume. Moscow: *Pravda*, 3, 1-310. ["Levsha. Collected works"]. Lewin, R. (2000). *Complexity: Life at the Edge of Chaos*. Chicago: University of Chicago Press, 1-242.

Lorenz, E. N. (1995). "Predictability: does the flap of a butterfly's wings in Brazil set off a tornado in Texas?" *139th Annual Meeting of the American Association for the Advancement of Science (29 Dec 1972).* New York: American Association for the Advancement of Science, 1972 in Essence of Chaos, appendix 1, 181.

Meadows, D. H. (1999). *Leverage Points: Places to Intervene in a System*. New York, The Sustainability Institute, 1-21.

Meadows, D. L. (1999). Ot sopernichestva k sotrudnichestvu: Praktich. rukovodstvo k aktivnym metodikam v ekologicheskom obrazovanii."

Moscow: RKhTU im. D. I. Mendeleeva Publ., 1- 237. [*From Rivalry to Cooperation: Pract. guide to active methods in environmental education*]. Moscow: RKhTU im. D. I. Mendeleeva Publ., 1- 237.

Mindell, E. (1997). "Psikhoterapiya kak dukhovnaya praktika." Moscow: *NF "Klass"*, 1-160. ["Psychotherapy as a spiritual practice"]. Moscow: *NF "Klass"*, 1-160.

Minigalieva, M. R. (1999). "Kognitivnye skhemy i evristicheskie protsessy v sotsial'nom poznanii." *Mir psikhologii*, *3*, 37 46. ["Cognitive patterns and heuristic processes in social cognition"]. *Mir psikhologii* [*World of Psychology*], *3*, 37 46.

Packard, V. (2001). "Psikhoanaliz v reklame." Samara: Bakhrakh-M, p. 415 443. ["Psychoanalysis in advertising"]. Samara: Bakhrakh-M, p. 415 443.

Pekar, V. (2010). "Raznotsvetnye miry." *Upravlenie personalom in Ukraina*, *10* (204), 56-67. ["Colorful Worlds"]. *Upravlenie personalom in Ukraina* [Personnel Management - Ukraine], *10* (204), 56 -67.

Prigozhin, I. & Stengers, I. (1986). "Poryadok iz khaosa: Novyy dialog cheloveka s prirodoy." ["Order from chaos: A new dialogue of man with nature"]. Moscow: *Progress*, 1-432.

Sangsawang, T. (2020). "An Instructional Design for Online Learning in Vocational Education according to a Self-Regulated Learning Framework for Problem Solving during the CoViD-19 Crisis. *Indonesian Journal of Science and Technology*, vol. *5*, no. 2, (March), 283–298.

Scheffer, M., Bascompte, J., Brock, W. A., Brovkin, V., Carpenter, S. R., Dakos, V., Held, H., van Ness, E. H., Rietkerk, M. & Sugihara, G. (2009). "Early-warning signals for critical transitions." *Nature*, vol. *461*, 53-59.

Ufimtsev, R. (2009). "Mertsayushchie zony." Kaliningrad: ["Flickering zones"]. Kaliningrad: *Atel'e ER*, 29.

Van Ray, V. "Zarozhdayushchiesya tendentsii i "dzhokery" kak instrumenty formirovaniya i izmeneniya budushchego." ["Emerging trends and "jokers" as tools for shaping and changing the future"]. *Foresight-Russia*. *6* (1), 60-73.

Zinkevich-Evstegneeva, T. D. (2012). *Master skazok.* [*Master of fairy tales*]. St. Petersburg: Rech' Publ. 1220.

Zinkevich-Evstigneeva, T. D. (1998). "Put' k volshebstvu (teoriya i praktika skazkoterapii)" ["The path to magic (theory and practice of fairy tale therapy)"]. *Workshop on fairy tales*. St. Petersburg: Piter Publ., 1 –140.

Zinkevich-Evstigneeva, T. D. (2013). "Put' k volshebstvu (teoriya i praktika skazkoterapii" [The path to magic (theory and practice of fairy tales)"]. *Praktikum po skazkoterapii* [*Workshop on fairy tale therapy*]. St. Petersburg: Rech' Publ. 1-230.

In: COVID-19 ISBN: 978-1-53618-903-2
Editors: A. B. D. Nandiyanto et al.

Chapter 8

COVID-19 POSSIBLE TREATMENT THROUGH EXERCISE AND NUTRITION

***Hamidie Ronald Daniel Ray*[*]**
and A. Firmansah Wargahadibrata
Universitas Pendidikan Indonesia, Bandung, Jawa Barat, Indonesia

ABSTRACT

In December 2019, a public health emergency was induced by an outbreak of novel beta coronavirus termed 2019-novel coronavirus (SARS-CoV-2) in Wuhan City, Hubei Province, China. Since May 20, 2020, in Indonesia, there were 20.162 cases confirmed as positive for COVID-19. COVID-19 prevention and mitigation actions are the keys to implementation in health and community services. This paper aimed to provide some possibilities treatment through exercise and nutrition in order to improve immune system as a prevention to COVID-19. A weak immune response will occur due to fewer nutrients. If the nutrients with sufficient energy and micronutrients are adequate then the body's immune system will be strong. A home exercise program using different safe, simple, and easily implementable exercises is suitable to avoid the airborne

[*] Corresponding Author's Email: hamidieronald@upi.edu.

coronavirus and preserve fitness levels due to the high risk of spread (by a person to person or contaminated surfaces.

Keywords: COVID-19, exercise, nutrition, prevention and mitigation actions.

1. INTRODUCTION

Virus disease is still emerging and is a serious public health problem. Several virus diseases include the severe acute respiratory syndrome coronavirus (SARS-CoV) from 2002 to 2003, and H1N1 influenza in 2009 was recorded. In December 2019, a public health emergency was induced by an outbreak of novel beta coronavirus termed 2019-novel coronavirus (SARS-CoV-2) in Wuhan City, Hubei Province, China, which is going to be a worldwide epidemic with high mortality and morbidity (Pradhan et al., 2020) and the World Health Organization (WHO) declared an official name for the new coronavirus disease as COVID-19 (Hamidah, Sriyono and Hudha 2020; Anggraeni et al., 2020).

Since May 20, 2020, in Indonesia, there were as many as 20.162 cases confirmed as positive for COVID-19. The numbers of fatalities are 1.278, while the number of recovered patients is 4.838 and these cases still increases until now. Based on scientific evidence, COVID-19 can be transmitted from human to human through coughing/sneezing (droplets). The people at the highest risk of developing this disease are people in direct contact with patients with COVID-19, including those who treat patients with COVID-19. Standard recommendations for preventing the spread of infection are regular hand washing with soap and clean water, applying the ethics of coughing and sneezing, avoiding direct contact with livestock and wild animals, and avoiding close contact with anyone who shows symptoms of respiratory illnesses such as coughing and sneezing. Also, implementing Prevention and Control Infection while in health care facilities, especially at the emergency departments.

COVID-19 prevention and mitigation actions are the keys to implementation in health and community services. The most effective preventive measures in the community include maintaining hand hygiene by washing hands with soap and using running water or with a hand sanitizer; avoiding touching eyes, nose and mouth; applying the ethics of coughing or sneezing by covering the nose and mouth with the inner upper arm or tissue, then throwing the tissue in the trash; wearing a medical mask if you have respiratory symptoms and doing hand hygiene after removing the mask; maintaining a distance (at least 1 meter) from people who experience symptoms of respiratory distress.

2. Prevention of Covid-19 Through Physical Activity

Keeping your physical condition fit is an important thing to do, especially for people who are at risk of non-communicable diseases. However, on the COVID-19 pandemic like this, physical activity and space are limited. How could we work around this? Previous studies have shown that moderate-intensity physical activity has positive enhancing effects on immune system responses against viral respiratory infections (Halabchi, Ahmadinejad, Selk-Ghaffari 2020; Martin, Pence, Woods 2009; Harris 2011).

People who exercise with moderate-intensity physical activity suggested to increase in neutrophil. Furthermore, natural killer (NK) cell counts are detected and salivary IgA concentrations are enhanced (Halabchi, Ahmadinejad, Selk-Ghaffari 2020; Martin, Pence, Woods 2009). Moderate-intensity physical activity increases stress hormones, which leads to a reduction in excessive inflammation (Harris 2011). This leads to a boost in immunity in order to against viral infections via a change in Th1/Th2 cell responses (Pradhan et al., 2020). Twenty to thirty percent reduction of upper respiratory tract infections is reported in individuals performing on moderate levels of physical activity in their daily life. However, prolonged high-intensity physical activity leads to immunosuppression (Pradhan et al., 2020; Ahmadinejad 2014). Moderate intensity physical activity boosts the immune system and the risk of respiratory track viral infections is reduced. However, high-intensity physical activity with long durations weakens the immune system for several hours following the exercise, and the risk of inspiratory track infection is increased in this period (Rondanelli, 2018).

3. Sport Health Characteristic to Prevent Covid-19

Sports Health is a form of sports activities for health purposes. As a sporting activity, it is clear that it is working on the body or the body - (physical aspects). General characteristics of sports health are:

1. Easy: the movements are easy, so that it can be followed by ordinary people, which can enrich and enhance the ability and basic movement skills, for example the motion needed for the implementation of daily living activities.
2. Cheap: very minimal equipment or even no equipment at all.
3. Festive: able to arouse excitement and not boring.
4. Beneficial and Safe:
   - The benefits can clearly be felt, and it is safe to be implemented by each participant with different age levels and dynamic healthy levels.
   - The intensity is sub-maximal and homogeneous, not maximal movements or maximal explosive movements (safety factor).

Terms of the benefits and safety of health sports require special technical-physiological characteristics, namely:

1. Homogeneous and submaximal in intensity or sports load:
   - Sports are carried out with ± flat / homogeneous intensity

- There are no movements with a load / intensity that is maximal,
- No deployment of maximal capabilities.

A homogeneous intensity is needed to make it easier to regulate exercise dosages appropriately, while submaximal intensity is needed as a safety factor. In health sports, people are not required to make a maximum appearance, except when undergoing physical fitness tests. Health sports consist of units of motion that can (deliberately) be made to reach all joints and muscles and can be assembled to become a continuous movement (non-stop), which is an important factor to be able to regulate the dose and intensity of health sports.

1. A unity of measure (dosage): - can be regulated both in intensity (by adjusting the load/strength and/or the speed of repetition/contraction repetition), as well as the duration (duration) of its implementation (by adjusting the number of repetitions).
2. Adequate:
   - There are certain minimum limits for the intensity and timing of the exercise of health to produce benefits, in particular, to increase the functional ability of the Supporting Motion Equipment, held 3-5x/week (minimum 2x/week).
   - It can reach intensities between 60-80% maximum pulse rate (Maximal Heart Rate / MHR) according to age. MHR according to age = 220 - age. It is good for each participant to know how to set and calculate the pulse of each exercise.
3. No Stress Conditions: done with ease, without emotional burden, not competing with each other

4. Sports Health Targets

There are three stages of health sports goals.

1. *Goal 1 - MINIMUM Targets*: In this first goal, the main goal is to at least maintain the ability of motion that is still there, and if possible

try to improve the ability of motion by seeking an increase in area movement of all joints to achieve flexibility, through stretching and relaxation training as much as possible, without any jerks or snaps, which means mobilizing all joints. For example, people who are attached to a wheelchair must maintain and improve the ability of movement that still exists in all their joints, as well as maintaining flexibility and coordination ability, through movements such as Aerobic Gymnastics. Basic abilities (physical abilities) and coordination skills can be improved by requiring participants/students to follow the movements exemplified by the instructor as intensely and accurately as possible following their abilities.

2. *Goal 2 - Goal BETWEEN*: The goal of health exercise at this stage is to maintain and enhance the ability of muscles to maintain and improve their mobility further. The exercise is conducted dynamically and statically. Training in a dynamic way is to perform movements that are fast, repetitive, and antagonistic accompanied by a jolt to further "fill" the movement (the plyometric principle). The exercise of health sports must always be gradual and not exceed the capabilities at that time. Static training is by performing isometric contractions, but breathing must continue as usual (may not suppress breathing/straining), because it should be done part by part. As an example, first, an isometric contraction is done both the upper extremity and then the two lower extremities. Isometric contractions are maintained for 4-6 seconds repeated 3-5 times with active breaks in between. Active rest is intended as an auto-massage. A mistake that can be dangerous is when an isometric contraction is carried out at the same time for the whole body so that there is a kind of Valsalva maneuver (= straining), which will increase blood pressure so that it can be dangerous for health sport participants who have high blood pressure or have heart disease. Health sports training which has reached the Goal 2 stage will naturally include the Gold 1 stage because to train the strength and endurance of the

muscles it must always go through joint movements. Therefore, the dynamic way is the most physiological.

3. *Goal 3 - MAIN Targets*: The main objective of health sports is to maintain adequate aerobic abilities or increase aerobic capacity to achieve a "medium" minimum category.

5. Body Immune Function and Micronutrients Requirement

The immune system is a system that works naturally in one's body. Immune system function is protecting the body against microorganisms, infections and harmful substances from outside the body. This self-protection system consists of three layers, namely:

- Physical (for example skin, epithelial layer along the airways and gastrointestinal tract) and biochemical (for example mucus and stomach acid),
- Various immune cells: granulocytes, CD4/CD8 T cells and B cells,
- Antibodies, e.g., immunoglobulin.

This first line of defense system is commonly referred to as innate immunity, which is a combination of physical and biochemical protection (Castelo-Branco and Soveral 2014). In the case of the COVID-19 which enters through the skin from a handshake, the body will respond by activating this first layer of self-protection system. When COVID-19 successfully passes this first tier, then will face various components of the second layer of T cell and B cell. In the case of the above there are two consequences that will occur, depending on the functioning condition of the immune system of the person, namely:

- First, when the immune system function is strong then the individual will be painless and there are no symptoms, or mild pain such as

mild cold symptoms, muscle aches, bloating and diarrhea, but a few days later back healthy.
- Secondly, if the immune system function is weak then the individual will experience the symptoms of COVID-19, even one to death.

Both systems also protect against cancerous or precancerous cells. The immune system function is also influenced by the age factor. In infants and children, the system is newly developed and has not been functioning. In adulthood, the body's immune system is already functioning maturely. In elderly people, the system will gradually experience a decline in function (Rondanelli et al., 2018). Common symptoms that are perceived when the immune system decreases are fever, colds, and diarrhea. Even in the age of adulthood, the function of the body's immune system is mature, its strong or weak condition is strongly influenced by the adequacy of energy and micronutrients, or nutrients, derived from food. If the nutrients with sufficient energy and micronutrients are adequate then the body's immune system will be strong, and conversely if less it will be weak. Energy supply can be obtained from foods with adequate carbohydrates, protein, and fat content. Whereas micronutrients that are important to enhance the body's immune system are vitamins A, C, D, E, B2, B6, and B12, folic acid, beta carotene, iron, selenium and zinc (Alpert 2017).

Aside from the adequacy of energy and micronutrients, other factors are also important for the immune system. This factor is emotional stress, which will increase cortisol (a type of stress hormone). Heavy stress and stress that occurs for a long time, will weaken the immune system. In this condition, the body will also need a micronutrient substance above in larger quantities, so that the immune system can function optimally. Emotional stress occurs as a result of a person's mindset that is fraught with fear, excessive anxiety, and often negative thinking. The COVID-19 pandemic condition is at risk of triggering the negative flavors above which ultimately cause emotional stress which is the consequence of weakening the body's immune system. This condition will cause a person's body to be a high risk for contracting and suffering from the symptoms of COVID-19.

There is a close relationship between nutrients, infections, and the body's immune system. A weak immune response will occur due to fewer nutrients. There is a contact history with infections, and a malnourished physical condition (Calder 2013). It is clear that optimal immunocompetence depends upon nutritional status (Watson, Zibadi, and Preedy 2010). It has been reported by researchers that micronutrient deficiency is a common factor in the world (Biebinger, Hurrell, and Ottaway 2008). Micronutrients are often not noticed by the layman, even by medical personnel, because of the enormous amount and need to be consumed in the long term, and the given effect is not realized in the improvement. For example, if we are rarely sick this is an extraordinary blessing of life, but many people are unaware of it. The use of micronutrients as primary therapy has not been a standardized medical procedure, whereas there have been some reports stating that therapy with micronutrients can provide a corrective effect on the health of a person, even in those who are experiencing certain diseases.

In one case, X, experiencing similar symptoms to that of autoimmune sufferers: weak muscles, bloating, and digestive tract body often not fit. Apparently, after being checked, X has a deficiency in blood levels of vitamin D. After being administered vitamin D for three months, the blood vitamin D levels gradually increased to normal, increased muscle strength significantly, bloating becomes rare and the body is more fit, becoming less flu pain. It is an example of a good case, to see the relationship between vitamins and the immune system. Until now, X is still a consume vitamin D and still performs a vitamin D blood test regularly and health conditions are better than before.

The following will display some types of micronutrients that are beneficial to the function of the immune system and various food sources. And it will be explained which micronutrients are somewhat difficult to digest and are processed by the body, so it needs to be considered obtained through the supplement.

Vitamin A, stand out from the color aspects of the food, is colorful. This colorful food source contains carotenoids. Food sources with high carotenoid content: carrots, yam, pumpkin, egg, and deep-sea fish. Our body can convert carotenoids into vitamin A which serves as an antioxidant and strengthens the immune system function of the body against infections. Vitamin B12 is a vitamin that helps the formation of energy in the body. Food source with vitamin B12 content: Red meat, clams, oysters, and eggs. The body needs carbohydrates, proteins and fats to form energy so that energy production can be optimal, hence this is the role of vitamin B12. If the body is deficient in vitamin B12, then the body will feel less energy and tired quickly.

Vitamin C is the most popular and well-known vitamins in society. It is known that vitamin C is essential for the functioning of the immune system. Food sources with high vitamin C levels are papaya, strawberry, orange, lemon, broccoli, kale, spinach, and green leaves. Furthermore, vitamin D is a vitamin commonly referred to as the sun's vitamin. It is generally known that sunbathing at 9 a.m. will increase vitamin D in the blood. Although it increases, not necessarily the level of vitamin D blood is sufficient to support the function of the immune system. This is because vitamin D obtained from the food and the sunbathing process should still be processed in the liver organ to be vitamin D active. Most Indonesians have problems digesting vitamin D food sources and also process problems in the liver organs, so it is necessary to check the blood level of vitamin D and consult the doctor. Food sources with high vitamin D content are deep-sea fish, salmon, sardines, tuna, fish oil, and krill shrimp oil.

Vitamin E is a vitamin that is already known for the health of our skin. It also works to help the body fight infections. Food sources with high vitamin E content spinach, broccoli, almonds, peanuts, cashews, and sunflower seeds. Folic acid, a vitamin that helps the formation of new cells, is essential for cells involved in the immune system. Food sources for folic acid are kidney beans, black beans, white beans, peas, and other foods added folic acid supplements. Iron is a blood-enhancer vitamin that has been well known by the people of Indonesia. Blood will bring oxygen and distributed to all parts of the body. Food sources for iron are chicken, duck, turkey, red meat, liver, kidney beans, black beans, broccoli, kale, and various seafood.

Additionally, selenium is an important vitamin in enhancing the functioning of the immune system. It includes for its effect on lowering the over-active response of the body in the case of terrorism, therefore selenium is also known as a vitamin for cancer. High-feeding sources of Selenium are Brazilian beans, broccoli, garlic, sardines, tuna, and barley. Zinc, a vitamin that helps the body's immune response and also lowers the inflammation that occurs in various diseases. Food sources are high in Zinc levels: oysters, clams, crabs, low-fat meats, chickens, ducks, red beans, and Arabic beans.

Conclusion

As a conclusion, moderate-intensity (and not high-intensity) exercise may be helpful for healthy asymptomatic people and should be recommended. However, as mentioned earlier, due to the high risk of spread (by a person to person or contaminated surfaces), an exercise in private environments (at home) with good ventilation and use of personal equipment may be more reasonable. A home exercise program using different safe, simple, and easily implementable exercises is suitable to avoid the airborne coronavirus and preserve fitness levels. This program may include aerobic (walking in the house), strengthening, stretching, and balance exercises, or a combination of these (Chen et al., 2020).

References

Ahmadinejad, Z., Alijani, N., Mansori, S., and Ziaee, V. 2014. "Common sports-related infections: a review on clinical pictures, management and time to return to sports." *Asian journal of sports medicine* vol. 5,1 (March): 1-9. doi:10.5812/asjsm.34174.

Alpert, P. T. 2017. "The Role of Vitamins and Minerals on the Immune System." *Home Health Care Management & Practice* 29, no. 3 (August): 199–202. doi:10.1177/1084822317713300.

Anggraeni, S., Maulidina, A., Dewi, M.W, Rahmadianti, S., Rizky, Y. P. C., Arinalhaq, Z. F., Usdiyana, D., Nandiyanto, A. B. D., Al-Obaidi, A. S.

M. (2020). The Deployment of Drones in Sending Drugs and Patient Blood Samples COVID-19. *Indonesian Journal of Science and Technology*, vol. 5, no. 2 (March):193–200.

Biebinger, R., Hurrell, R., and Ottaway, P. 2008. *"Vitamin and mineral fortification of foods, Food fortification and supplementation: technological, safety and regulatory aspects."* oca Raton, Fla.: CRC Press. p (2008) 27-40.

Calder, P.C. 2013. "Feeding the Immune System." *Proceeding of the Nutrition Society* vol. 72, no. 3 (August): 299-309. https://doi.org/10.1017/S0029665113001286.

Castelo-Branco, C., and Soveral, I. 2014. "The immune system and aging: a review." *Gynecological endocrinology: the official journal of the International Society of Gynecological Endocrinology* vol. 30, no1: 16-22. doi:10.3109/09513590.2013.852531.

Chen, P., Mao, L., Nassis, G. P., Harmer, P., Ainsworth, B. E., & Li, F. 2020. "Coronavirus disease (COVID-19): The need to maintain regular physical activity while taking precautions." *Journal of sport and health science* vol. 9,2 (March): 103-104. doi: 10.1016/j.jshs.2020.02.001.

Halabchi, F., Ahmadinejad, Z., and Selk-Ghaffari, M. 2020. "COVID-19 Epidemic: Exercise or Not to Exercise; That is the Question!" *Asian Journal of Sports Medicine* vol. 11, no.1 (March): e102630. doi: 10.5812/asjsm.102630.

Hamidah, I., Sriyono, S., & Hudha, M. N. (2020). A Bibliometric Analysis of COVID-19 Research using VOSviewer. *Indonesian Journal of Science and Technology*, vol. 5, no. 2 (March):209-216.

Harris, M. D. 2011. "Infectious disease in athletes." *Current sports medicine reports* vol. 10, no. 2: 84-9. doi:10.1249/JSR.0b013e318214 2381.

Martin, S. A., Pence, B. D., and Woods, J. A. 2009. "Exercise and respiratory tract viral infections." *Exercise and sport sciences reviews* vol. 37, no.4 (October):157-64. doi:10.1097/JES.0b013e318 1b7b57b.

Pandya, P. H., Murray, M. E., Pollok, K. E., and Renbarger, J. L. 2016. "The Immune System in Cancer Pathogenesis: Potential Therapeutic Approaches." *Journal of immunology research* vol. 2016: 4273943. doi:10.1155/2016/4273943.

Pradhan, P., Pandey, A.K., Mishra, A., Gupta, P., Tripathi, P.K., Menon, M.B., Gomes, J., Vivekanandan, P., and Kundu, B. 2020. "Uncanny similarity of unique inserts in the 2019-nCoV spike protein to HIV-1 gp120 and Gag." bioRxiv. doi: https://doi.org/10.1101/2020.01.30.927871.

Rondanelli, M., Miccono, A., Lamburghini, S., Avanzato, I., Riva, A., Allegrini, P., Faliva, M. A., Peroni, G., Nichetti, M., and Perna, S. 2018. "Self-Care for Common Colds: The Pivotal Role of Vitamin D, Vitamin C, Zinc, and *Echinacea* in Three Main Immune Interactive Clusters (Physical Barriers, Innate and Adaptive Immunity) Involved during an Episode of Common Colds-Practical Advice on Dosages and on the Time to Take These Nutrients/Botanicals in order to Prevent or Treat Common Colds." *Evidence-based complementary and alternative medicine: eCAM* vol. 2018 5813095. 29 Apr. 2018, doi:10.1155/2018/5813095.

Watson, R.R., Zibadi, S., and Preedy, V.R. 2010. *"Dietary Components and Immune Function."* Humana Press. 1st Ed. Springer Science & Business Media2010.

In: COVID-19 ISBN: 978-1-53618-903-2
Editors: A. B. D. Nandiyanto et al.

Chapter 9

CHANGES AND TRANSFORMATIONS IN HUMAN AND SOCIAL LIFE: ANTICIPATION AND UNDERSTANDING OF EVENTS AND STRESSES

Asnul Dahar Minghat[1,*], Mariam R. Arpentieva[2], Danat Zh. Zhanatayev[3] and Gulzhaina K. Kassymova[4,5]
[1]Razak Faculty of Technology and Informatics,
Universiti Teknologi Malaysia,
University College of Islam Melaka, Malaysia
[2]Department at the Development and Education Psychology,
Tsiolkovskiy Kaluga State University, Russian Federation
[3] Al-Farabi Kazakh National University, Kazakhstan
[4]Abai Kazakh National Pedagogical University, Kazakhstan,
[5]Institute of Metallurgy and Ore Beneficiation, Satbayev University

* Corresponding Author's Email: asnul@utm.my.

Abstract

The stress of change is comprehended, experienced, and passed by a person depending on the sociocultural situation, especially facing corona virus disease 2019 (COVID-19) pandemic. This pandemic influence how people lives, changing traditions and stage of development of society. Scenarios and human life stories in the COVID-19 pandemic include many points of change and transformation, including changes associated with external and internal deformations and dangers, such as bodily somatic and other diseases and disorders. These points form narratives - a multidimensional and multicomponent phenomenon. The aim of the study was an integrative analysis of anticipation and minimization of the stress of changes in the life of a person (patient) in the context of the analysis of sociocultural changes. The research method was a systematic theoretical understanding of the problems of anticipating and minimizing the stress of changes in the life of a person (patient) in the context of the analysis of sociocultural changes. The main results of the study showed that archetypes and role models are of great importance in the analysis of the sociocultural aspects of understanding, experiencing and undergoing the stresses of change. Moreover, role models, unlike archetypes, according to researchers, can be classified based on a comparison with the basic motives of life. In addition, human communities go through developmental levels, which manifest themselves as different approaches to solving the problems that reality poses for them.

Keywords: archetypes, narrative psychotherapy, markers of change, stress of change, triggers for change, weak signals

1. Introduction

Scenarios and human life stories include many points of change and transformation, including changes associated with external and internal deformations and dangers, such as bodily somatic and other diseases and disorders. These points form narratives a multidimensional and multicomponent phenomenon. Participants or heroes of narratives (narratives of change or narratives of stress of change) live in a number of spaces and times, a number of worlds intersecting with each other, changing their understanding of themselves, others and situations of interaction

(Arpentieva 2015; Jung 2003; Khlebnikova 2013; Meadows 1999; Meadows 1999). Therefore, in working with stresses of changes) and narratives describing them, aimed at understanding and anticipating ("foresight") stresses of changes in order to minimize them, special attention should be paid to combinations of diachronic and synchronous analysis. One of the incidents currently occurring is the Corona Viruses Diseases 2019 (COVID-19) pandemic (Anggraeni et al. 2020), which made online learning papular in the education system worldwide; it is discussed that not all teachers were ready to provide online lessons during this COVID-19 pandemic time (Arlinwibowo et al, 2020). However, online education has certain advantages for both teachers and students. Teachers should focus on its benefits in order to develop educational process and students' competences (Asnul Dahar Minghat et al., 2020; Kassymova et al, 2019).

COVID-19 is a disease caused by the corona virus. This virus first hit China in the city of Wuhan. This virus can infect the human body and cause death (Maryanti et al. 2020a, Maryanti et al. 2020b). Currently, the COVID-19 virus pandemic is hitting various countries in the world. The spread of COVID-19 does not only have an impact on health problems (Machmud and Mighat 2020). The spread of this virus has implications for problems in other aspects of human life and the country (for example, education, economy and social). The government has made various policies on preventing the transmission of COVID-19. The community limits various social activities outside the home (Putra and Abidin 2020). The danger of COVID-19 has made a large part of the community experience fear. In addition, the education process creates tangible level of stress by itself. Espesially, when academic assignments are too much to be completed in a short period of time (Kassymova, 2018). However, there are different stress management techniques for students to cope (Kassymova et al., 2018). In fact, most people experience stress with the various changes that are made. This results in most of the illnesses suffered by them because of the suggestion of fear they have. They need an understanding of how to deal with and respond to various problems caused by this pandemic.

Changing patterns of behavior and the essence of the actions of participants at different stages of their life paths, in different worlds and times. Particularly great attention in this context should be given to metaphors - denoting worlds and times, as well as - accomplished or emerging transitions between worlds and times. Metaphors act as bright signals and triggers of change (Forrester et al. 1977; Loveridge 2009; Van Ray 2011). Each metaphor is a germ or designation of intention, which the heroes follow on their way to themselves, to each other and to God, to happiness and the resolution of the crisis.

2. Purpose and Method

The aim of the study was an integrative analysis of anticipation and minimization of the stress of changes in the life of a person (patient) in the context of the analysis of sociocultural changes. The research method was a systematic theoretical understanding of the problems of anticipating and minimizing the stress of changes in the life of a person (patient) in the context of the analysis of sociocultural changes.

3. Results of the Study

The stress of change is comprehended, experienced and passed by a person depending on the sociocultural situation in which he lives, on traditions and stage of development of society.

3.1. Archetypal Metaphors in the Work of a Narrative Therapist

Despite the huge variety of narratives, they highlight the main stages and moments inherent in any life narrative and form an algorithm (Zinkevich-Evstegneeva 2012; Zinkevich-Evstegneeva 1998; Zinkevich-Evstegneeva 2013).

The algorithm of life stresses or changes usually includes:

- Life in the "father's home" (appropriation of parental experience, understanding the world, building relationships with worlds, people - life support),
- Parting with the home (voluntary or forced start of the path),
- Choice of road (crossroads and a choice corresponding to the goal of the path),
- Verification (for "good" or "evil heart" - selfishness or mutual assistance),
- Meeting with future helpers (friends who can help),
- Struggle and victory (achieving the goal of the path and fighting with personified evil, as a result which man becomes stronger and wiser or, on the contrary, succumbs to evil, weakens),
- Returning home (difficulties of going back, meeting a hidden evil, death when applying the old experience),
- Rebirth (death of the past, illusions, infantilism, discovering new creative abilities, strength and wisdom, help from friends, victory inside and out),
- Arrival home (a changed home, changed relationships, help from friends and the last trials, restoration of justice and roots that will serve as a support for him in further adulthood), a new image (change about Faces - Transformation: forgiveness, acceptance of the world, the path to a new future with an "open heart"),
- A wedding or a coronation (victory celebration, new social status, objectives, greater responsibility).

Each stage is important, meaning, forming stages, each of which has its own meaning, which can be revealed by asking the patient a series of questions (Beytson 2000; Zinkevich-Evstegneeva 2012, Zinkevich-Evstegneeva 1998). The description and problems of choosing behaviors are well demonstrated by archetypal and other typologies of personality development and its relations. These personal models describe the development of a person and human communities in terms of their belonging to certain generations, their social myths and archetypal figures and scenarios (narratives). The theory of archetypes, created by K. G. Jung on the basis of mythological narratives, was abroad. It developed in the typologies of J. Myers-Briggs, E. Schwartz, E. Bern, and others (Beck and Cowan 2005; Beck and Cowan 2010; Graves, Cowan and Todorovic 2005; Frants 1998; Fromm 2010; Jung 1996). Currently, the theory of archetypes is an effective and efficient tool for creating successful brands and advertising, as well as developing innovative areas of psychotherapeutic care. Based on their work, practitioners and theorists often distinguish a number of basic models of behavior and archetypes as systems of partially conflicting basic needs (intentions), as well as combinations that implement them. Often distinguished archetypal figures and scenarios can also be classified (Briggs-Myers 1998; Jung 2003; Lewin 2000; Meadows 1999; Jung 2003).

In Russia, a detailed typology of the archetypes of A. V. Chernyshov deserves special attention. Studying and analyzing fairy narratives, he revealed a number of characters corresponding to archetypes: Mother (Stepmother), Bogatyr, Lefty/Craftsman, Tsar/King, Koschey, Goldfish, Soldier, "Beautiful Vasilisa", "Fool Ivan", Prince Ivan, Damn, Baba Yag/ Witch (Chernyshov 2011). Many of these archetypes are similar to the archetypes of C. Jung et al. A. V. Chernyshov analyzes the ancient Russian folk tales and myths. However, he did not find complete coincidences of all archetypes and names; in particular, he did not find a clearly defined archetype (ideal image) that would correspond to the archetype of Creativity. The archetypes of the Goldfish and the magical qualities of Beautiful Vasilisa, creating the world and wonders, are somewhat similar to him.

Creativity acts as a process of implementing a project, a dream, a representation, the process of transforming an unstable imaginary object into some materials. This is reflected in a much later fairy tale tradition, in an author's fairy tale. This is personifying in such images of Russian craftsmen from the people as Levsha/Craftsman of the N.S. Leskov (Jung 1996 or Master Danila of P. P. Bazhov (Bazhov1993). When analyzing narratives, "fabulous" archetypes help to expand identity and balance different intentions in the patient's relationship with himself and the world. However, not all archetypes are combined, which sometimes causes an internal go or even an external conflict, a misunderstanding of the need for a particular type of behavior/attitude, and the need for change (Chernyshov, 2011). The archetype can become a design, a way of realizing significant or probably significant for the subject of intentions: changes, attitudes or understanding (Chernyshov, 2011, Jung 1996; Jung 2003).

At the very beginning of their research, K. G. Jung wrote that the field of archetypes is not limited, archetypes pass into each other, and the archetype itself is a definite "tendency to form a representation of motive" (Jung 2003). At the same time, archetypal structures include both positive and negative traits, which is quite consistent with the reality of human life, but can form obstacles for people to understand each other, for changes, making what is happening between patients and the therapist, patient and other people ambiguous and blurred. Moreover, the archetype as a super cultural concept is characteristic of all humankind, for each person in one way or another. Therefore, appeal to archetypes does not guarantee that their use will be effective, and the use of archetypes in themselves in psychotherapy is sufficiently motivating to transformations.

However, it is impossible and unproductive to ignore the cultural context. Narrative therapy can be quite successful, productive, and effective if you use not so much the archetypes as support and transformation, but role models — some reference (unambiguous) sets of behavioral patterns that have typical characteristics and act as role models. The role model, like the archetype, has super cultural significance, however, it is not necessarily addressed to the collective unconscious and is included in the process of socialization of a person to one degree or another fully and intensively, depending on the characteristics of the cultural context.

In each culture, role models have special and common features. The main thing in them is the possibility of forming a reference sample and an important, from the point of view of the psychotherapeutic process, design of the stereotype of the carrier of other role-playing behavior. The role model is significant as a specific way of implementing a motive, and, more broadly, of a person's self-expression, designation of his life beliefs in a specific context of life. The role model applicable in psychotherapy can be considered as a potential image that a person may have a desire to play, that is, demonstrate to people around. And it can become the basis of a new way of life. Moreover, role models, unlike archetypes, according to researchers, can be classified based on a comparison with the basic motives of life. Role models correspond to different situations of life and, importantly, do not have conflicts with the cultural context, as they can be used as specific, and as super cultural, but with a specific embodiment in a specific cultural environment.

3.2. The Development of Metaphors - Models for the Development of Archetypes

The archetype or role model, with all its "timelessness" and "super culturalism," is more or less specific, representing in the conscious and unconscious patient certain aspects depending on the time and space of his life. One of the interesting approaches to taking into account the diachronic and synchronous aspects of role models, understanding the cultural and historical features of their forms and contents, their relevance and realization, is provided by the so-called "spiral dynamics", which is based on the work of the American psychologist and philosopher of the 60s of the XX century Cl. W. Graves (Beck and Cowan 2005; Beck and Cowan 2010; Graves, Cowan and Todorovic 2005; Ufimtsev 2009). He investigated the "emergent cyclical levels of existence" that "adult biopsychosocial systems" are subject to, believing that human communities go through developmental levels, which manifest themselves as different approaches to solving the problems that reality poses to them.

At the same time, the models of behavior described by him change depending on the cultural and historical space into which a person falls (Hamidah et al. 2020; Dirgantari et al 2020). Each stage of its development in this space is characterized by a specific system of values, different cognitive attitudes ("cognitive points" or strategies for understanding oneself and the world) and different behaviors. At the same time, each next level is not so much crowding out the previous one as it is superimposed on it: all previous levels of development continue to exist along with the most recent one. Cl. Graves argued that in usually societies one or another paradigm prevails, which is the “cognitive glasses” through which society looks at the world. It is subject to change, because, helping society to solve some problems, it raises others before it, the solution of which requires a paradigm shift. This process is not accidental and the following paradigm is in certain dialectical relations with the previous one, hypothetically described as a spiral of two turns, on which there are a number of nodal points. Each paradigm does not completely replace the other; it only supplants it from a dominant position. This transition is not just “rebranding”, but the process of changing identities that are not related to each other as levels of development (Graves, Cowan and Todorovic 2005).

Later D. Beck and Cl. Cowan (Beck and Cowan 2005; Beck and Cowan 2010; Graves, Cowan and Todorovic 2005) noted that communities of people are carriers of memes (cognitive structures), among which a special, decisive role is played by “valuememes” - in their designation, v-memes (values-memes). Value memes or “supermemes” attract lower-order memes that define cognitive habits, as well as actions as methods for solving life tasks and problems accepted in a given community, at a given age, etc. (that is, in fact, role-playing models). The prevailing supermem gives rise to a new supermem, which gradually replaces the previous one, moving to the “shadow” or marginal areas of mass and individual consciousness. Usually a movement is realized from one level to the next, located higher on a spiral, but a downward movement, “degradation” to lower-level values is also possible. Each level is associated with its own supermem, endowing a person with its worldview and values. Each level is characterized by its own understanding of itself and the world, which affects more or less conscious aspirations (intentions) and the choice of behavior patterns (response to problems) (Ufimtsev 2009; Van Ray 2010).

A change of levels occurs when a person or society accumulates tasks that cannot be solved within the framework of the current level (Graves, Cowan and Todorovic 2005; Pekar 2010; Scheffer et al. 2009). D. Beck and C. Wilber introduced the concept of “spiral masters” - people and communities who have reached the “highest level” of the spiral and have the ability to control all other communities. However, still Cl. Graves warned that his levels are no more advanced among less developed people and groups, but simply different value systems and ways to solve problems. That is, “spiral masters”, including in psychotherapy, are people who are able to reflect and use the potential of each stage and changes in the community for the development of man, his relations with himself and the world (Beck and Cowan 2005; Graves, Cowan and Todorovic 2005; Wilber 2013). Described by Cl. Graves and colleagues, the particulars of understanding the world and the intentions of changes at each level, as well as the theory of generations, can serve as the direct basis for the development of role models.

4. Discussion

A similar model of the behavior patterns of different types of people, their development over time, in different historical and political periods, is presented in the theory of generations developed by W. Strauss and N. Howe (Howe and Strauss 1997). They believe that there are “generational cycles” that reflect a repeating pattern of behavior of different types of generations in which one or another “age identity” dominates. People of each separate age group (cohort) tend to share a special set of relationships and values, perceptions (“cognitive points”) and patterns of behavior and communication, insofar as they grew up in the same historical conditions.

At the same time, representatives of each generation experience a sense of belonging to their generation and subjectively share one historical era: they are faced with the same historical events and social trends, being in the same phases of life; they share certain general ideas and relationships, as well as patterns of behavior and communication. Since each generational period lasts 20–25 years, four periods make up a complete cycle lasting approximately 80–90 years: it is called sakuala (saeculum) - the “natural age”. According to the survey of centenarians, a new cycle or “natural age” begins at the age of 90: the cycles tend to repeat, reproducing in the individual development the stages of youth-adulthood-old age. In addition, in some cultures, people predominate whose psychological age does not rise above that of children (many “primitive” cultures“), and in some (Tibet, India) there are many psychologically” old “people. Therefore, the result of various processes and layers of a person's relationship with the world is very diverse, although it is not devoid of trends, the consideration of which can help resolve development crises, intergenerational conflicts and development crises of civilization as a whole.

In general, researchers identify a number of generational archetypes that are repeated sequentially, creating and maintaining the rhythms of the crisis/awakening cycle: idealist, responsive, civic and adaptive (Howe and Strauss 1997). Work with people of different generations, therefore, must take into account generational intentions and models, those problems that are associated with the birth, life and death of a person in certain periods of time. At each moment in time in the inner space - the time of man - there are several alternative "paradigms" or models at the same time. In turn, each of them gives rise to a family of templates, which together form an understanding and attitude to various life problems. During the life cycle of each model or paradigm, it gives rise to several other models and paradigms that go through their shorter life cycle - from the stages of ascension to the stages of decline. The psychotherapist's task is to connect the patient with the myths or models that are at the apogee stage and regularly "transplant" it with the "descending" one, which has demonstrated its limitations and errors, the paradigm on another, "upward", giving a more developed, complete and accurate understanding of oneself and the world.

Understanding archetypal and more specific metaphors, including role models implemented by a person in his life, allows us to evaluate the direction of the patient's internal movement towards the realization of a particular motivation, intention, support upward and/or slow down downward intentions, reduce the level of negative impact of stress of changes (Arpentieva 2015; Meadows 1999; Meadows 1999; Ufimtsev 2009). Turning to the study of patient's narratives and metaphors, with all its external simplicity, requires a specialist to have a good knowledge of himself, highly qualified: an individual approach, empathy and intelligence of the psychotherapist himself, his willingness and ability to see the "truth" of a person, life, himself (Arpentieva and Terentiev 2006). In addition, the idea of "weak", intertextual and intertextual signals can be laid in the basis of psychotherapeutic stories/fairy tales (Arpentieva 2015; Arpentieva and

Terentiev 2006). In them, "weak signals" take on their own names (Bakurova 2015; Harris and Zeisler 2002; Hilborn 2004). The simplest and most common concept becomes a metaphor for another concept or a whole group of concepts. These are metaphors of Path, Light, Love, Change, etc. they are fill the space of fairy tales in such a way that, in fact, they act, along with the main characters. Thanks to such stories, the patient, as a reader or even as the author of the story, tunes in to the fact that the story he will study has much more meanings than it might seem he himself becomes a seeker and conceptualizer of the metaphors with which he resonates in the process narrative psychotherapy.

CONCLUSION

Classical predictions of a person's development, changes in his life, including changes in psychotherapy, are based on the quite logical idea that small, weak changes usually produce small results. They underestimate or simply ignore weak signals, focusing on indicators of the strength of trends and probabilities. However, many phenomena do not fit into statistical trends. Oscillations on the border of chaos is a rich environment in which weak signals can most often be detected (Minigalieva 1999; Minigalieva 1999). If you teach a person or group to recognize the border and balance between areas of order, structure and randomness, uncertainty, they gain the advantage of understanding to see and take into account weak signals and those trends that stand behind them. The richest source of weak signals is the periphery of culture: 1) interdisciplinary, inter-traditional; 2) kitsch and simulated, pseudo-art and pseudoscience; 3) extra-traditional, cultural, anti-science and anti-art. That is, rejected and forbidden, unusual and rare, devoid of price - worthless and priceless, and magical, fabulous, which is why narrative therapy has the most significant psychotherapeutic potential among other types of psychotherapy.

REFERENCES

Anggraeni, S., Maulidina, A., Dewi, M. W., Rahmadianti, S., Rizky, Y. P. C., Arinalhaq, Z. F., Usdiyana, D., Nandiyanto, A. B. D. & Al-Obaidi, A. S. M. (2020). "The Deployment of Drones in Sending Drugs and Patient Blood Samples COVID-19." *Indonesian Journal of Science & Technology*, vol. 5, no. 2, 193–200.

Arlinwibowo, J., Retnawati, H., Kartowagiran, B., Kassymova, G.K. (2020) Distance learning policy in Indonesia for facing pandemic COVID-19: School reaction and lesson plans. *Journal of Theoretical and Applied Information Technology*, 98(14), 2828-2838

Arpentieva, M. R. (2015). *Vzaimoponimanie kak fenomen mezhlichnostnykh otnosheniy (na materiale psikhologicheskogo konsul'tirovaniya.* Diss. ...grand dokt. psikhol. nauk. Moscow: Lomonosov Moscow state university, 1-497. [*Understanding as a phenomenon of interpersonal relationships (based on psychological counseling)*]. Diss. ...grand doctor of the psychol. Sciences. Moscow: Lomonosov Moscow State University, 1-497.

Arpentieva, M. R. & Terentiev, A. A. (2016). *Skazkoterapiya v razvitii ponimaniya sebya i mira*. Kaluga, 1-792. [*Fairytale therapy in the development of self-understanding and peac*e]. Kaluga: KGU Publ., 1-792.

Asnul Dahar Minghat, Mustakim Siti Salina, A. Ana, G.K. Kassymova, Suparman (2020). Measuring Technical and Vocational Education and Training (TVET) Teacher's Technical Competency and the Development of Programme-Specific-Directory. *International Journal of Psychosocial Rehabilitation*, Vol. 24, Issue 8, 3730-3735.

Bakurova, O. N. (2015). Chuvstvitel'nost' k probleme: psikhologicheskie podkhody k opredeleniyu i izucheniyu. [Sensitivity to the problem: psychological approaches to the definition and study]. *Vestnik Kaluzhskogo universiteta* [*Bulletin of the Kaluga University*], *3*, 82-90.

Bazhov, P. P. (1993). *Ural'skie skazy*. [*Ural tales*]. Moscow: Zenit, 1-336.

Beck, D. E. & Cowan, C. C. (2005). "Spiral dynamics: mastering values, leadership, and change." New Jersey: Blackwell Publishing, Inc, 1-335.

Beck, D. & Cowan, C. C. (2010). *Spiral'naya dinamika. Upravlyaya tsennostyami, liderstvom i izmeneniyami v XXI veke* [*Spiral dynamics. Managing values, leadership and change in the 21st century*] Moscow: Otkrytyy Mir; Best Business Books, 1-424.

Beytson, G. (2000). *Ekologiya razuma* [*Ecology of the mind*]. Moscow: Smysl Publ., 1-476.

Briggs-Myers, I., McCaulley, M. H., Quenk, N. L. & Hammer, A. l. L. (1998). *Manual: A Guide to the Development and Use of the Myers-Briggs Type Indicator*. Palo Alto, Calif: Consulting Psychologists Press, 1-420.

Chernyshov, A. V. (2011). *Russkie arkhetipy v brendinge i effektivnost' telereklamy.* [*Russian archetypes in branding and the effectiveness of television advertising*. Abstract. PhD in sociology]. Nizhniy Novgorod: N. I. Lobachevskiy Novgorod State University Publ., 1-22.

Dirgantari, P. D., Hidayat, Y. M., Mahphoth, M. H. & Nugraheni, R. (2020). "Level of Use and Satisfaction of E-Commerce Customers in Covid-19 Pandemic Period: An Information System Success Model (ISSM) Approach." *Indonesian Journal of Science and Technology*, vol. *5*, no. 2, (March), 261–270.

Forrester, Dzh., Render Yu., Medouz, D. & Bekhrens, V. (1977). "Sovremennye problemy kibernetiki: Sb. Statey Znanie. Ser. Matematika i kibernetika". ["Modern problems of cybernetics"], *Knowledge. - Ser. Mathematics and cybernetics*, 1-45.

Frants, fon M. L. (1998). *Proritsanie i sinkhroniya. Psikhologiya znachimogo sluchaya.* [*Divination and synchrony. Psychology of a significant case*]. St. Petersburg: B.S.K. Publ., 107.

Fromm, E. (2010). *Zabytyy yazyk. Vvedenie v nauku ponimaniya snov, skazok, mifov* [*Forgotten language. Introduction to the science of understanding dreams, fairy tales, myths*]. Moscow: AST, 624.

Graves, c. w., cowan, c. c. & todorovic, n. (2005). *The never ending quest: dr. Clare w. Graves explores human nature: a treatise on an emergent cyclica*. Santa barbara, c: eclet publishing, 1-570.

Hamidah, I., Sriyono, S. & Hudha, M. N. (2020). "A Bibliometric Analysis of COVID-19 Research using VOSviewer." *Indonesian Journal of Science and Technology*, vol. *5*, no. 2, 209-216.

Harris, D. & Zeisler, St. (2002). "Weak signals: Detecting the next big thing." *The Futurist*, vol. *36*, no. 6, 21-29.

Hilborn, R. C. (2004). Sea gulls, butterflies, and grasshoppers: A brief history of the butterfly effect in nonlinear dynamics. *American Journal of Physics*, *72* (4), 425 427.

Howe, N. & Strauss, W. (1997). "The Fourth Turning." New York: Broadway Books, 1-400.

Jung, K. (1996). *Dusha i mif. Shest' arkhetipov.* [*Soul and myth. Six archetypes*]. Kiev, Kiev Publ., *236*.

Jung, K. G. (2003). *Sinkhroniya* [*Synchrony*]. Moscow: "Refl-buk" Publ, Kiev: Vakler Publ, 1-320.

Jung K. G. (2003). *Sinkhroniya* [*Synchrony*]. Moscow: "Refl-buk" Publ, Kiev: Vakler Publ, 1-320.

Kassymova G.K. (2018) Stress management techniques recommended for students. *International Practical Internet Conference "Challenges of Science*", 22 November 2018. https://doi.org/10.31643/2018.008

Kassymova G.K., ArpentievaR. M., KosherbayevaA N., TriyonoB. M., Sangilbayev O. S., Kenzhaliyev B. K. (2019) Science, education & cognitive competence based on e-learning. *Bulletin of the National academy of sciences of the Republic of Kazakhstan*, Volume 1, Number 377, 266-275. https://doi.org/10.32014/2019.2518-1467.31

Kassymova G.K., Kosherbayeva A. N., Sangilbayev O. S., Schachl H., Cox N. R.B.C. (2018) Stress management techniques for students. *Advances in Social Science, Education and Humanities Research*, volume 198, 47-56. https://doi.org/10.2991/ictppfms-18.2018.10

Khlebnikova, S. A. (2013). "Ispol'zovanie arkhetipov K.-G. Yunga v tselyakh pozitsionirovaniya territorial'nykh brendov." ["The use of archetypes K.-G. Jung for the positioning of territorial brands"]. *Fundamental'nye issledovaniya*, 10-11, 184187.

Lewin, R. (2000). *Complexity: Life at the Edge of Chaos*. Chicago: University of Chicago Press, 1-242.

Loveridge, D. (2009). *Foresight: The Art and Science of Anticipating the Future*. New York: Routledge., 1-420.

Machmud, A. & Mighat, A. D. B. (2020). "The Price Dynamics of Hand Sanitizers for COVID-19 in Indonesia: Exponential and Cobweb Forms. *Indonesian Journal of Science and Technology*, vol. *5*, no. 2, 176 - 184.

Maryanti, R., Hufad, A., Sunardi, Nandiyanto, A. B. D. & Manullang, T. I. B. (2020a). "Understanding Coronavirus (COVID-19) as a Small Particle to Students with Special Needs." *Horizon*, vol. *2*, no. 1, 121-130.

Maryanti, R., Hufad, A., Sunardi., Nandiyanto, A. B. D. & Al-Obaidi, S. M. (2020b). "Understanding COVID-19 particle contagion through aerosol droplets for students with special needs." *Journal of Engineering Science and Technology*, vol. *15*, no. 3, 1909-1920.

Meadows, D. H. (1999). *Leverage Points: Places to Intervene in a System*. New York the Sustainability Institute, 1-21.

Meadows, D. L. (1999). *Ot sopernichestva k sotrudnichestvu: Praktich. rukovodstvo k aktivnym metodikam v ekologicheskom obrazovanii*. [*From Rivalry to Cooperation: Pract. guide to active methods in environmental education*]. Moscow: RKhTU im. D. I. Mendeleeva Publ., 1- 237.

Minigalieva, M. R. (1999). "Kognitivnye skhemy i evristicheskie protsessy v sotsial'nom poznanii." ["Cognitive patterns and heuristic processes in social cognition"]. *Mir psikhologii* [*World of Psychology*], *3*, 37 46.

Minigalieva, M. R. (1999). "Kognitivnye skhemy i evristicheskie protsessy v sotsial'nom poznanii". ["Cognitive patterns and heuristic processes in social cognition"] *Mir psikhologii* [*World of Psychology*], *3*, 37 46.

Pekar, V. (2010). "Raznotsvetnye miry" ["Colorful Worlds"]. *Upravlenie personalom in Ukraina* [Personnel Management - Ukraine], *10* (204), 56 -67.

Putra, Z. A. & Abidin, S. A. Z. (2020). "Application of SEIR Model in COVID-19 and The Effect of Lockdown on Reducing The Number of Active Cases." *Indonesian Journal of Science & Technology*, vol. *5*, no. 2, 185 - 192.

Scheffer, M., Bascompte, J., Brock, W. A., Brovkin, V., Carpenter, S. R., Dakos, V., Held, H., van Ness, E. H., Rietkerk, M. & Sugihara, G. (2009). "Early-warning signals for critical transitions." *Nature*, vol. *461*, 53-59.

Ufimtsev, R. (2009). "Mertsayushchie zony." ["Flickering zones"]. *Kaliningrad: Atel'e ER, 29.*

Van Ray, V. (2012). "Zarozhdayushchiesya tendentsii i "dzhokery" kak instrumenty formirovaniya i izmeneniya budushchego." ["Emerging trends and "jokers" as tools for shaping and changing the future"]. *Foresight-Russia.*, *6* (1), 60-73.

Wilber, K. (2013). *Integral'naya dukhovnost: Novaya rol' religii v sovremennom i postsovremennom mire*. [*Integral Spirituality: A New Role of Religion in the Modern and Post-Modern Wor*ld]. Moscow: Aypraktik, 1-34.

Zinkevich-Evstegneeva, T. D. (2012). *Master skazok*. [*Master of fairy tales*]. St. Petersburg: Rech' Publ. 1220.

Zinkevich-Evstigneeva, T. D. (1998). Put' k volshebstvu (teoriya i praktika skazkoterapii ["The path to magic (theory and practice of fairy tale therapy"] [*Workshop on fairy tales*]. St. Petersburg: Piter Publ., 1–140.

Zinkevich-Evstigneeva, T. D. (2013). "Put' k volshebstvu (teoriya i praktika skazkoterapii" [The path to magic (theory and practice of fairy tales)"]. *Praktikum po skazkoterapii* [*Workshop on fairy tale therapy*]. St. Petersburg: Rech' Publ. 1-230.

In: COVID-19 ISBN: 978-1-53618-903-2
Editors: A. B. D. Nandiyanto et al.

Chapter 10

Adjustment of Thai Curriculum and Instruction in the COVID-19 Crisis

Sutthiporn Boonsong*
Faculty of Technical Education,
Rajamangala University of Technology Thanyaburi,
Khlong Hok, Khlong Luang District,
Pathum Thani, Thailand

Abstract

The crisis from COVID-19 has a big impact on the education sector both in Thailand and abroad. Educational institutions, including tutoring schools and various skill schools, were closed. During this stage, both the schools and many universities have begun to consider postponing the entrance exam, changing the curriculum, and making the online examination to reduce the risk of student gatherings. This includes the graduation ceremony as well.

Therefore, educators or educational policy administrators under the emergency situation of COVID-19 should consider not only accessing to online teaching but also changing other teaching methods during the

* Corresponding Author's Email: sutthiporn_b@rmutt.ac.th.

COVID-19 crisis. Traditional methods might be used to support local areas that cannot access online education effectively. The person responsible for Thai education must also concern the context of inequality and disadvantaged children in society. Thailand is not the only country in the world that has this problem. Many countries face with this problem together and are able to learn lessons and solutions together.

Keywords: COVID-19, education adjustment, Thai curriculum

1. INTRODUCTION

A crisis happens from the COVID-19 pandemic after the World Health Organization (WHO) declared it a serious pandemic (Anggraeni et al. 2020).

One way to deal with an outbreak is through social distancing or maintains physical distance in society in order to break the chain of COVID-19 spread from person to person.

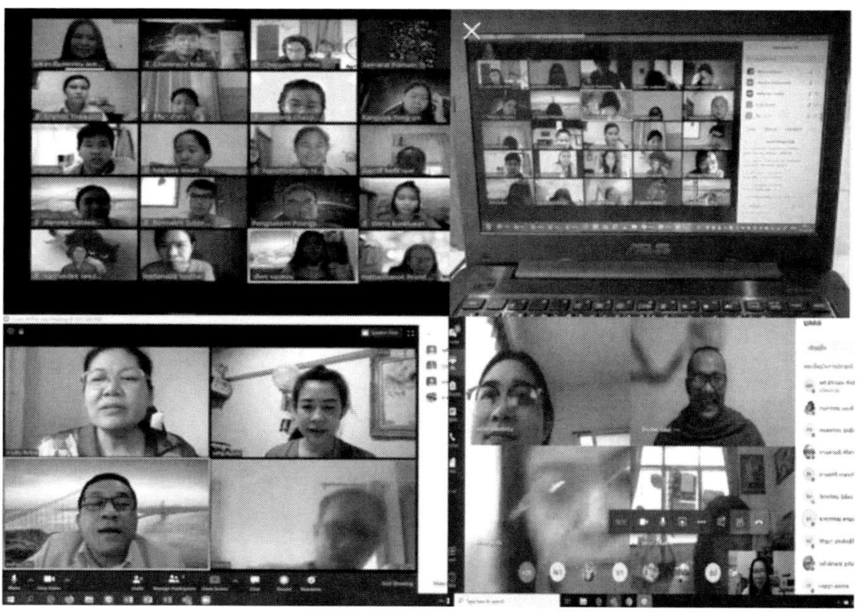

Figure 1. Online teachers meeting and instructions in the COVID-19 crisis.

The social distancing has a significant impact on all levels or sectors (Hashim et al. 2020). Adaptation to survive has been happening both in Thailand and abroad. The pandemic has influenced the education sector as well. Online teaching system has been adopted in order to conduct teaching and learning (Figure 1). Schools and universities have started to consider postponing the exam and switching regular to online classes to reduce the risk of student gatherings on the test day. It also includes the adjournment of the graduation ceremony as well. The state declared tutoring schools and vocational schools to also start providing online education (Bangkok Busyness 2020).

Activities to promote skills and knowledge such as a science camp and summer camps in foreign countries are also affected. Postponing travel is also considered to be the safest under unprecedented situation and to reduce the risk of virus infection.

2. Adaptation of the Thai Education Segment

As mentioned earlier that COVID-19 has affected education sector, therefore, the Ministry of Higher Education, Science, Research, and Innovation (MHESRI) of Thailand announced the request for cooperation with educational institutions affiliated with MHESRI. The cooperation includes (Margetingoop 2020):

1. Reducing the rental fee for small business operators in the university.
2. Reducing student tuition in this upcoming semester.
3. Reducing other expenses which is not urgent in order to increase the employment of students and general personnel.
4. Preparing online learning and teaching (Mulyanti et al. 2020).
5. Reducing various service fees charged by Small-Medium-Sized-Enterprises, startup, and the general public as special case.
6. Higher education institutions consider and assess suitable steps to support those impacted by the additional incidents.

In addition, Thai universities have released different initiatives to respond to the COVID-19 crisis. As an example, "Srinakharinwirot University" has announced guidelines for teaching and learning to prevent the spread of COVID-19. At the end of the announcement stated that:

1. Teaching and learning management help teachers to adapt the assessment and evaluation of teaching styles as necessary.
2. Final examination allows teachers to adapt appropriate and effective methods of measurement and evaluation that can use the original format test or other methods.
3. Examination at the graduate level can be adjusted using the online examination or teleconference program.
4. All non-urgent tasks should be postponed, but, if a justification is required, the faculty should plan the screening/prevention/control of infectious diseases (COVID-19).
5. Implementation of the teaching and learning model adjustment and final exams to avoid the spread of COVID-19 are exempted from checking the number of courses attended by at least 80%.
6. Implementation of the teaching and learning model adjustment and graduation final exam and other activities.

Therefore, teaching and learning in the COVID-19 era is one of the challenges for teachers encountered. They have to find ways to transfer knowledge through new channels as the traditional lecture in the classroom is no longer available (Sangsawang 2020). One approach is to build online lessons using internet technologies and different software, but the key issue is the infrastructure. In some countries, as we know, the digital basics are not quite excellently-supported to all teachers. According to the 'Teacher Tapp' survey, which surveyed the teaching of more than 6,000 teachers in the UK, it is found that teachers in public schools can publish less online lessons than that in private schools.

Taking into account for 40 to 69% of respondents indicates that the availability of tools in public schools is much slower than in private schools (Thanalerdsomboon 2020).

In addition, some teachers do not have enough knowledge or expertise to use technology. Some subjects, such as physical education, are not familiar with tools which are not suitable for online teaching. Therefore, it is difficult to adjust the design of new teaching methods to keep things up to date. In regards, some students are not able to access online lessons effectively due to the lack of equipment and the quality of the network signals. Furthermore, it is still found that most students continue to show less ability when studying online, so learning online may not be the best option for long-term studies. Unless, the curriculum designed for this type of teaching approach has been prepared from the outset. However, problem-solving strategies for changing educational problems will have to consider important issues such as the World Economic Forum projected that the world of education will change in the future schools (Thanalerdsomboon 2020).

1. We will see educational development and changes in the lifestyle of learning
   In the past, almost all educational structures around the world stayed in the classroom and had schools was the main center. However, many educational institutions will continue to implement new technologies in the future to replace classroom teaching. Within a short time, there will be several developments for education, and there will be different types of access to information. Resulting in a learning lifestyle outside the classroom, we do not adhere to the conventional school hour schedule which may mean that 'Learn Anywhere, Anytime' is one of the everyday practices.
2. We will see cooperation from many parties to improve education.
   COVID-19 crisis phenomenon allows us to see cooperation in developing educational systems from many sections. In addition to teachers and educational stakeholders, there are governments, media, scholars, and various service providers of communication networks, technology developers, in which they help build a platform database system. Many interactive learning platforms considered a positive indication that the education system would be

able to progress much far from brainstorming and collaboration like this condition in the future.

3. We must reduce the inequality of access to digital technology for equal education.

   In the future, online classrooms (that play a greater role in the classroom) create a secure comprehensive infrastructure,and enhance access to technology. All aspects of innovations that the education system is currently using such as 5G will help all groups of children to have equal education or at the very least causing most children to have a better education.

3. Conclusions to Be Considered for Education Management to Support the COVID-19 Crisis

According to data collected in 2018 by The Organization for Economic Co-operation and Development (OECD) (Margetingoop 2020), it is found that Thailand still has an inequality access online learning, such as in-house study sites, computer, notebook, and tablet. Particularly, it happens when comparing between rich and poor families. In terms of digital divide, there may be exceptions for accessing television, mobile phones, and smartphones. It seems that all families can access these digital devices. This information can be used as sources of knowledge for educators or policy executives regarding the emergency COVID-19 crisis in order to address the online access to make teaching and learning (Margetingoop 2020).

However, Thailand is not the only country in this world facing the same problems. Many countries also encounter a similar problem, so each country should learn from each other and work together to find solutions. Therefore, the conclusions that could be considered in order to handle education during the COVID-19 crisis (Tongliemna 2020) are written as follows.

3.1. The Use of Radio and Newspapers

The use of radio and newspapers are the most traditional method in the United States. Schools were closed because of the polio outbreak in 1937, causing 325,000 elementary school students to leave the school. In that era, the use of broadcasting on the radio with homework questions sent to the newspaper every morning. There were qualified teachers to check the lesson contents, and experts were invited to broadcast and used the hotline system so parents could call for consultations. There were about 20 teachers waiting to answer the call with parents interested in calling on all the time to make comments. Parents were given support to help children to do homework by taking lessons with children. However, there were also problems. As an example, some houses did not have a good radio signal, so they had to move from outside the city where radio signals. Another problem was uneven learning speeds that are not much different from the era of Internet use. Despite being more convenient, unequal access has problems.

In countries where students have difficult situations for accessing communication devices as during the Ebola crisis in 2014. During that time, West African region shut down schools and delivered the education via radio. They also used text messaging where they shared educational news via mobile phone using Short Message System or short video transmission that uses less internet signals.

3.2. Television Use

During school holidays, China has a television program for students at different levels to learn on the screen by dividing the channel, channel schedule, date, time by grade level and by different subjects. It is considered the most accessible method for students without internet or computers. Although it is one-way communication, many countries use television as one of the educational channels, such as Greece, New Zealand, Educational TV channels in some U.S. states and British BBC television Discovery television station that focused on education. In Thailand, the teaching system via satellite television (DLTV) has long been used, and there is a fairly complete database and operating system.

3.3. Using a Document System (Learning Box Set)

Using the learning document method by using a series of books or lessons and various activities are the traditional way. Students can study on their own or combining it with other methods, such as providing homework and then having time to ask questions or discuss online. In Portugal, the documents are sent to students by mail including the homework. In China, parents who worry their children spend too much time on the screen could learn to read or work by typing documents. In New Zealand, when the school is closed the printing and distribution on educational materials has increased because they send it to students.

3.4. The Context of Inequality and Disadvantaged Children in Society

Regardless of the method used in the teaching and learning during the COVID-19, it is important to choose the appropriate approach according to the context and readiness of the learners and instructors. Apart from academic concerns, the main concern is that school should be cautious and helpful to the students who might be absent for a long time due to the closure of the school. In times of COVID-19 crisis, school should be giving importance to the mental, emotional, and social conditions of the students as well. Teachers and schools should make students feel comfortable, feel they are not abandoned by the teacher, and in times of crisis, they are still part of the school.

Furthermore, Thai education should continue to think about students in special education classes, people with disabilities, people with learning disabilities, students whose parents or guardians cannot support them because they must work to earn money, students in a poor environment, and students live in domestic violence. How are the government and schools going to better assist those students? This is because children need special support in these communities and simply cannot wait for such a long crisis.

Conclusion

The crisis from COVID-19 has a big impact on the education sector. Therefore, educators or educational policy administrators under the emergency situation of COVID-19 should consider not only access to online teaching but also other teaching methods during the COVID-19 crisis. Traditional methods might be used to support local areas that cannot access online education effectively. The person responsible for Thai education must also consider the context of inequality and disadvantaged children in society. Thailand is not the only country in the world that has this problem. Many countries faced with this problem together and are able to learn lessons and solutions together.

References

Anggraeni, S., Maulidina, A., Dewi, M. W., Rahmadianti, S., Rizky, Y. P. C., Arinalhaq, Z. F., Usdiyana, D., Nandiyanto, A. B. D. and Al-Obaidi, A. S. M. 2020. "The Deployment of Drones in Sending Drugs and Patient Blood Samples COVID-19". *Indonesian Journal of Science and Technology,* vol. 5, no. 2: 193 - 200.

Bangkok Busyness. 2020. *The effect of COVID-19 on the semester*. https:// www.bangkok iznews .com/news/detail/872053.

Hashim, S., Masek, A., Abdullah, N. S., Paimin, A. N. and Muda, W. H. N. W. 2020. "Students' Intention to Share Information via Social Media: A Case Study of COVID-19 Pandemic". *Indonesian Journal of Science and Technology,* vol. 5, no. 2: 236 - 245.

Marketing Oops! 2020. *'COVID-19' Education reform around the world! Use of new learning technology - 'Thai University' taught online.* Marketingoops.com. https://www.marketingoops.com/exclusive/business-case/covid-19-reinvent-global-education-system-with-educational-technology/, retrieved on July 1, 2020.

Mulyanti, B., Purnama, W. and Parwinanto, R. E. 2020. "Distance Learning in Vocational High Schools during the COVID-19 Pandemic in West Java Province, Indonesia". *Indonesian Journal of Science and Technology,* vol. 5, no. 2: 271 - 282.

Sangsawang, T. 2020. "An Instructional Design for Online Learning in Vocational Education according to a Self-Regulated Learning Framework for Problem Solving during the CoViD-19 Crisis". *Indonesian Journal of Science and Technology,* vol. 5, no. 2:283 - 298.

Thanalerdsomboon, B. 2020. "Closing the school, changing the future: an educational world after the virus COVID-19". *The101world.com.* April 7, 2020. https://www.the101.world/covid19-school-closure/.

Tongliemna, P. 2020. "Cope with education in the COVID-19 era: inequality and student resources will be even more importan"t. *The101world.com.* April 16, 2020. https://www.the101.world/covid-19-and-inequality-in-education/.

In: COVID-19 ISBN: 978-1-53618-903-2
Editors: A. B. D. Nandiyanto et al.

Chapter 11

EDUCATION AND INFORMATION ABOUT COVID-19 FOR IMPROVING STUDENTS WITH SPECIAL NEEDS KNOWLEDGE IN INDONESIA

Rina Maryanti, Asep Bayu Dani Nandiyanto, Achmad Hufad and Sunardi
Universitas Pendidikan Indonesia, Bandung, Jawa Barat, Indonesia

ABSTRACT

Students with special needs have several challenges in various developments and academics aspects. They need special treatments and ways to understand realistic conditions. At the time this research conducted, an outbreak of the coronavirus diseases 2019 (COVID-19) is spreading in Indonesia. Providing information and education about the COVID-19 is very important, especially for students with special needs in Indonesia. It is very crucial since special needs students are easily infected with the COVID-19. Most of them have low self-development skills (for example, rarely washing their hands, weak immune system, and not keeping the body and the environment clean). They need guidance on how to against the COVID-19 and how to improve their awareness, as well as how to avoid and reduce virus transmission. They can get education and information about the COVID-19 from the family, school, and community. Various questions were asked to students to find out the level of student knowledge about the COVID-19. Most students with special needs can understand COVID-19 through education and getting information from their environment. They understand COVID-19 through habituation, appropriate methods, and media, as well as simple and concrete explanations.

Keywords: COVID-19, education, information, knowledge, students with special needs

1. INTRODUCTION

COVID-19 stands for Coronavirus Diseases 19, and this pandemic was first discovered in 2019 (Ana 2020, 246-260). At the time this research conducted, Indonesia is experiencing problems because COVID-19 outbreak has hit people in Indonesia. Patients infected by COVID-19 in Indonesia continue to grow (Martina et al. 2020). We need efforts to prevent the spread of COVID-19. Giving education and information about COVID-19 is very important to students, especially for students with special needs. Students with special needs are students who have problems in both developmental and academic aspects. They need teaching, guidance, and special services. Students with special needs have difficulties in understanding information (Maryanti et al. 2020). They need methods and media that suit their needs. Students with special needs have difficulties understanding abstract phenomena (Maryanti et al. 2020, 1909-1920). They need concrete media to understand.

COVID-19 is a virus that can infect the human body. This virus has a very small size and invisible (Maryanti et al. 2020). We need an electron microscope to observe this virus. The small form of the virus makes it easy for viruses to enter the human body (Li et al. 2020). For students with special needs having knowledge of COVID-19 is very important. They have a greater potential for being infected with the COVID-19 virus compared to normal students. That is because they have a weak immune system, low awareness of hygiene (Giust and Valle Riestra 2017), and limited knowledge about the dangers of COVID-19.

At present, there are many papers or news that contain information (Hashim et al. 2020), the form (Sahin et al. 2020), the size (Yunus and Rezki 2020), the transmission (Windhiyana 2020), symptoms (Razon 2020), the impact (Putra and Abidin 2020), and the efforts to prevent the COVID-19 (Telaumbanua 2020). However, until now there has been no paper or book that explains education and information about COVID-19 knowledge for students with special needs.

Students with special needs can get education and information from their environment (Kurniawan 2017). Education and information about the COVID-19 are not only obtained through education from teachers in the formal environment. However, students can obtain education and information from the family and the community. Students understand information through habituation, appropriate methods, and media, as well as simple and concrete explanations. This study was one of the efforts to prevent the spread of the COVID-19 in Indonesia.

2. Theory

2.1. COVID-19

The COVID-19 is a virus originated from animals (Maryanti et al. 2020). This virus first spreads in the city of Wuhan, China. The virus can infect the human body through the nose, mouth, and eyes, causing shortness of breath as it damages the lung organs. This virus is very dangerous and even causing death (Angraeni et al. 2020).

The small size of the virus makes it easy to enter the human body (Hamidah et al. 2020). We can prevent the spread of this virus in several ways, including keeping a distance, maintaining the cleanliness of the body, washing hands, and wearing a mask when leaving the house. COVID-19 pandemic does not only affect public health problems but also economic, social, and educational fields, especially in Indonesia.

2.2. Students with Special Needs in Indonesia

Students with special needs are students who have problems in their developments and it affects their academic performance (Hermawan et al. 2020). There are several categories of students with special needs including visual impairment, hearing impairment, intellectual disabilities, physical impairment, autism, and down syndrome. The classifications are simply explained as follows:

1) Students with visual impairments known as blind people are students who have problems in their visual senses (Purwati et al. 2020).
2) Students with hearing impairments have problems with hearing organs or nerves resulting in hearing disability (Hidayat et al. 2020). They usually have difficulties in understanding and communicating verbally.
3) Students with intellectual disabilities are often referred to mentally disabled (Sari and Kustiawan 2020). They have below-average intelligence, problems in adaptive behavior, and independence.
4) Students with physical disabilities in Indonesia are called *tunadaksa* (Munir and Aljauhari 2020). Students with physical disabilities have problems in their physical aspects, one of which relates to gross and fine motor movements.
5) Students with autism are students who have problems with interaction and communication (Ayunungtyas et al. 2020). They have difficulties in establishing eye contact and communicating their needs.
6) Students with down syndrome are students who have the same facial characteristics, short thick tongue, and short fingers (Keen et al. 2020). They have problems in the aspect of intelligence, usually included in the classification of mentally retarded children.

2.3. Education for Students with Special Needs

Education for children with special needs is different with the education in general (Hernawati 2007). Educating children with special needs requires special methods, strategies, media, and services based on their needs that impacted by their conditions. There are several principles of educational services that must be considered in an effort to educate children with special needs such as compassion, individual service, readiness, advocacy, motivation, learning, working in groups, skills, and the cultivation and refinement of attitudes (Abdullah 2017).

3. METHOD

This research used descriptive qualitative method. The subjects in this study were students with special needs (visually impaired, deaf, intellectually impaired, physically impaired, autistic, down syndrome) in special schools in Indonesia. We obtained data through a number of questions given to students. The aim was to determine the level of students' understanding of the COVID-19. We made 15 polar questions, and the analysis of a score of 0 (no) and 1 (yes) with a total score of 100 for all questions answered with 'yes'. We made questions through Google Form and distributed the questions through social media. Parents and teachers played an important role in helping the process of obtaining data in the field. Table 1 shows the 15 polar questions given to students.

4. STUDENTS DEMOGRAPHIC

Figure 1 displays student data about the types of challenges they encountered. 7% of students were students with visual impairments. Students had obstacles in orientation and mobility, understanding abstracts, and auditory learning. 18% of students had hearing impairments resulting challenges in language, speech, and communication. They also had visual learning characteristics and difficulties in socializing and behaving. Furthermore, 45% of students were children with intellectual disabilities. They had problems with concentration, adaptive behavior, and intelligence. Students with intellectual disabilities generally are easy to forget, easily bored, difficult to focus, difficult to understand abstract concepts, and problems in independence. 8% of students were children with physical disabilities. They had problems in the perception of motion, gross motor, and fine motor.

Table 1. COVID-19 knowledge question instrument for students with special needs

No	List of questions	Answer	
		Yes	No
1	Do you know what COVID-19 is?		
2	Do you know the size of the COVID-19?		
3	Do you know the form of the COVID-19?		
4	Do you know that the COVID-19 originated from animals?		
5	Do you know how the COVID-19 is transmitted?		
6	Do you know how COVID-19 enters the human body?		
7	Do you know the symptoms of COVID-19 infection?		
8	Do you know the danger of the COVID-19?		
9	Are you aware of the efforts to prevent the transmission of the COVID-19?		
10	Do you know that physical distancing can prevent COVID-19 transmission?		
11	Do you know that washing your hands can prevent COVID-19 transmission?		
12	Do you know that social distancing can prevent COVID-19 transmission?		
13	Do you know that wearing a mask can prevent COVID-19 transmission?		
14	Do you get information about the COVID-19 from your parents?		
15	Do you get information about the COVID-19 from the teacher?		

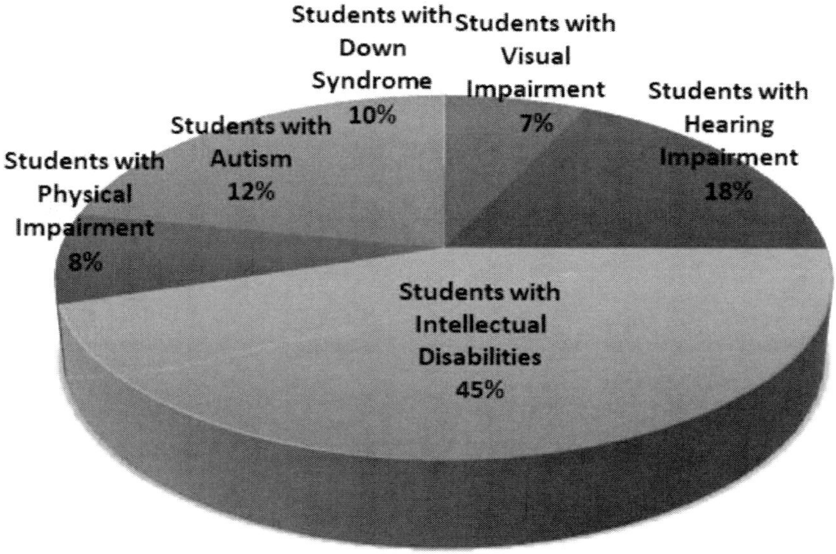

Figure 1. Types of Disabilities that Subjects have.

In the cognitive aspect, some of students did not experience obstacles and were able to participate in learning like children in general. 12% of students were students with autism who had obstacles in interaction and communication. They had difficulties in making eye contact, interacting, and often raging. 10% of students were students with down syndrome. Students with down syndrome have characteristics of unclear pronunciation, thick short tongue, and fingers, motor resistance, lack of concentration, and have below-average intelligence.

5. Educational Process and Provision of Information about COVID-19 for Students with Special Needs

For students with special needs, it is very important to obtain education and information about COVID-19 and how it is transmitted because they have difficulties when studying the COVID-19 (Maryanti et al. 2020).

Providing education and information about the virus for students with special needs can increase their knowledge.

In providing knowledge and support, we must pay attention to many issues including students' challenges, the opportunities, and students' needs. They have difficulties in understanding complicated and abstract concepts. As for students with visual impairments, they need learning media that can optimize their hearing and tactile capacities. Furthermore, children with hearing impairments need visual learning media and students with intellectual disabilities, autism, and down syndrome need interesting and fun media.

Basically, providing education and information about COVID-19 for students with special needs requires simple explanations and concrete examples. The role of family is also essential to increase students' knowledge. Collaboration between parents, families, teachers, and the community is needed in educating students with special needs. They can learn through habituation in daily life. As they often get education and information about the COVID-19 from the surrounding environment, their level of knowledge will improve (Abdullah 2017). In an effort to find students' improvement in understanding COVID-19, several questions about the virus were given to students with special needs from easy to difficult questions.

6. Data Analysis

Table 2 shows the percentage data analysis of students knowledge about COVID-19 before and after given education and information. A few students with special needs knew COVID-19. After given information and education, their knowledge increased.

Students with special needs require education and information to improve their knowledge. They get the knowledge and information from their families, teachers, and community. However, a few students with special needs only receive education from one party. This is one of the reasons why the level of student understanding is low. Environmental factors greatly affect students' knowledge improvement besides the obstacles they have. Building good collaboration between various parties to provide education and information will increase the level of student knowledge.

Table 2. Subject knowledge before and after the provision of education and information about COVID-19

No	Subject	Total	Before Providing Education and Information		After Providing Education and Information		COVID-19 Knowledge Enhancement
			K	NK	K	NK	
1	Students with Visual Impairment	7%	2%	5%	5%	2%	3%
2	Students with Hearing Impairment	18%	6%	12%	15%	3%	9%
3	Students with Intellectual Disabilities	45%	10%	35%	30%	15%	20%
4	Students with Physical Impairment	8%	3%	5%	6%	2%	3%
5	Students with Autism	12%	2%	10%	7%	5%	5%
6	Students with Down Syndrome	10%	2%	8%	7%	3%	5%
Percentage Amount		100%	26%	74%	70%	30%	44%

Note: K= know; NK= Not Know

Figure 2 explains the percentage of efforts made by parents and teachers in providing education and information about COVID-19. About 35% of parents and 65% of teachers gave education about COVID-19 to students with special needs.

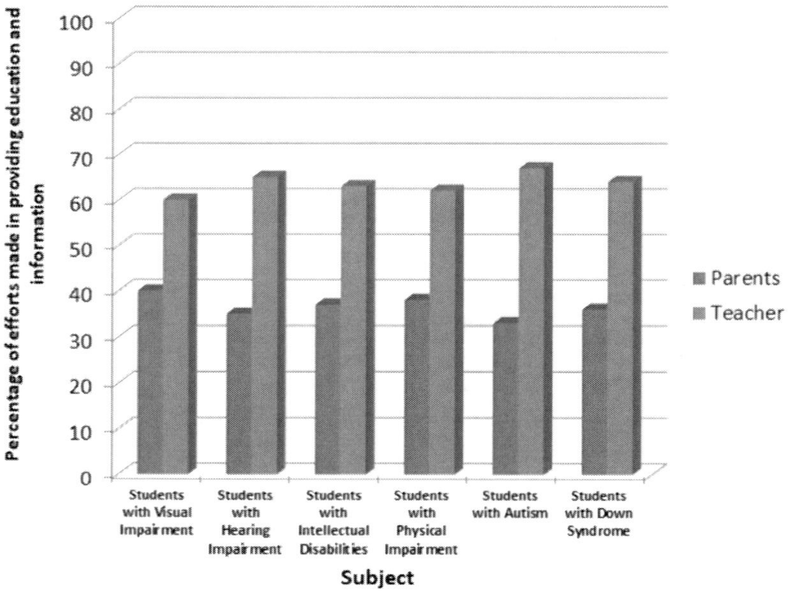

Figure 2. Efforts made in providing education and information about COVID-19.

Students with special needs are also vulnerable towards COVID-19. Most of them have low self-development skills (rarely washing hands, weak immune system, and poor hygiene). The education and information provided must be adjusted to their needs and conditions. Habituation, simple explanations, and concrete examples help students to understand education and information about the COVID-19. The balanced participation among parents and teachers makes students' knowledge increase.

CONCLUSION

Providing information and education about the COVID-19 is essential to students with special needs in Indonesia. It is important because students with special needs are very much easily infected by the COVID-19. They need education and information about the virus so their knowledge increases. They can get education and information about the virus from the family, school, and community. 70% of students with special needs can understand COVID-19 through education and information they get from their environment. They understand the concepts through habituation, appropriate methods and media, simple explanations, and concrete examples.

ACKNOWLEDGMENT

We would like to acknowledge Sekolah Pasca Sarjana Universitas Pendidikan Indonesia for supporting this research. This study was supported by Bangdos Universitas Pendidikan Indonesia. We would also like to thank teachers at Sekolah Luar Biasa in Indonesia for assisting this study.

REFERENCES

Abdullah, N. 2013. "Get to know children with special needs". *Magistra,* vol. 25, no. 86: 1 - 10.

Ana, A. 2020. "Trends in Expert System Development: A Practicum Content Analysis in Vocational Education for Over Grow Pandemic Learning Problems". *Indonesian Journal of Science and Technology,* vol. 5, no. 2: 246 - 260.

Anggraeni, S., Maulidina, A., Dewi, M. W., Rahmadianti, S., Rizky, Y. P. C., Arinalhaq, Z. F., Usdiyana, D., Nandiyanto, A. B. D. and Al-Obaidi, A. S. M. 2020. "The Deployment of Drones in Sending Drugs and Patient Blood Samples COVID-19". *Indonesian Journal of Science and Technology,* vol. 5, no. 2: 193 - 200.

Ayuningtyas, F., Venus, A., Suryana, A. and Yustikasari, Y. 2020. "Communication Patterns of People with Special Abilities: Ethnographic Studies of Communication on Social Interaction of People with Special Needs at Autistic Homes, Depok Branch". *Ekspresi Dan Persepsi: Jurnal Ilmu Komunikasi,* vol. 3, no. 2: 23 - 34.

Giust, A. M. and Valle-Riestra, D. M. 2017. "Supporting men-tors working with students with intellectual disabilities in higher education". *Journal of Intellectual Disabilities,* vol. 21, no. 2: 144 - 157.

Hamidah, I., Sriyono, S. and Hudha, M. N. 2020. "A Bibliometric Analysis of COVID-19 Research using VOSviewer". *Indonesian Journal of Science and Technology,* vol. 5, no. 2: 209 - 216.

Hashim, S., Masek, A., Abdullah, N. S., Paimin, A. N. and Muda, W. H. N. W. 2020. "Students' Intention to Share Information via Social Media: A Case Study of COVID-19 Pandemic". *Indonesian Journal of Science and Technology,* vol. 5, no. 2: 236 - 245.

Hermawan, B., Hufad, A., Rochyadi, E., Nandiyanto, A. B. D., Maryanti, R. and Sunardi. 2020. "Teaching "Changes in Electrical Energy to Light" to Students with Intellectual Disabilities in Junior High School". *International Journal of Psychosocial Rehabilitation,* vol. 24, no. 8: 3658 - 3675.

Hernawati, T. 2007. "Pengembangan kemampuan berbahasa dan berbicara anak tunarungu". *Jurnal JASSI_anakku,* vol. 7, no. 1: 101 - 110.

Hidayat, D. S., Rakhmat, C., Fattah, N., Rochyadi, E., Nandiyanto, A. B. D. and Maryanti, R. 2020. "Understanding Archimedes Law: What the Best Teaching Strategies for Vocational High School Students with Hearing Impairment". *Journal of Technical Education and Training,* vol. 12. No. 1: 229 - 237.

Keen, C., Hunter, J. E., Allen, E. G., Rocheleau, C., Waters, M. and Sherman, S. L. 2020. "The association between maternal occupation and down syndrome: A report from the national Down syndrome project". *International journal of hygiene and environmental health,* vol. 223, no. 1: 207 - 213.

Kurniawan, I. 2017. "Implementasi Pendidikan Bagi Siswa Tunanetra Di Sekolah Dasar Inklusi". *Edukasi Islami: Jurnal Pendidikan Islam,* vol. 4, no. 08: 16 - 26.

Li, R., Pei, S., Chen, B., Song, Y., Zhang, T., Yang, W. and Shaman, J. 2020. "Substantial undocumented infection facilitates the rapid dissemination of novel coronavirus (SARS-CoV-2)". *Science,* vol. 368, no. 6490: 489 - 493.

Martina, A., Muhtarulloh, F., Awalluddin, A. S. and Cahyandari, R. 2020. *Build a multivariate Markov transition opportunity matrix and analyze it on COVID-19 data in Indonesia.* Lecturer Scientific Writing of UIN SGD Bandung at the time Work from Home. Online: http://digilib.uinsgd.ac.id/30865/1/Naskah%20KTI%202020%20%28Annisa%2C%20Fahrudin%2C%20Asep%20Solih%2C%20Rini%29.pdf.

Maryanti, R., Hufad, A., Sunardi. and Nandiyanto, A. B. D. 2020. "Experimental Demonstration of Colligative Properties of Solution on Material Phase Transition to Students with Intellectual Disabilities". *International Journal of Psychosocial Rehabilitation,* vol. 24, no. 8: 3610 - 3623.

Maryanti, R., Hufad, A., Sunardi., Nandiyanto, A. B. D. and Al-Obaidi, S. M. 2020. "Understanding COVID-19 particle contagion through aerosol droplets for students with special needs". *Journal of Engineering Science and Technology,* vol. 15, no. 3:1909 - 1920.

Maryanti, R., Hufad, A., Sunardi., Nandiyanto, A. B. D. and Manullang, T. I. B. 2020. "Understanding Coronavirus (COVID-19) as a Small Particle to Students with Special Needs". *Horizon,* vol. 2, no. 1:121 - 130.

Munir, M. and Aljauhari, A. M. S. 2020. "Prayer Learning Strategies by Islamic Religious Education Teachers against Children with Disabilities at SDLB Negeri Pangkalpinang". *Journal of Islamic Education Research,* vol. 1, no. 02: 67 - 79.

Purwati, Y., Utomo, D. W., Utomo, F. S. and Baihaqi, W. M. 2020. Windows Communication Foundation untuk Audiobook Dongeng bagi Anak Penyandang Tunanetra". *Jurnal Teknologi Informasi dan Ilmu Komputer,* vol. 7, no. 2: 339 - 348.

Putra, Z. A. and Abidin, S. A. Z. 2020. Application of SEIR Model in COVID-19 and The Effect of Lockdown on Reducing The Number of Active Cases". *Indonesian Journal of Science and Technology,* vol. 5, no. 2:185 - 192.

Razon, B. C. 2020. "COVID 19: Impetus for "Community Spirits" among Filipinos". *Indonesian Journal of Science and Technology,* vol. 5, no. 2: 201 - 208.

Sahin, A. R., Erdogan, A., Agaoglu, P. M., Dineri, Y., Cakirci, A. Y., Senel, M. E. and Tasdogan, A. M. 2020. 2019 novel coronavirus (COVID-19) outbreak: a review of the current literature. *EJMO,* vol. 4, no. 1: 1 - 7.

Sari, G. S., Huda, A. and Kustiawan, U. 2020. "Media Quiet Book to Improve the Skills of Caring for Minor Wounds of Children with Disabilities". *Jurnal Ortopedagogia,* vol. 5, no. 2: 81 - 84.

Telaumbanua, D. 2020. "The Urgency of Establishing Regulations Related to the Prevention of COVID-19 in Indonesia". *QALAMUNA: Jurnal Pendidikan, Sosial, dan Agama,* vol. 12, no. 1: 59 - 70.

Windhiyana, E. 2020. "The impact of COVID-19 on online learning activities at a Christian university in Indonesia". *Perspektif Ilmu Pendidikan,* vol. 34, no. 1: 1 - 8.

Yunus, N. R. and Rezki, A. 2020. "Lock Down Enforcement Policy in Anticipation of Corona Virus COVID-19 Spread". *Salam: Jurnal Sosial dan Budaya Syar-I,* vol. 7, no. 3: 227 - 238.

In: COVID-19 ISBN: 978-1-53618-903-2
Editors: A. B. D. Nandiyanto et al.

Chapter 12

INCREASING THE SCIENCE PROCESS SKILLS USING VIRTUAL SCIENCE LABORATORY DURING THE COVID-19 PANDEMIC

Ida Hamidah
Universitas Pendidikan Indonesia, Bandung, Jawa Barat, Indonesia

ABSTRACT

One of the science learning's main goals is to provide students with skills in the science process. Typically, these skills are acquired when students do an experiment in the laboratory. However, laboratory experiments have become difficult to conduct in the current corona virus disease 2019 (COVID-19) pandemic. This study aimed to examine all forms of learning that could be applied to improve the science process skills of the students. Types of learning that could be performed for this purpose include virtual science laboratory, problem-based gaming, open-ended science experiment, mobile scientific inquiry, and project-based learning. Based on the characteristics of each learning, it is suggested that the most effective learning during this pandemic is virtual science laboratory. This learning has features that offer students the ability to analyze, describe, anticipate, collect, prepare and answer questions.

Keywords: COVID-19 pandemic, science process skills, virtual science laboratory, problem-based gaming, open-ended science experiment, mobile scientific inquiry, project-based learning

1. INTRODUCTION

The corona virus disease 2019 (COVID-19) pandemic has now spread across the world since it first emerged in Wuhan, China in December 2019 (Hamidah, Sriyono, and Hudha 2020). On 11 February 2020, the WHO named the disease as "COVID-19," an acronym of "coronavirus disease 2019" (Razon 2020). This pandemic naturally affects all sectors of human life, from the manufacturing, health, transport, government, maritime affairs, to education (Ng and Peggy 2020). Education plays a key role in shaping people into being resilient people to face the changing challenges of real life. By education, we will prepare students to have certain skills that are aligned with the demands of the workforce. Scientific process skills are one of the skills they need.

Scientific process skills are skills that allow students to observe, explain, predict, pose questions, plan, and communicate (Harlen 1999). Typically, these skills are incorporated into the curriculum when performing laboratory experiments. Students are divided into different groups, then work together to accomplish an experiment with a particular topic, discuss data analysis and report results. It can be identified that there are additional benefits to the students during the experimental activities. Students feel inspired and enjoy doing it, because these practices help students grasp a concept in the same way as a scientist discovers the theory (Elfeky, Masadeh and Elbyaly 2020). Unfortunately, this practice could not be performed during this pandemic because almost all countries implement lockdown to prevent wider spread of coronavirus. The implementation of quarantine is also supported by the findings of scientists by conducting analysis based on Reduced-Space Gaussian Process Regression, which states that new quarantine measures with more restrictions for the implemented containment strategy can be successful, but in a late period (Arias Velásquez and Mejía Lara 2020).

However, learning must continue. There is no way we can let students go through the day without a lesson. During this pandemic, various ways can be taken to keep students involved in learning, including virtual science laboratory, problem-based gaming, open-ended science experiment, mobile scientific inquiry, and project-based learning.

Among the learning models listed above, it is prudent for a teacher to be able to choose one that is in line with the characteristics of science learning. In Indonesia, the fourth core competency of the 2013 curriculum notes that students must be able to process, view, and reason in the concrete realm (use, interpret, organize, modify, and make) and the abstract realm (writing, reading, counting, drawing, and composing) according to what is learned from the same perspective or theory in school and other sources (Kemendikbud 2014). These core competencies are consistent with the scientific method, namely the acquisition of knowledge through observation, questioning, testing, reasoning, analysis, presentation and creation, which are carried out in deep discussion or group practice through classical activities.

Acquiring knowledge through practicum group activities will train critical thinking and problem-solving skills as one of the skills of the 21st century. Therefore, there are several ways to improve science process skills. It can be obtained through virtual science laboratory, problem-based gaming, open-ended science experiment, mobile scientific inquiry, and project-based learning.

2. SCIENCE PROCESS SKILLS

Practicum group activities, as described previously, may provide students with skills in the science process. Science process skills are a wide range of transferable skills, applicable for many disciplines and representing the scientists' behavior. Science process skills can be divided into two levels as basic and integrated. Basic science process skills consist of observation, communication, classification, measuring with numbers, inference, prediction, and using the space-and-time relationship. Integrated process skills consist of interpreting data, controlling variables, defining operationally, making hypotheses, and experimenting. Those two science process skills are essential cognitive skills for the success of primary school science learning, specifically at the pre-school or early childhood level because children do not have sufficient cognitive competence. Therefore, science processing skills for them do not need to be overemphasized. Nonetheless, the teaching of basic skills that will lead them to higher-order skills should also be guided. The active role of students to play, discover, solve problems and conduct research needs to be explored in the learning curriculum developed by the teacher. (Bati, Ertürk and Kaptan 2010).

Experts recommend that each stage be evaluated through a series of questionnaires to ensure the effectiveness of providing students with any measure of science process skills. The questions can include the students' findings related to their initial questions, the comparison to their findings with their earlier predictions, the associations between changes in one variable and another, the patterns or trends against all the evidence, the conclusion that students summarize and also students' recognition that any conclusions may have to be changed in the light of new evidence (Harlen and Jelly 1997; Harlen 1999). To provide science process skills with each indicator, the following describes several learning models or strategies that correspond to its characteristics.

3. Virtual Science Laboratory

Initially, the virtual science laboratory was intended to improve students' understanding of science concepts that have abstract phenomena (for example, the concept of electric fields, electricity flow and fluid flow) or to overcome the limitations of experimental equipment in schools that lack complete practical tools. However nowadays, in accordance with the rapid advancement of information and communication technology (ICT), virtual science laboratories can be applied to various subjects outside of science, for example mathematics, engineering, and languages. In general, the virtual science laboratory module must provide various information or instructions before students carry out a science experiment project, namely:

1 Course and content introduction
2 Problem or question introduction
3 Discussion and Collaborative Learning
4 Links to other learning resources and case studies
5 In-house three-dimensional virtual laboratory
6 Online scaffolding (Klentien and Wannasawade 2016)

Virtual science laboratory is a term used to refer to a digital environment designed to meet research needs. A significant contribution to many research domains, facilitating more efficient, open and reproducible research in new ways possible through virtual laboratories (Barker et al., 2019). Specifically, virtual science laboratories refer to integrated access to a variety of resources including software, databases, collaboration tools, workflows, instrumentation, and high-performance computing, usually via websites and mobile applications. Thus, the virtual science laboratory requires an internet connection when operating it. However, during difficult times like we experiencing nowadays, every virtual science laboratory developer is required to produce programs that can also be accessed offline.

There is a wide variety of applications available on the market for building virtual laboratories, from basic to complex, from free to purchased applications (Bilgehan, et al., 2016). All of this software is useful for producing various kinds of simple simulations to more sophisticated virtual laboratories. The subject matter can be presented to students in an integrated way with its web-based and mobile application-based characteristics. Virtual science laboratories can be used effectively in the classroom as well as outside the classroom, even at home if some further work may be required. What needs to be addressed when developing content in a virtual science laboratory is the pedagogical aspect that is integrated with the content that enables students to construct an easy-to-understand learning environment (Esquembre 2015).

A more sophisticated virtual laboratory model, for example, can be created with unique characteristics into a 3-dimensional interactive virtual laboratory. Due to its design, this model is the first of its kind which allows multi-admin, multi-user, special software compatible to run on iPad, iPhone, android and other smartphone platforms. This 3-dimensional virtual laboratory is ideal for the use of all student-centered active learning models (problem-based learning, cooperative learning, project-based learning, inquiry-based learning, research-based learning, invention-based learning and structuralist learning), due to its multi-user nature and accessible through the Internet (İnce et al., 2015).

Several research findings have shown the acceptance of the virtual science laboratory, including that student acceptance of this technology is focused on levels of performance, enjoyment and student satisfaction. Efficiency and fun are factors that positively influence student adoption of this technology. As a result, virtual activities and practices must be well designed to provide a successful educational environment for students. Additionally, virtual tools should be built with a playful approach, since fun and enjoyment are essential to involve students in the subject matter and learning process, as well as to increase the motivation and acceptance of these tools (Estriegana, Medina-merodio and Barchino 2019).

In contrast to science subjects, in the engineering field, virtual laboratory applications are less meaningful if the students' desired skills are hands-on especially if it is applied to distance or online learning. The reason for this difference lies in the fact that engineering often requires laboratory training to provide effective skill acquisition and hands-on experience. Real laboratory still needs to be activated or replicated as a virtual laboratory that is completely software-based (Potkonjak et al., 2016). In line with the virtual science laboratory, virtual learning is also being promoted in various countries (Almarzooq, Lopes, and Kochar 2020; Jowsey, Foster, Cooper-Ioelu, and Jacobs 2020) because during pandemic like this time, face-to-face learning is less likely to be implemented.

4. Problem Based-Gaming

Teachers often have to think that learning must be enjoyable for students, so that they can acquire knowledge in a more meaningful way. Games are a medium that can be used for this purpose, like puzzles or simulations. Games could become simple solution games or complex multi-solution paths that require inquiry skill and all dimensions of science process skills to complete. Games are proven to be able to meet the challenges of strategic and logical thinking as well as challenges to win the game (Rahmani and Abbas 2014). Other researchers also mentioned that problem-based gaming can improve student programming skills (Topalli and Cagiltay 2018). This is because problem-based gaming can increase student motivation to introduce programming concepts. In addition, because they can see the big picture of the software development cycle and the place of coding in that cycle, their understanding of programming concepts can most likely be conceptualized thereby enabling them to better integrate other concepts in their programs. Specifically, for increasing learning motivation, the same thing is also revealed that with problem-based gaming in the English course, student learning motivation can be further improved compared to conventional learning. (Hwang et al., 2017).

5. Open-Ended Science Experiments

The open-ended experiments are designed to enable students to explore and create. This method allows students to select experimental equipment, obtain and interpret data, and to determine results. Therefore, with the open experimental method it is hoped that students can develop psychomotor skills and behaviors such as thinking, deciding, making original implementations according to their decisions, and deducing the results obtained (Aydoğdu, Buldur, and Kartal 2013). The results of other studies show that with an open-ended experiment, students are able to better design and carry out experiments, analyze and interpret experimental results and work in groups (Haron et al., 2013). They are also able to design their own procedures, analyze and interpret experimental results, and work in teams (Mahmoud, Hashim and Sunarso 2020).

6. Mobile Scientific Inquiry

Mobile scientific inquiry is defined as a scientific investigation application that is supported by mobile devices in the science process skills. The development of mobile scientific inquiry is based on the fact that the use of mobile devices has become an integral part of our daily lives, and this has great potential for educational applications. With a storage unit, camera, sensors, and internet connection, it allows students to use their cellphones for more meaningful learning. Regarding science process skills, technology-based inquiry activities need to be designed. Developing better science process skills, which are not only related to science but also with problem solving and critical thinking, will help students to develop higher order thinking skills that can be generalized for the life of students (Ekici and Erdem 2020). Learning using mobile scientific inquiry is also suitable for fostering student curiosity and motivation. It helps learners to develop their ability to work in complex and unpredictable environments that can make them critical thinkers and agentic learners (Suárez et al., 2018).

7. Project-Based Learning

Project-based learning is a learning that refers to an inquiry-based learning method that involves students in knowledge construction by asking them to complete meaningful projects and develop real-world products (Guo et al., 2020). Project-based learning can also increase student motivation and problem-solving abilities (Chiang and Lee 2016). Through project-based learning, students are trained to challenge driving abilities focus on learning goals, participation in educational activities, collaboration among students, the use of scaffolding technologies, and the creation of tangible artifacts. Of all these measures, the most relevant is the development of tangible objects which can authentically solve the problem. This indicator differentiates project-based learning from other student-centered learning, for example problem-based learning (Helle, Tynjälä and Olkinuora 2006). This creation process requires students to work together to find authentic problem solutions in the process of integrating knowledge, application, and construction. Instructors and community members (clients), usually as facilitators, provide feedback and support for students to help their learning process.

Project-based learning with its indicators is a powerful teaching method that can achieve the following results: (1) motivating students, (2) preparing students for college, careers and becoming good citizens, (3) helping students meet expectations and perform well on tests that allow students to demonstrate knowledge and deep thinking skills, (4) enable teachers to teach in a more satisfying way, and (5) providing opportunities for schools and governments to find new ways to communicate and connect with parents, the community and the wider world (Larmer, Mergendoller, and Boss 2015).

For all the characteristics of each defined model or learning media, teachers are required to be able to sort, select and develop content that is integrated for pedagogical aspects to improve students' skills in the science process. Particularly in the current situation, where face-to - face learning is difficult to do, students need the psychological touch of a teacher that is represented in every learning model or media that teacher develops.

CONCLUSION

Being based on the five learning models or media outlined, the authors argue that the Virtual Science Laboratory is one of the most likely strategies to be implemented to equip science process skills in the current COVID-19 pandemic situation. It is because, in the virtual science laboratory learning, all the necessary experimental stages have been properly incorporated into the module. Then, by utilizing ICT which is very advanced and familiar to students, teachers can further develop learning programs that are in line with the current situation (contextual) and students can also be creative in exploring their environment in the search for scientific concepts like a scientist. Hopefully, everyone's creativity would be strengthened so that it can produce something useful for all especially during the COVID-19 pandemic which no one expected or want.

REFERENCES

Almarzooq, Z., Lopes, M., and Kochar, A. 2020. "Virtual Learning during the COVID-19 Pandemic: A Disruptive Technology in Graduate Medical Education." *Journal of the American College of Cardiology*, vol. 75, no. 20 (May). https://doi.org/https://doi.org/10.1016/j.jacc.2020.04.015.

Arias Velásquez, R. M., and Mejía Lara, J. V. 2020. "Forecast and evaluation of COVID-19 spreading in USA with reduced-space Gaussian process regression." *Chaos, Solitons and Fractals*, 136 (July). https://doi.org/10.1016/j.chaos.2020.109924.

Aydoğdu, B., Buldur, S., and Kartal, S. 2013. "The Effect of Open-ended Science Experiments based on Scenarios on the Science Process Skills of the Pre-Service Teachers." *Procedia - Social and Behavioral Sciences*, vol. 93 (October): 1162–1168. https://doi.org/10.1016/j.sbspro.2013.10.008.

Barker, M., Olabarriaga, S. D., Wilkins-Diehr, N., Gesing, S., Katz, D. S., Shahand, S., … Costa, A. 2019. "The global impact of science gateways, virtual research environments and virtual laboratories." *Future Generation Computer Systems*, vol. 95 (June): 240–248. https://doi.org/10.1016/j.future.2018.12.026.

Bati, K., Ertürk, G., and Kaptan, F. 2010. "The awareness levels of pre-school education teachers regarding science process skills." *Procedia - Social and Behavioral Sciences*, vol.2, no. 2: 1993–1999. https://doi.org/10.1016/j.sbspro.2010.03.270.

Bilgehan, M., Kiraz, A., Eski, H., Çiftçi, Ö., and Kubat, C. 2016. "A conceptual framework for cloud-based integration of Virtual laboratories as a multi-agent system approach." *COMPUTERS & INDUSTRIAL ENGINEERING*, vol. 102 (December): 452-457. https://doi.org/10.1016/j.cie.2016.04.011.

Chiang, C. L., and Lee, H. 2016. "The Effect of Project-Based Learning on Learning Motivation and Problem-Solving Ability of Vocational High School Students." *International Journal of Information and Education Technology*, vol.*6*, no.9:709–712. https://doi.org/10.7763/IJIET.2016. V6.779.

Ekici, M., and Erdem, M. 2020. "Developing Science Process Skills through Mobile Scientific Inquiry." *Thinking Skills and Creativity*, *36*(April): 1–12. https://doi.org/10.1016/j.tsc.2020.100658.

Elfeky, A. I. M., Masadeh, T. S. Y., and Elbyaly, M. Y. H. 2020. "Advance organizers in flipped classroom via e-learning management system and the promotion of integrated science process skills." *Thinking Skills and Creativity*, vol.35 (March). 100622. https://doi.org/ 10.1016/j.tsc. 2019.100622.

Esquembre, F. 2015. "Facilitating the Creation of Virtual and Facilitating the of Creation Creation Virtual Science Science Science Engineering." *IFAC-PapersOnLine*, vol.48, no.29: 49–58. https://doi. org/10.1016/ j.ifacol.2015.11.212.

Estriegana, R., Medina-merodio, J., and Barchino, R. 2019. "Student acceptance of virtual laboratory and practical work : An extension of the technology acceptance model." *Computers & Education*, vol. 135 (July): 1–14. https://doi.org/10.1016/j.compedu.2019.02.010.

Guo, P., Saab, N., Post, L. S., and Admiraal, W. 2020. "A review of project-based learning in higher education: Student outcomes and measures." *International Journal of Educational Research*, 102. https://doi.org/ 10.1016/j.ijer.2020.101586.

Hamidah, I., Sriyono, S., and Hudha, M. N. 2020. "A bibliometric analysis of COVID-19 research using vosviewer." *Indonesian Journal of Science and Technology*, vol. 5, no. 2 (March): 34–41. https://doi.org/ 10.17509/ijost.v5i2.24522.

Harlen, W. 1999. "Purposes and procedures for assessing science process skills." *Assessment in Education: Principles, Policy & Practice*, vol.6, no. 1 (June):129–144. https://doi.org/10.1080/09695949993044.

Haron, Z., Mohammad, S., Sam, A. R., MushairryMustaffar, and JamaludinMohdYatim. 2013. "The Implementation of an Open-ended Experiment in the Civil Engineering Laboratory." *Procedia - Social and Behavioral Sciences*, no. 102 (November): 548–559. https://doi.org/10.1016/j.sbspro.2013.10.771.

Helle, L., Tynjälä, P., and Olkinuora, E. 2006. "Project-based learning in post-secondary education - Theory, practice and rubber sling shots." *Higher Education*, vol. 51, no.2 (March): 287–314. https://doi.org/10.1007/s10734-004-6386-5.

Hwang, G. J., Hsu, T. C., Lai, C. L., and Hsueh, C. J. 2017. "Interaction of problem-based gaming and learning anxiety in language students' English listening performance and progressive behavioral patterns." *Computers and Education*, vol.106 (March): 26–42. https://doi.org/10.1016/j.compedu.2016.11.010.

İnce, E., Kırbaşlar, F. G., Güneş, Z. Ö., Yaman, Y., Yolcu, Ö., and Yolcu, E. 2015. "An Innovative Approach in Virtual Laboratory Education: The Case of "IUVIRLAB" and Relationships between Communication Skills with the Usage of IUVIRLAB." *Procedia - Social and Behavioral Sciences*, vol.195 (July):1768–1777. https://doi.org/10.1016/j.sbspro.2015.06.377.

Jowsey, T., Foster, G., Cooper-Ioelu, P., and Jacobs, S. 2020. "Blended learning via distance in pre-registration nursing education: A scoping review." *Nurse Education in Practice*, vol. 44(March). https://doi.org/10.1016/j.nepr.2020.102775.

Kemendikbud. Indonesia. 2014. Konsep dan Implementasi Kurikulum 2013. *Kementrian Pendidikan Dan Kebudayaan*: 1–118. https://www.kemdikbud.go.id/kemdikbud/dokumen/Paparan/Paparan%20Wamendik.pdf.

Klentien, U., and Wannasawade, W. 2016. "Development of Blended Learning Model with Virtual Science Laboratory for Secondary

Students." *Procedia - Social and Behavioral Sciences*, vol. 217, no. 2 (February): 706–711. https://doi.org/10.1016/j.sbspro.2016.02.126

Larmer, J., Mergendoller, J., & Boss, S. 2015. *Setting The Standard For Project Based Learning*. Alexandria: ASCD.

Mahmoud, A., Hashim, S. H., and Sunarso, J. 2020. "Learning permeability and fluidisation concepts via open-ended laboratory experiments." *Education for Chemical Engineers*, vol.*32* (July): 78–81. https://doi.org/10.1016/j.ece.2020.05.008.

Ng, Y., and Peggy, P. L. 2020. "Coronavirus disease (COVID-19) prevention: Virtual classroom education for hand hygiene." *Nurse Education in Practice*, vol.45 (May):102782. https://doi.org/10.1016/j.nepr.2020.102782.

Potkonjak, V., Gardner, M., Callaghan, V., Mattila, P., Jovanovi, K., Guetl, C., and Petrovi, V. M. 2016. *Virtual laboratories for education in science, technology, and engineering: A review*, vol. *95* (April): 309–327. https://doi.org/10.1016/j.compedu.2016.02.002.

Rahmani, R., and Abbas, M. 2014. "The Influence of Single-gender Peer Scaffolding in Problem-based Gaming on Performance in Double-loop Learning and Sub-dimensions of Science Process Skills." *Procedia - Social and Behavioral Sciences*, vol.116 (February): 4103–4107. https://doi.org/10.1016/j.sbspro.2014.01.898.

Razon, B. C. 2020. "COVID 19: Impetus for "Community Spirits" among Filipinos." *Indonesian Journal of Science and Technology* vol.5, no. 2 (March): 201-208.

Suárez, Á., Specht, M., Prinsen, F., Kalz, M., and Ternier, S. 2018. "A review of the types of mobile activities in mobile inquiry-based learning." *Computers and Education*, vol. 118 (March): 38–55. https://doi.org/10.1016/j.compedu.2017.11.004.

Topalli, D., and Cagiltay, N. E. 2018. "Improving programming skills in engineering education through problem-based game projects with Scratch." *Computers and Education*, vol. *120* (May): 64–74. https://doi.org/10.1016/j.compedu.2018.01.011.

In: COVID-19 ISBN: 978-1-53618-903-2
Editors: A. B. D. Nandiyanto et al.

Chapter 13

POST COVID-19 COMPETENCIES OF TEACHERS

***Sujin Nukaew*[1,*]*, Sangrung Poolsuwan*[2] *and Rossarin Jermtaisong*[3]**
[1]Faculty of Education, Nakhon Si Thammarat Rajabhat University
Tha Ngio, Mueang Nakhon Si Thammarat District,
Nakhon Si Thammarat, Thailand
[2]Aksorn Education Pub Co.,Ltd, Thailand
[3]Faculty of Technical Education, Rajamangala University
of Technology Thanyaburi Khlong Hok, Khlong Luang District,
Pathum Thani, Thailand

ABSTRACT

As the COVID-19 pandemic spread around the world, most educational institutions have been temporarily closed and it affects the student learning process. A competent and skilled teacher is one of the most important inputs in the education system, but teachers are often unprepared

* Corresponding Author's Email: sujinnukaew@gmail.com, sangrung20@yahoo.com, rossarin_j @rmutt.ac.th.

for teaching in crisis and post-emergency settings. They are stressed since they cannot attain responsibility as their roles. It seems that some competencies in the 21st century do not efficient enough to the crisis settings. This crisis teaches a lesson to the educator to rethink the teacher efficiency competences. Research claims that a relationship and cooperation with communities for learning organization is the competency that significantly helps student learning in the crisis-affected setting. Moreover, technology literacy is advantaged to help students learning in and out the classroom. Teachers with limited qualified for technology have to be trained. To prepare the new generation student for the fast-changing world and in times of emergency, the teachers should have more efficient and competent. The competent teacher can shape the best student.

Keywords: COVID -19, 21st century competencies, teacher competencies

1. Introduction

COVID -19, an emergency pandemic presents the big experience for the global citizen and all the organizations, including education. There are no schools, no exams, but teachers. The crisis is highlighting the teacher to play the roles outside the school because of the closure of schools. How could they be responsible for this challenging role, outside-school teachers? In Thailand, there are nearly 13 million students, which are out of school and 600,000 teachers are unable to teach in their classes until at least 2020; however, education has to continue as soon as possible through alternative learning pathways (Rattana Lao 2020). Online learning and distance learning program are the responses for teaching and learning within the urgent condition (Saripudin et al., 2020). This means Thailand maintains the learning and ensures that all the students retain knowledge and skills. Although that is just the action in the short term, it causes bitter stress to teachers, students, and even the parents. Not all teachers can use technology to teach. Some of them are just trained whereas the students especially those who are in the rural area are out of necessary technological tools for learning. Worst yet, some parents, who are unemployed during the crisis or have low-wage jobs, have no time to fill in the temporary teachers for their kids nor have the financial resources to afford outside support (John DaSilva 2020).

Due to the big impact of the crisis to the education sector around the world, educators have to rethink what the education and teacher competencies for emergency settings in the future should be.

2. Teacher Competencies and the Student Success

Being a teacher at any level requires a significant amount of knowledge and skill. Teachers are key to success in education. The competent and skilled teachers make learning possible whether during times of crisis or not. Research confirms this common perception that all factors under the control of schools, the maximization of student success relates to the powerful influence of teacher the most (Babu and Mendro 2003). The competencies address the ability to do something successfully or efficiently. Competencies are not skills, but competencies are inherent qualities an individual possess – combining skills, knowledge, and ability. What are teacher competencies? They are a combination of skills, knowledge, behavior, and attributes that enable effective or better job performance. To fulfill student learning, teachers must have expertise and good competencies with the changing educational context where hundreds of critical decisions are required (Jakson 1990).

According to the importance of the teacher, paying attention to the competencies for teachers helps to ensure that all teachers are prepared to make school a positive experience for students and their families. The strong set of competencies that every competent teacher also needs to possess are knowledge, skills, and values. What core competencies do the modern effective teachers in the 21st need for preparing their students and equip them with the essential skills required for the future? UNESCO (2011) defines that the teacher competency in 21st Century consisted of five core competencies which are knowing and applying technology; deep understanding education policies, curricula and be updated on national, regional, and global developments, what to teach, assessment, flexibility in teaching, instructional skill for problem-solving; building the knowledge of learning process, learning strategies, Information and Communication

Technology (ICT) instruction, ICT community designing to promote the continuous learning skill; being a leader of the colleagues and community; and developing teacher profession as well as applying ICT for the professional learning community. That is the big picture of teacher competencies in the global level. Similarly, in the Southeast Asia region, the eleven Ministries of Education realize that schools today operate in a complex and constantly changing world of knowledge and information. Thus, the Teachers' Council of Thailand (TCT), in partnership with the SEAMEO Secretariat (SEAMES) and the SEAMEO Regional Center for Educational Innovation and Technology (SEAMEO INNOTECH), initiated the development of the Southeast Asia Teacher Competency Framework (SEA-TCF) in April 2017. The SEA-TCF consists of four essential competencies and twelve general competencies that high performing teachers in the region must possess. Four essential competencies are:

1. *Know and understand what to teach*. This is the ability of teachers to deepen and broaden their knowledge on what to teach, understand education trends, policies, and curricula and be updated on local, national, regional, and global developments.
2. *Help students learn*. It is the ability to know their students, use the most effective teaching and learning strategy and assess and give feedback on how students learn.
3. *Engage the community*. This is the ability to partner with parents and caregivers, involve the community to help students learn, and encourage respect and diversity.
4. *Become a better teacher every day*. This is the ability to know oneself and others, practice human goodness and then master the teaching practice. (Teacher Council of Thailand 2018).

However, the competencies listed in the framework can be interpreted based on local context and specific needs. For Thailand, the teacher competencies included five core competencies and six functional competencies. The core competencies consisted of an achievement in performance, self-development, teamwork, ethics, and teacher profession conducts, while the functional competence consisted of a curricular administration and learning management, a learner development, a classroom organization, an analysis, synthesis, and research for a learner development, a teacher leadership, a relationship and cooperation with communities for learning organization (Chatchai Wangmeechongmee 2017). It seems that the competencies defined are able to enhance the student 21st Century skills - learning skills, literacy skills, and life skills, but some are inadequate for the emergency setting.

3. What Kind Teacher Competency in Post- Crisis?

In this crisis situation, the risk-control decision of government led the students to study at home with the distance learning program or online learning. This causes a degree of inconvenience and problem. Students lack technology tools. Although they are the digital age citizen, they cannot learn. Besides, some cannot access the online system. Some teachers and parents lack of technology implementation potential and problem-solving skills. To provide technology to support the students learning opportunity and to imply technology to enhance students' knowledge, learning is essential for the 21st Century teachers. In fact, some teachers cannot operate a computer as well. Because of the sudden COVID-19 crisis, the educators evidently perceive that teacher is incompetent in technology. The question is if the others are efficient enough for the current rapidly changing world, especially in the emergency setting.

To continue the student learning during the crisis, the educators have to emphasize on the access to learning and the quality of education as well. There is a strong evidence supported that the use of community-based education is the valuable channel to increase access to education, including accelerated learning programs, and approaches to distance learning for primary, and secondary students. For the quality of education, community-based education and community participant monitoring are needed to increase academic achievement for the primary school students related to one of the 21st century competencies (Burde et al., 2015), as well as a relationship and cooperation with communities for the learning organization. Therefore, to build a strong relationship with the community, one success key is to make strong education. Besides the community supporting, remote education in the midst crisis is the other success key.

Digital learning television, online learning, and distance learning program are the alternative nation educational pathways. Although learning through TV is user-friendly and particularly for vulnerable students, it is a one-way communication. Online learning is "the most ideal" for the current situation in Thailand because of its ability to accommodate a two-way communication and a real-time response, so digital literacy competence is also essential for the teacher in this crisis (Kertbundit 2020) UNESCO defines that knowing and applying technology is one of the 21st-century competence; nevertheless, some teachers are still inadequate in this competency. How are about students? They will be no problem for the digital age generation, but some families do not either have access to the same technology tools (internet, computer, television, smartphone) nor have the same level of knowledge and skills in using technology. It is impossible for online learning. It is crucial for the teacher to follow up and identify the specific needs of the vulnerable students to maintain their appropriate learning which reflects that learning management and learner development are also practical competencies.

The spread of COVID-19 is the great opportunity to reform the education system, including the teacher profession development (Sangsawang 2020). What should the competent teacher in post- crisis setting be? Are the teacher competencies today sufficient for tomorrow world? As the responsibility in shaping the students and community, development of the competent and skilled teachers is the most considering factor. Unfortunately, the professional teacher development in Thailand is not as successful as the expectation level. One way to develop the effective professional teacher is to develop teacher competency. Undoubtedly, there are some 21st Century teacher competencies are relevant to the research finding competence in crisis: a relationship and cooperation with communities for learning organization, learning management and technology literacy.

Right now, the educators have to learn that both pre-service teacher and in-service teachers have to be retrained some essential competencies to be more effective, especially technology literacy. Not only those competencies in 21st century are the emergency response but also some renew ones. The recently crisis teaches the educator a new lesson for preparing the better students for what the future might hold. The lessons are to educate citizens in an interconnected world, redefining the role of the educator, teaching life skill needed for the future, and unlocking technology to deliver education. Similarity, some researchers (Helen Soulé and others (2014)) stated their researches that project based and inquiry-based learning (PBL) instructional 21st century learning practices is proven to produce positive student outcomes. They also claim that "PBL and other instructional practices that promote student engagement, real-world experiences, the acquisition of 21st-century skills, and transform the role of the teacher from lecturer to guide/facilitator have been shown to produce the desired student outcomes (Soulé, et al., 2014, https://www.hanoverresearch.com/insights-blog/bringing-21st-century-skill-development-to-the-forefront-of-k-12-education/, retrieved on July 1, 2020)." According to the research, the practical instructions reflect a very different role for teachers and require significant changes in behavior, pedagogy, and practice. The significant competence for the unpredicted future, emergency setting should be:

1. Pedagogy competency, including ability to design learner centered methodology, organize instructional management related to the learner requirement, the contexts, and the situations (Mulyanti et al., 2020, 271-282).
2. Flexibility and adaptability competency, including the ability to adjust profession planned work by gathering relevant information and applying critical thinking to address multiple demands and necessary priorities in a changing environment and emergency setting.
3. Social competency, including the ability to deal with social condition, get more sensitive to the problem around, access to the

society well, take another's perspective, or idea concerning a situation.

4. Critical decision competency, including the ability to critical analyze the education situations and problems, as well as to make a critical decision to solve the conflict and problem based on the information analyzed in specific context.
5. Lifelong learning competency, including the ability to gain knowledge and skills continuously to develop professional job, and to provide quality learning.

The teacher is the most important factor indicating the quality of education; therefore, they need strong and efficient professional competencies. COVID-19 is the catalyst to reform the education system and the teacher competency in managing the quality outcome, so teachers' competencies must be reviewed and redefined depending on the fast-changing world and the unexpected crisis (Ana 2020). A relationship and cooperation with communities for learning organization the competency related to the research findings, showing that community-based education and community participant monitoring are increasing academic achievements for the primary school students related to one of the 21st-century competencies (Burde et al. 2015). The competent teachers are the ones who can collaborate well with the community in order to build a learning organization. This is necessary for the crisis setting for the closure school and students have to study at home. Some parents have no time and lack of knowledge and digital skill which put them a lot of pressure. The teachers collaborate with the community to continue student learning it reflect the teacher's proficiency in learning management. In addition, the alternative pathway in the pandemic is online learning and distance learning. Online learning is "the most ideal" for the emergency situation in Thailand, the interrupted education could be progress if the teachers and parents are potential resources.

The educators have to rethink what the other necessary competencies are required for the fast-changing global. The responses are pedagogy competency, flexibility and adaptability competency, social competency, critical decision competency, and lifelong learning competency. As the education needs a competent teacher, the professional development (both pre-service teachers and the in-service teacher) must be a priority and carefully prepared in order to shape the best teacher that they can be. To support the success of the student, government initiatives to maintain student learning cannot be effective without the use of an invaluable educational resource.

CONCLUSION

A competent and skilled teacher is one of the most important inputs in the education system, but teachers are often unprepared for teaching in crisis and post-emergency settings. This crisis teaches a lesson to the educator to rethink the teacher efficiency competences. The relationship and cooperation with communities for learning organization is the competency that significantly helps student learning in the crisis-affected setting and technology literacy is also advantaged to help students learning in and out the classroom. Teachers with limited qualified for technology have to be trained to prepare the new generation students for the fast-changing world and in times of emergency.

REFERENCES

Rattana Lao. 2020. *Pandemic is exposing the gaps in Thai education.* https://www.bangkokpost.com/opinion/opinion/1910956/pandemic-is-exposing- the- gaps-in-thai-education.

DaSilva, John. 2020. *Three consequences of COVID-19 on Thai Education.* https://www.kenan-asia.org/covid-19-thai-education/.

Babu, S., and Mendro, R. 2003. "Teacher accountability: HLM-based teacher effectiveness indices in the investigation of teacher effects on student achievement in a state assessment program." In *American*

Education Research Association Annual Meeting. https://scholar.google.com/scholar?hl=en&as_sdt=0%2C5&q=Teacher+accountability%3A+HLbased+teacher+effectiveness+indices+in+the+investigation+of+teacher+effects+on+student+achievement+in+a+state+assessment+program.&btnG=.

Jackson, P.W. (1990). *Life in classrooms*. New York, NY: Teachers College Press.

Teacher Council of Thailand. 2018. *Southeast Asia teachers competency framework*. Bangkok: Thailand.

Chatchai Wangmeechongmee. 2017. *Competency of Thai teacher in 21st century: wind of change*. http://www.journalhri.com/pdf/1202_03.pdf.

Burde, D., Guven, O., Kelcey, Z., Lahman, H., and Al-Abadhi, K. 2015. What work to promote children's educational access, quality of learning, and wellbeing in crisis-affected contexts. *UKAID: INEE*. https://s3.amazonaws.com/inee-assets/resources/Education-emergencies-rigorous-review-2015-10.pdf.

Kertbundit, B. 2020. "COVID-19 presents big challenges for schooling." *The Times,* April 16, 2020. https://www.bangkokpost.com/opinion/opinion/1900890/covid-19-presents-big challenges-for-schooling.

Sangsawang, T. 2020. "An Instructional Design for Online Learning in Vocational Education according to a Self-Regulated Learning Framework for Problem Solving during the CoViD-19 Crisis." *Indonesian Journal of Science and Technology* vol.5, no.2: 283–298.

Soulé, Helen., Fischer-Tubbs, Tracy., Hart., and Katie. 2014. *Bringing 21st century skill development to the forefront of K-12 education*. https://www.hanoverresearch.com/insights-blog/bringing-21st-century-skill-development-to-the-forefront-of-k-12-education/.

Mulyanti, B., Purnama, W., and Parwinanto, R. E. 2020. "Distance Learning in Vocational High Schools during the COVID-19 Pandemic in West Java Province, Indonesia." *Indonesian Journal of Science and Technology* vol.5, no.2: 271–282.

Ana, A. 2020. "Trends in Expert System Development: A Practicum Content Analysis in Vocational Education for Over Grow Pandemic Learning

Problems." *Indonesian Journal of Science and Technology* vol.5: no.2: 71-85.

Saripudin, S., Rohendi, D., and Abdullah, A. G. 2020. "Developing Information Technology in OpenCourseWare: From Movements to Opportunities in Asia." *Indonesian Journal of Science and Technology* vol.5: no.2: 308-320.

In: COVID-19 ISBN: 978-1-53618-903-2
Editors: A. B. D. Nandiyanto et al.

Chapter 14

PERSPECTIVES OF THAI PARENTS ON COVID-19 OUTBREAK THAT EFFECTS STUDENTS LEARNING

Sutthiporn Boonsong[1] and Klairung Rabieboat[2]
[1]Faculty of Technical Education, Rajamangala University of Technology Thanyaburi, Khlong Hok, Khlong Luang District, Pathum Thani, Thailand
[2]Faculty of Business Administration, Rajamangala University of Technology Thanyaburi, Khlong Hok, Khlong Luang District, Pathum Thani, Thailand

ABSTRACT

The COVID-19 outbreak has caused a big problem for Thai students and parents because most of the education systems have not yet entered the world of learning. By using program for International Student Assessment digital devices, the data showed that teachers and schools are well-equipped with technology and support online teaching. In the aspect of students' access to the internet, Thailand still has students who are in unfortunate and unfavourable environment. Qualified online knowledge is essential and various fundamentals should be taken into account in order to ensure that all Thai students receive quality learning. The COVID-19 Adult Digital Technology helps students to acquire quality knowledge. However, it is a costly education learning system and paying special attention to the suitability of applications that maintain the relationships of teachers and students, including family members' relationships is needed.

Keywords: COVID-19, crisis problems, Thai parents' perspectives

1. Introduction

The advent of the COVID-19 crisis reveals that most education systems have not been ready to enter the world of learning using digital devices. Based on the data collected from 15-year-old students and school administrators at Program for International Student Assessment (PISA) 2018 in 79 educational systems around the world, it was found that many opportunities and access to online learning begin with the basic necessities of online learning. Having a quiet place is the first thing that students should have in order to concentrate on learning. PISA 2018 found that only 15% of students in Organization for Economic Cooperation and Development (OECD) countries do not have a quiet place in their home to use for learning and up to 30% in Indonesia, the Philippines and Thailand (Boonsu, 2020).

In Thailand, there are students who come from schools with inferior socioeconomic status, reporting that there are no more quiet places in the house for learning than students from schools with socioeconomic status who obviously have a distinct advantage. In Thailand, important information from PISA 2018 shows that Thai students still lack important factors for online learning at home, including quiet places in the house for computer learning and internet connection. A comparison between students from disadvantaged schools and students from advantageous schools including Thailand shows the gap of having computers at home between these two groups is more than 50%, which shows the inequality of educational opportunities. Furthermore, Thailand has about 80% of students accessing the internet from home, in which the difference between students from advantageous schools and students from disadvantaged schools is approximately 30% (Institute for the Promotion of Teaching Science and Technology 2020; OECD 2020; OECD 2020b).

1.1. Thai Parents' Opinion on the Student Studying Problems

The situation of the COVID-19 outbreak affects the teaching and learning of Thai students who have to study online. However, the readiness and family status are different. Some families may be in a position to have everything, and some parents are able to access the learning media when needed, whereas other families may not be able to afford it at all and it is a huge issue that affects them. During the outbreak, students should study at home in online learning. It means the learning must be compatible with the Wi-Fi contract system including communication devices such as computers, laptops, and tablets that can be used to efficiently access the online program. Besides, the place for studying and sending the assignments to their teacher or lecturer must be a private space or a quiet room such as private bedrooms. Another problem for a university student where the student requires to follow real time online class so the student has the responsibility to a certain extent. However, in a primary or secondary school student's case, there must be a guardian to monitor them especially primary school students. They need close guardians to help them in their learning. As some comments from Thai families are as follows:

> " ...Since our family has two members who are students in a university and junior high school the effects found are different. In March, when the COVID-19 outbreak began in Thailand, it has impacted the exam study, which was close to the end of the semester. The government has encouraged schools to accelerate the learning and give tests faster and stop learning once the exam is completed. The regulation did not give much impact to primary and secondary schools because the school holiday is closer. However, for the student studying at the university level the student still needs lecture, therefore, the learning has changed to teaching and testing online because the student is an English language student. It is still a mid-term study and will continue to study and have exam. This may cause

problems in online learning because either students or teachers have never had this type of teaching before and are not ready. The problem occurs as well as adaptation for online learning at home or on the internet via wi-fi using a laptop or tablet should also be taken. Our family is ready to promote necessary learning media equipment and support the arrangement of the health care readiness in our area, useful food discussions for encouragement…" (Taipae 2020).

" … As a parent, I wish the director of every school and the Ministry of Education help to review the teaching online learning as well. As I see the hardships of many parents and they have come to discuss to share our varied challenges and the reasons behind them. Therefore I would like to give examples below:

1 In order to have online learning, it is very important for students to have a computer and internet connection. If they do not have those facilities at home, they cannot learn. Consequently, parents have to buy them in order to support the children learning but computer is quite expensive. On the other hand, at this time, parents have less work and make a living is difficult, find extra money is challenging and it is also difficult for to findmoney for food or buy a daily. If a family has two or three children, they have buy two or three devices because the children must study online at the same time. Some parents do not want their children to be inferior to others. As a result, parents must borrow money to buy computers so their children can learn like other students. Moreover, they must find money to pay for tuition, books, clothes, school supplies in each semester and it has already been difficult. Why should we find more money to pay for the computer?
2 Regarding online learning, if there are no adults sitting near children, do you think the children will not open other pages like Youtube, games, and other websites? Will each student study hard? And if the parents have to sit and watch over the course, when will they work to pay for the newly purchased computer?
3 For young children, such as kindergarten 1-3, is it appropriate to allow children to sit and study in front of the screen for such a long time? It affects their eyesight and also they do not have long attention span to endure sitting and listening until the class over.

4 Parents must pay tuition, but they must sit and teach all of their children. The point is why parents would pay the tuition if parents must sit and teach children. Paying tuition does not mean we will teach our children or we cannot raise children. During the online learning, the schools do not lower the tuition but still pay the same amount of tuition. And if parents have many children, the parents may not be able to take care of all the children's learning, because they study online at the same time.

5 If parents do not let the children study online for their own reasons, will children be embarrassed?When they are embarrassed, as a result children do not want to go to school the next day, suppressing various things and children will ask parents to buy a computer that every child wants. However, many students, instead of studying they play games or see the movies. Do you think most kids will do what more than each other?

Therfore, for the aforementioned reasons, I would like to ask the director of every school and the Ministry of Education consider them as well because I think it affects parents in many ways, and these are just some examples to understand. There are still many reasons that impact how hard parents have to fight with the online education policies you have created now". (Boonsuk 2020)

Problems in online learning have also been encountered by university students since March 2020. Initially, the modifications on the learning made quite suddenly causing students and professors had not much time to prepare or adjust. It has causes problems that emerged both from teachers and students. Some teachers are old who lack information and technology skills, creating difficulties with the use of programs and instructional materials when they conduct online courses. It takes time to solve the problem or call someone to help and it takes almost an hour of study time (Mulyanti et al. 2020). Regarding the issues with the study time, as in the past, one subject took three hours but was changed to just two hours.

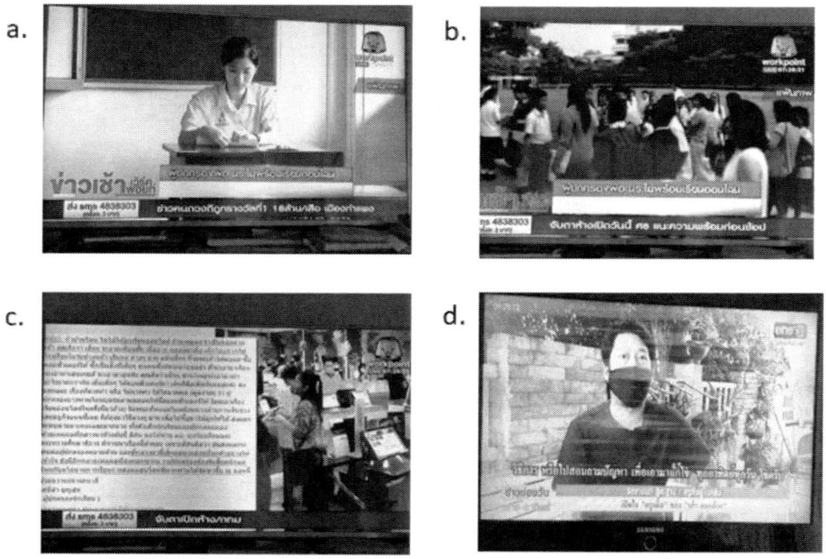

Figure 1. News in television about Thai parents and teachers concern about online study (Television Station Channel 23 2020a; Television Station Channel 23 2020b).

Other challenges include difficulties in understanding the content and learning styles, questions and also answers are not clear and distinct from the classroom. The instructors sometimes let the students study from the recorded clip. Consequently, when they do not understand the lecture, they cannot ask immediately. Additionaly when doing groupwork, students encounter problems especially when they need to coordinate with peers specifically when submitting work to the teacher. The fact that students have to present their work online is also difficult (Ana 2020). Students are unable to solve problems as good as while learning in the classroom and most importantly, the problem of inter-connected signals that sometimes gets stuck or fails.

Furthermore, concentration span is also an issue as studying at home is different from studying at school (Sangsawang 2020). At home, other family members accidentally might disturb the student. Students commented that online learning was not as effective as studying in a classroom which was more understandable and merrier. During the online learning, some parents are willing to accommodate the learning and help solve the problem, while some families are willing to provide the tools needed for the learning. However, there are still many families who are not able to support students at all (Figure 1).

New semester and opening of schools and universities in Thailand arrive in July. The government announced the semester would be started, however, there is a requirement for educational institutions to manage online teaching along with studying at school by alternating days to study online. Most teachers and parents agree that for elementary and junior high school students studying online for 2-3 are plausible because this group of students still have fairly limited self-control. During school hours, parents should closely monitor the students to help them particularly on certain sections that they do not understand.

Furthermore, students may not have a lot of concentration studying outside classroom because they have never previously encountered this situation. Students may think of their peers, wonder when they could meet in school again, and think of when they start school. This condition affects the students' development. During the online study the family member who would take care of the students would then help to make the learning more efficient.

Online education requires a lot of adaptation from parents and students because each family prepares differently. Most people in Thailand are relatively in the middle level although there are still many people who are in low economic level. Thus, many families will encounter a variety of obstacles in online education. Opinions from some of the parents are:

1 Each family may have two to three children who are at the school age and does not have enough money. Each child studying at different levels, causing problems such as a place to learn at home and insufficient equipment for learning.
2 There are serious problems if a family has children in kindergarten and elementary school years. It means adults or parents should always help and closely control all the time.
3 Parents mostly have to work. Some parents have their own business while others work in public or private agencies. They may not have

time to look after children and some poor families will get more problems.

4 Some families do not live with their parents and some live with grandparents or elderly people. If they have to support children education, this is very complicated because some people do not know much about education or uneducated.

5 Families will have to spend more in school supplies if they have more than one child and they will have to pay more for the monthly internet charge that allows the fast Wi-Fi signal speed that helps students to learn well.

6 Education for children is not as effective as studying in school because children may not be concentrated for a long time and lack of motivation because the learning is different from the class in the real classroom.

7 Children will become bored because it is not as fun as studying with friends in the class that has the interactive talk and have fun activities together.

8 Some students may not attend classes online at the time the teacher teaches. It can definitely happen or some students are addicted to games and the might play games instead of studying when their guardian or parents are not around.

The aforementioned are just some of the problems that many families have encountered and they are still worried. Therefore, coping with what has been happening and working on the adjustment together with the parents and students are essential. According to us, below are things that parents might need to prepare:

1. A place to study which is private and no noise, such as a children's bedroom.
2. Sufficient educational materials and equipment at leas for two children in order to minimize the educational hurdles they might encounter and they can send the assignments punctually.

3. Schedule for children such as when to wake up take a shower, eat, and study online.
4. Studying time and understand the each course hour together with the children, as well as taking care of learning activities with teachers and friends while online.
5. Monitoring children homework, lesson review and others.
6. Providing children with relaxation from studying to avoid excessive tension.
7. Discussions and communication between parents and class teachers or subject teachers about various problems.
8. Allocating time to take care of the children, although parents are not sure how much they can do.

CONCLUSION

The COVID-19 oubreak has caused a big problem for Thai students and parents because the education mostly served through online classes. In the aspect of students' access to the internet, Thailand still has students who are in unfortunate and unfavourable environment. Online learning is a costly education learning system. Therefore, paying special attention to the suitability of applications (that maintain the relationships of teachers and students, including family members' relationships) is needed in order to provide continuous learning for our students and expand the home school collaboration.

REFERENCES

Ana, A. 2020. "Trends in Expert System Development: A Practicum Content Analysis in Vocational Education for Over Grow Pandemic Learning Problems." *Indonesian Journal of Science and Technology* vol.5, no.2: 246–260.

Boonsuk, R. 2020. Rossanisa Boonsuk's online post, *Television Station Channel 23*, retrieved on May 14, 2020.https://www.google.com/search?safe=strict&client=firefoxd&q=Television+Station+Channel+23.+(2020+a).+Morning+news&spell=1&sa=X&ved=2ahUKEwihlb_Lu7rrAhWVF3IKHYA5DA4QBSgAegQIDRAn&biw=1366&bih=654.

Institute for the Promotion of Teaching Science and Technology. 2020. *How well are schools and students equipped with online education: PISA findings.* https://pisathailand. ipst.ac.th/issue-2020-51/, retrieved on May 13, 2020.

Mulyanti, B., Purnama, W., and Parwinanto, R. E. 2020. "Distance Learning in Vocational High Schools during the COVID-19 Pandemic in West Java Province, Indonesia." *Indonesian Journal of Science and Technology* vol.5, no.2: 271–282.

OECD. 2020a. Learning remotely when schools close: How well are students and schools prepared? Insights from PISA, PISA, OECD Publishing: Paris.

OECD. 2020b. A framework to guide an education response to the COVID-19 Pandemic of 2020, *PISA*, OECD Publishing: Paris.

Sangsawang, T. 2020. "An Instructional Design for Online Learning in Vocational Education according to a Self-Regulated Learning Framework for Problem Solving during the CoViD-19 Crisis." *Indonesian Journal of Science and Technology* vol.5, no.2: 283–298.

Taipae, K. 2020. Interview, retrieved on May 6, 2020.

Television Station Channel 23. 2020a) *Morning news.* retrieved on May 17, 2020. https://www.google.com/search?safe=strict&client=firefoxd &q= Television+Station+Channel+23.+(2020+a).+Morning+news&spell=1 &sa=X&ved=2ahUKEwihlb_Lu7rrAhWVF3IKHYA5DA4QBSgAeg QIDRAn&biw=1366&bih=654.

Television Station Channel 31. 2020b. *Channel 1 Sunday-news*, retrieved on May 17, 2020. https://www.google.com/search?safe=strict&client=firefox-b-d&q=Television+Station+Channel+23.+(2020+a).+Morning+news&spell=1&sa=X&ved=2ahUKEwihlb_Lu7rrAhWVF3IKHYA5DA4QBSgAegQIDRAn&biw=1366&bih=654.

In: COVID-19 ISBN: 978-1-53618-903-2
Editors: A. B. D. Nandiyanto et al.

Chapter 15

CHALLENGES AND CHANCES IN LEARNING MANAGEMENT FOR THAI STUDENTS DURING THE COVID-19 OUTBREAK

Rossarin Jermtaisong[1], Sangrung Poolsuwan[2] and Sujin Nukaew[3,*]

[1]Faculty of Technical Education, Rajamangala University of Technology Thanyaburi, Khlong Hok, Khlong Luang District, Pathum Thani, Thailand

[2]Aksorn Education Pub Co., Ltd, Thailand

[3]Faculty of Education, Nakhon Si Thammarat Rajabhat University, Tha Ngio, Mueang Nakhon Si Thammarat District, Nakhon Si Thammarat, Thailand

ABSTRACT

Coronavirus disease 2019 (COVID-19) is a new deathly contagious disease that poses tremendous threats to the human race. It was announced by the World Health Organization as a global pandemic. The spread of the

[*] Corresponding Author's Email: sujinnukaew@gmail.com.

virus is the urgent crisis which affects the educational management in Thailand and around the world both in a direct and indirect way. This is considered a big challenge for the opportunity to develop new learning channels and blend online materials or digital technology devices with various instruction in order to broaden the teaching and learning experience on both offline and online platforms so that learners are able to learn continuously, effectively, and efficiently. In Thailand, On Site, On Air, and Online are the keys for every student, either who is able or unable to access online learning, to be able to keep up with the study during the implementation of the semi-lockdown and social distancing measures for preventing the spread of the pandemic by encouraging people, and to limit travel and refrain from participating in activities that involve a lot of people. Regarding this condition, what needed to be taken into consideration is educational inequality, resource management, readiness and cooperation of parents and family, the adaptation of teachers, and changing behaviors of learners. It is required that a strategic plan on educational management must be implemented in order to draw up short-term, medium-term, and long-term respond plans as well as seek cooperation from various sectors: educational, governmental, and private to support, develop, and exchange instruments or new techniques for successfully overcoming the obstacles of teaching and learning during the COVID-19 pandemic.

Keywords: COVID-19, learning management, Thai students

1. Introduction

In the history of Thailand's education, there have always been problems since the founding of Thailand 800 years ago. The first Thai alphabet was invented to protect the nation from losing territories to neighboring states that had already owned a written language (Office of the Education Council. Ministry of Education 2017). Until today when a large number of crises emerged due to different factors such as those relating to public health, the economy, politics, society and Thailand once again works on the crises.

The spread of the Corona Virus Disease 2019 (COVID-19) pandemic has posed a series of impacts to people involved in Thailand's educational sector, ranging from students, parents, teachers, as well as the state and future educational management. COVID-19 pandemic is a serious issue, and combating viral diseases has always been a serious challenge for many aspects, including health authorities throughout the world (Mulyanti, Purnama and Parwinanto 2020).

This COVID-19 pandemic seems to "disrupt" Thailand's instructional management since Thailand's education system has been driven mainly by schools and universities through educational intervention, interaction, and cooperation. In fact, those who are responsible for and play a role in Thailand's education have tried so hard to seek appropriate approaches to move the education system forward.

This is considered the opportunity that lies in the crisis which transforms the education system into a new form, especially the application of "technology" to the instructional system to a greater extent as identified in the Strategy for Promoting and Developing Digital Technology Systems for Education of the 12th National Education Plan (2017 – 2036), which aims at providing Thai people with the opportunity for continuous learning through information technology throughout life. This corresponds to the development in terms of access to equal and efficient services (Office of the Permanent Secretary Ministry of Education 2016). The blending of "technology" with teaching and learning enables the system to run continuously and allows both learners and teachers to access education regardless of places or locations as shown by the analysis of Jeanne Allen, the founder and CEO of The Center for Education Reform, in Forbes indicating that there is always opportunity lying in the midst every crisis.

2. Opportunity in the Crisis: Educational Transformation

Based on the aforementioned challenges and opportunity, information technology is considered the tool for improving and driving Thailand's education forward. The application of "Educational Technology" to teaching and learning allows learners who are encouraged to keep learning at home during the COVID-19 pandemic be able to keep up with lessons.

As for Thailand Minister of Education, Nataphol Teepsuwan, has proposed three plans for basic education teaching and learning management as follows:

1. On Site refers to the normal operations of schools based on the discretion of public health agencies.
2. On Air refers to the teaching and learning approach applied in case schools cannot return to normal operations and the social distancing measure is still implemented. This can be carried out by different means; including Distance Education which are conducted through Distance Learning Television (DLTV), Distance Learning Information Technology (DLIT).
3. Online is the teaching and learning approach applied in case schools cannot return to normal operations as mentioned in point 2 above. Therefore, the teaching and learning activities are carried out by connecting DEEP (Digital Education Excellence Platform) with other platforms such as Google Slide, Google Docs, Google Sheets, Google Jamboard, or Microsoft Teams in which many features such as Chat, Hub, and Microsoft Office are used. In regard to this, the systems proposed in point 2 and 3 above require a test before the next academic semester starts (OBEC Chanel 2020; Silpakorn University 2012.

Generally, there are two parts to online instructional management. First, to which a lot of technologies are applied on which the implementation of the channel currently known as "Live Streaming" which engages teachers and learners in real-time activities as seen in Figures 1 and 2; and synchronous learning which is based on time conditions, teaching (learning schedules), the volume of learning content, and direct transference of knowledge from teachers through technology according to the established curriculum framework. This can be conducted using Facebook Live or Zoom Meeting application.

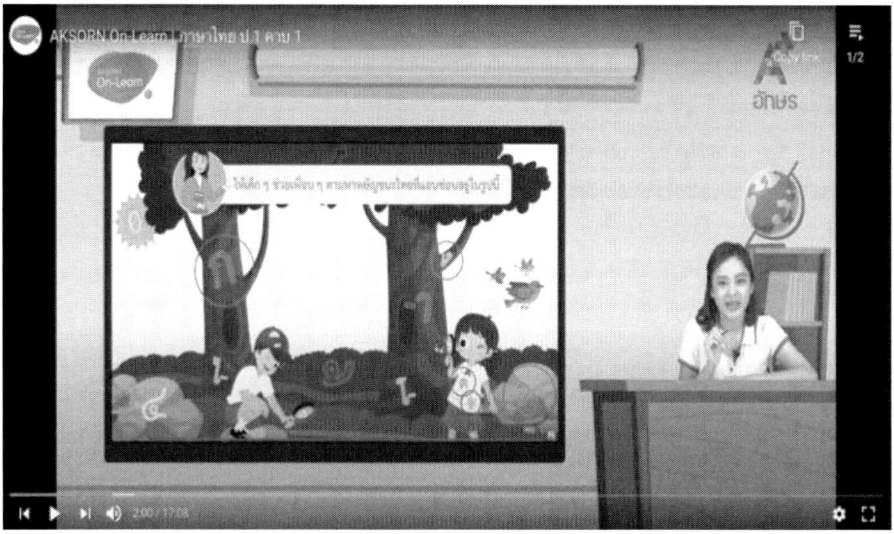

Figure 1. Live Streaming for teaching and learning.

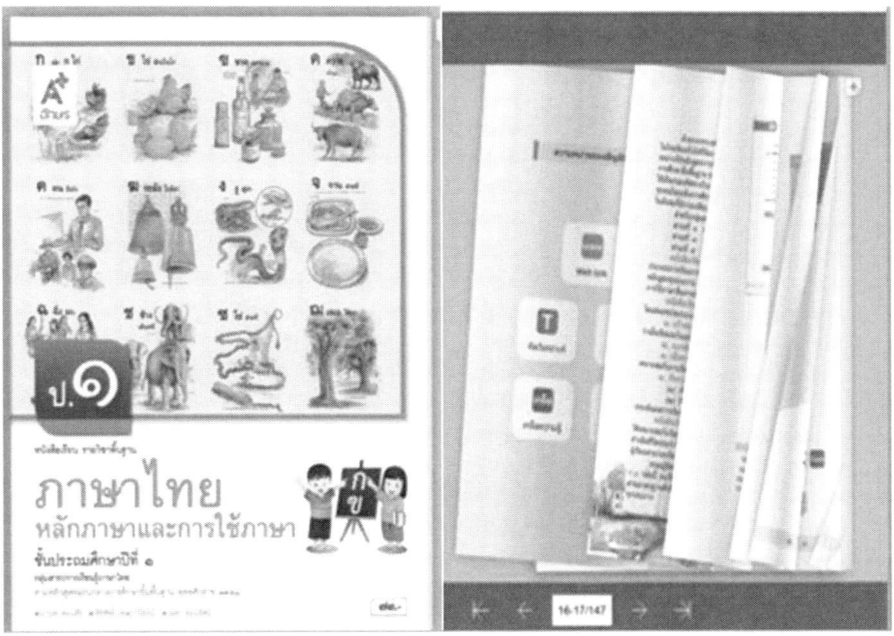

Figure 2. e-Books are education media on learning platform.

Second, the Asynchronous Learning Network (ALN) can also be used to enable the teaching and learning anywhere and anytime based on learners' needs with teachers to provide on-demand consultation. Through ALN (Figure 3) teachers who are accustomed to the conventional teaching approach may also take on other roles in the education system, such as mentors, counselors, and curriculum counselors. In addition, the content will be posted on media or sent to learners through various platforms, allowing learners to manage the amount of content and then be able to make choices about new knowledge information whenever they want. However, both teachers and learners need to keep up with each other through the use of blogs and social media, such as MOOC, COURSERA, OpenLearnership (Silpakorn University 2012).

As for higher education (Higher Education, Science, Research and Innovation 2020) instructional management, a lot of precautionary measures against the COVID-19 pandemic have been implemented with the aim of reducing the spread of the virus by encouraging people to limit travel and refrain from participating in the activities that involve a large number of people. There are three practices which are related to higher education teaching and learning management introduced as follows:

1. Stop all forms of teaching and learning activities except those conducted across online platforms. It aims to complete the transition of formal education into 100 percent online learning before 1 April 2020. As for some programs that require the assignments to be completed through practices and operations, each higher educational institution can use discretion to take a careful look for appropriate approaches that encourage learners to spend as much time as possible at home as approved and considered acceptable by the president of each higher educational institution.
2. Consider canceling, postponing, or replacing all kinds of internships with more appropriate activities.
3. Adjust or replace the normal examination and assessment practices with a more efficient one that is appropriate for the online teaching and learning style created.

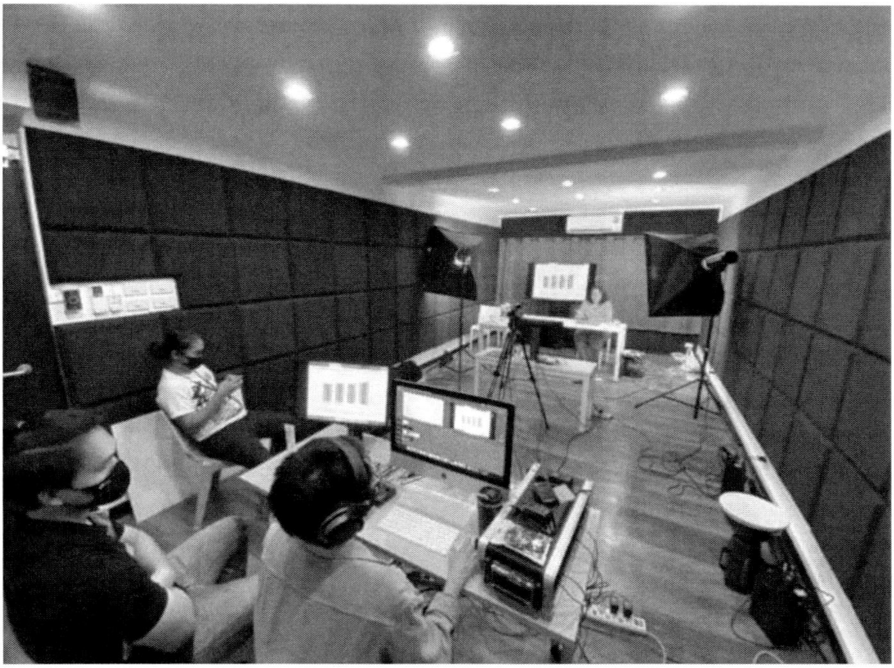

Figure 3. Teaching recording to provide content to students by asynchronous learning platform.

The management of education could not perform without teachers and students engaged in teaching and learning a certain subject, as its vital elements. Educational innovations can be implemented in instructional management based on the conditions of each particular process or in a mixed form that supports durations, opportunities, conditions, variables, readiness, or the ability to access learning sources primarily available in both classroom approaches or other teaching and learning methods.

Taking into account the acceptance of educational technology among stakeholders at basic education and higher education level, it is found that teachers, parents and all stakeholders in the basic education sector had to adjust slightly to optimize their application of technology due to various related factors such as parental economic disparity, school size, and technical devices. On the other hand, lecturers in the higher education sector are able to immediately apply the innovation. In conclusion, the university can manage their instruction in the new pathway in a short period. This is in line with the Innovation Decision Process Theory proposed by Roger (Rogers 1995) which stated that this process takes a certain period of time and is composed of the five steps to get through, namely knowledge, persuasion, decision, implementation, and confirmation.

This theory reflects the competence of higher education lecturers and students who may have adequate knowledge, skills, and opportunity to utilize innovations. Consequently, they have a higher level of technology acceptance than basic education teachers. However, every related sector needs to handle education inequality as the primary challenge. It is mostly caused by economic inequality, particularly the gap between the quality of education in rural and urban areas as shown below (Bangkok Department of Education 2016);

1. In rural and urban areas, school administrators do not have adequate resources to plan facilities and technical tools to serve every student.
2. Most teachers might lack adequate knowledge and skills in technology utilization.
3. The economic inequality makes most parents unable to provide their children with access to technology in general.
4. A lot of students lack technology access opportunity due to economic inequality.

Based on the above-mentioned challenges, if the responsible sectors recognize the importance of using technology that promotes deep and wide-ranging learning, as well as equipping learners with other critical skills that technology can help, it is important to implement the following preparatory steps and instructional guidance during the COVID-19 pandemic:

1. Build an understanding and create educational readiness for school infrastructure and the development of teacher skills, use of technology to support teaching, and learning against every kind of challenges (Ana 2020).
2. Introduce guidelines as well as instructional management styles that promote the learners' development of the balance skills in all

aspects and emphasize the development of practical skills and other necessary characteristics apart from those related to knowledge development.

3. Develop the required competence of teachers and the ability to connect technology with other approaches to instruction so they can design instructional management styles and provide instructional management then technology can be used as the primary, supplementary, and alternative media. In this context, the media needs to be adjusted and adapted to fit into the schools' context and readiness which take part in creating teachers' learning innovations (Maryanti et al., 2020).
4. Develop learners' competence to support the utilization of technology and promote their Media, Information, and Digital Literacy (MIDL) which is considered the necessarily desired characteristic for learners in the future and a primary factor contributing to the success in online teaching and learning.
5. Adjust and introduce a more flexible curriculum structure and learning areas that are appropriate for the COVID-19 period, and promote the development of the curriculum in which different learning areas are integrated, the loosening of the structure, and the learning approach that prevents and reduces the spread of coronavirus.
6. Use technology to yield educational measurements and assessments with the utmost efficiency. Reflect the actual competence of the learners at a degree equivalent to those measured by an ordinary method of assessment and evaluation, and in the manner suitable for online teaching and learning. This can be conducted through Assessment of Learning (AoL), Assessment for Learning (AfL), and Assessment as Learning (AaL) which cover the precise and assured assessment of all learners' competence.
7. Create a network of cooperation among public and private sectors to support technology-based teaching and learning (Hashim 2020).
8. Build an online Professional Learning Community (PLC), centered on technological usage, in which teachers gather to support each

other in order to establish effective teaching and learning strategies for learners during the pandemic by sharing teaching and learning experiences, setting learner goals, evaluating and reflecting each other's personal performance along with teaching and learning consequences.

Conclusion

COVID-19 is challenging, however, it creates opportunities for every country to seek guidance for solving and promoting learners to keep up with their education during the pandemic under the friendly, reliable, indiscriminate, and learning-promoting environment. The blending of technology with teaching and learning to the fullest extent within a short period of time leads to new teaching and learning styles that bring about changes in the role of teachers, students, and other educational personnel or even parents. Therefore, the spread of the COVID-19 pandemic has become a valuable lesson to learn, and post-COVID-19 planning must be started so as to prepare the nation for future unexpected threats and risks.

References

Ana, A. 2020. "Trends in Expert System Development: A Practicum Content Analysis in Vocational Education for Over Grow Pandemic Learning Problems. "*Indonesian Journal of Science and Technology* vol.5, no. 2: 246–260.

Bangkok Department of Education. 2016. *Research report: A course of educational technology development affiliated to Bangkok Metropolitan schools.* http://www.bangkok.go.th/upload/user/0000 0116/4-techno/maew/vijai/resche.pdf.

Hashim, S., Masek, A., Abdullah, N. S., Paimin, A. N., and Muda, W. H. N. W. 2020. "Students' Intention to Share Information Via Social Media:

A Case Study of COVID-19 Pandemic." *Indonesian Journal of Science and Technology* vol.5, no. 2: 236-245.

Higher Education, Science, Research and Innovation. 2020. *3nd Announcement of Ministry of Higher Education, Science, Research and Innovation subject: Vigilant measures against the spread of Coronavirus* (COVID-19). https://www.ops.go.th/main/index. php/ news-service/announcement/1983-covid-19, retrieved on July 1, 2020.

Maryanti, R., Hufad, A., Sunardi., Nandiyanto, A. B. D., and Al-Obaidi, S. M. 2020. "Understanding COVID-19 particle contagion through aerosol droplets for students with special needs." *Journal of Engineering Science and Technology* vol.15, no.3:1909-1920.

Mulyanti, B., Purnama, W., and Parwinanto, R. E. 2020. "Distance Learning in Vocational High Schools during the COVID-19 Pandemic in West Java Province, Indonesia." *Indonesian Journal of Science and Technology* vol. 5, no. 2 (March):271–282.

OBEC Chanel. 2020. "Directors Online Conference for Distance learning management During COVID-19." *The Times,* April 29, 2020. https://www.youtube.com/watch?v=NKw4PTy371g.

Office of the Education Council. Ministry of Education. 2017. *Education in Thailand*. Bangkok: OEC. https://www.bic.moe.go.th/images/ stories/pdf/EDUCATION_IN_THAILAND_2017.pdf.

Office of the Permanent Secretary Ministry of Education. 2016. *The National Scheme of Education B.E. 2560-2579 (2017-2036).* Bangkok: Thailand. https://planipolis.iiep.unesco.org/en/2017/national-scheme-education-be-2560-2579-2017-2036-thai-6635.

Rogers, E.M. 1995. *Diffusion of Innovations (4th ed)*. New York: Free Press.

Silpakorn University. 2012. *How to Development E-learning for Education Institute in Thailand*. Nakorn Pathom, Thailand. http://www.educ.su. ac.th/images/research/57/03.pdf.

In: COVID-19 ISBN: 978-1-53618-903-2
Editors: A. B. D. Nandiyanto et al.

Chapter 16

THE ROLE OF MALAYSIAN SCHOOL ADMINISTRATORS IN FACING MOVEMENT CONTROL ORDER DURING COVID-19

***Nazeri Mohammad*[1] *and Siti Ilyana Mohd Yusof*[2]**
[1]Department of International Education Cooperation and Relation, National Institute of Educational Management and Leadership, Genting Highlands, Malaysia
[2]Department International Education Cooperation and Relation, National Institute of Educational Management and Leadership, Genting Highlands, Malaysia

ABSTRACT

Corona Virus Disease 2019 (COVID-19) crisis may amend our world and our global outlook, it may also teach us about how education needs to change to be able to better prepare our young learners for what the future might hold. As for now, educators around the world are talking about the need to rethink how we can educate future generations. This might just a disruption that the sector needs us to rethink how we educate, and question what to be taught and what are we preparing our students for. Successful people in the coming decades need to be able to understand this interrelatedness and navigate across boundaries to leverage their differences and work in a globally collaborative way. So, as educators grapple with the new ways of communicating with students away from our classrooms, it is a good time to reflect on how this disruptive crisis can help us to define what learning should look like. What changes would need to occur in the preparation of school administrators if the focus of their training shifted to help them more consciously select the lenses that guided their school change efforts.

Keywords: COVID-19, Malaysia, pandemic, school administrator and movement control order

1. INTRODUCTION

Coronavirus Disease 2019 (COVID-19) has changed how students are educated around the world. Those changes give us a glimpse at how education could change for the better and the worse in the long term (Rodriguez and Rodriguez 2015; Cosner 2014). In fact, the COVID-19 pandemic is fast-forwarding the changes in the scope of the job landscape as predicted by the World Economic Forum (WEF). WEF estimated that 65 percent of children entering primary schools today will end to keep on delivering up working in completely new job types that have yet to exist (Penton and Pettersson 2019).

In Malaysia, we still have time to start preparing ourselves in case the situation worsens and the ministry has to enforce mitigation measures (Dohlan and Ishak 2017). By all means, stock up on non-perishable items to last for about two weeks, however, we need to avoid excessive hoarding of goods, which can cause a shortage of these goods and create panic in the community. Those on regular prescription drugs for chronic diseases like diabetes, heart conditions, liver disease, kidney disease, cancer, and chronic respiratory illnesses should get additional supplies of their medication sufficient for an extra month (Bernama 2020) and stock up on face masks and hand sanitizers are top in the list as well. This is very disruptive of social life and requires the cooperation and commitment of the public (Bernama 2020; Davis 2019; Doyle 2020).

2. COVID-19 IN SCHOOL: NEW NORM

COVID-19 pandemic is revealing new layers of inequity that may end up setting us back even further. Education leaders are tackling the unexpected challenge of providing distance learning as the primary mode of instruction for weeks, months, and possibly the remainder of the school year (Bernama 2020; Azmy et al., 2016; Ana 2020). Rescheduling the school academic calendar and public exams as an immediate measure is reasonable but this action plan must be reviewed for the coming school session. Public exams will have to be examined thoroughly, and appropriate alternate assessment has to be the new norm in schools and institutions of higher learning (Bernama 2020; Azmy et al., 2016; Dohlan and Ishak 2017; Mulyanti et al., 2020).

The conventional written test has to go and assessments must be revamped. The Minister of Education (MOE) has announced that if schools are to reopen in the near future, each class should only accommodate 16 to 17 students at any one time (Bernama 2020). This is to ensure social distancing to prevent the possible spread of the COVID-19 virus. While it is good to hear that the ministry is making plans to bring students back to school, it must ensure that the schools, the teachers and other staff are fully prepared to operate under the new norm (Rodriguez and Rodriguez 2015; Cosner 2014). The new conditions and new norms should include the following:

1. Utmost consideration must be given to ensure that the ministry is able to ensure the safety and health of all students before sending them back to school;
2. As social distancing is going to be the practice, teachers must be better prepared to teach in a new norm environment. New ways and

methods of teaching are required. Teachers must be consulted on this and a new schooling pedagogy based on the sop may need to be rolled out;

3. In addition to social distancing in classrooms, the schools must ensure students who return to school have their body temperature retaken and be provided with hand sanitizers and face masks, shoes must be sanitized before students enter classrooms; and
4. Teachers should be able to explain to students the necessity for social distancing while emphasizing that it is not the same thing as being anti-social. They must explain why this is necessary and that it is only meant to be a temporary measure.

3. COVID-19 in Learning: Innovative Norm

The primary challenge is to ensure adequate access and readiness of the stakeholders, students and teachers to the digital world that "real" teaming maybe missed out for the lack of learners' "readiness" for independent self-learning as well as teachers' wellbeing and readiness for online teaching (Mansaray 2019; Khan et al., 2014; Naseri 2019). Hence, education 4.0 strategy is perfectly befitting in the new normal, even in potential emerging pandemics in near or far future (Kilber et al., 2014; Kemp 2019). However, there are challenges (Kapur 2018). Education 4.0 strategy includes but is not limited to:

1. Encouraging more remote learning where theoretical knowledge will be disseminated through virtual communications while practical skills will be taught face to face;
2. Project based learning targeted to ensure wide set of skill roles; and
3. Personalized teaching based on students' independence and unique approach to studying and the ability to learn.

COVID-19 pandemic has changed education dramatically as it has increased the use of personal telecommunications gadgets such as smartphones which prior to this were prohibited from school grounds, for learning and teaching purposes (Khan et al., 2014; Naseri 2019). Teachers should develop their skills in terms of online teaching and home-based learning which would be the new normal in the teaching field as e-learning is the future of education (Abu 2016; Hall and Hord 2014; Hallinger 2018). Teachers need to improve their knowledge, competency, change of attitude and be ready to embrace the new normal in education especially those which are related to online learning. This preparation will be reflected in teaching, assessment, and dissemination of knowledge (Kilber et al., 2014).

Throughout the Movement Control Order (MCO) and the Conditional Movement Control Order (CMCO), teachers continue to impart knowledge via online platforms. Teachers need to have a paradigm shift to be able to accept the new scenario in global education in order to build a generation with digital literacy which is very important to face the challenges brought forth by the Fourth Industrial Revolution (IR 4.0) (Drucker 2017; Helmi et al., 2017). This global crisis has made an impact on the conventional teaching and learning as well as on the responsibilities of educators, rendering it more challenging and they have to adapt to the new normal condition that requires the process to be conducted online (Khan et al., 2014; Naseri 2019). Online tools such as Google Meet and Zoom allowed us to keep meetings running, we came to terms with the concept of working from home, as opposed to the cubicle layout we have grown accustomed to. Schools and higher learning education are resorting to online and virtual classes, and teachers are finding ways to teach from home while taking care of their own children (Ng et al., 2008).

4. Role of School Administration in COVID-19: New Norm vs. New Normal

Over the past few months, we have experienced an unprecedented shift in our way of life due to COVID-19. One phenomenon that is certain, we know that adjusting to change can be challenging: be it planned or unplanned, gradual or sudden, change is inevitable and very much part of being human (Al-alawi et al., 2019; Drucker 2017). School administrators can play an outsized role in providing the ultimate pressure test of an organization position and purpose, as what is decided today will define the future (Haris et al., 2017). Looking into the future, some of the most important skills that employers will be looking for will be creativity, Communications, and collaboration, alongside empathy and emotional Intelligence, and being able to work across demographic lines of differences to harness the power of the collective through effective teamwork (Naseri 2019).

Throw in a pandemic, along with changes to routines and plans for the weeks and months ahead in 2020, and it is more important than ever to acknowledge the challenges and difficulties that we face in light of COVID-19. Developing an awareness and sensitivity in the school leader to these perspectives requires an attention to the process by which schools change themselves and to the interpersonal facets of school organizational life (Mansaray 2019). Professional preparation would need to focus on introducing aspiring school leaders to the different epistemologies underlying their administrative practice, to help them understand how different constructions of reality can facilitate or thwart successful change (Drucker 2007; Helmi et al., 2017; Yulk 2013). Rather than considering the relative strengths and constraints of each lens, with an eye to deciding one set of lenses is inherently superior to another (Rodriguez and Rodriguez 2015; Cosner 2014).

The COVID-19 pandemic has resulted in educational institutions across the world being compelled to suddenly harness and utilize the suite of available technological tools to create content for remote learning for students in all sectors. This pandemic and its aftermath test the stamina of organizations to preserve, to endure, and to be resilient. In this new millennium that prioritizes life-long learning, the way forward is by utilizing technology and online education (Haris et al., 2017). The current context of education demands educators to have advanced literacy on the information technology (Azmy et al., 2016). Therefore, today's leaders need a careful preparation that extends beyond the boundaries of education and civilization. In addition, leaders need to be flexible with their current and future needs in line with current world demands (Mansaray 2019). Collaboration and support from various stakeholders are essential as the leader's rise lies in the support of his environment (Naseri 2019, 35-40, Maryanti et al., 2020). Furthermore, aspects related to risk management need to be implemented effectively in order for leaders to be prepared and actionable at all levels of MOE.

CONCLUSION

In conclusion, the ideas discussed here suggest that as we seek to restructure and change schools and redefine the role of the school administrators in those efforts, there is much we can learn during COVID-19. COVID-19 pandemic has merely hastened the arrival of what experts in the human resource and management fields have predicted is going to happen in the future anyway. Undeniably, there is an overall reevaluation of the significance and nature or everyone's work especially to the role of school administrators.

REFERENCES

Abu, F. B. 2016. *A Study on Adoption of Technology in SMEs Food Industry: UTAUT Model*. Malaysia: Universiti Teknologi Malaysia.

Al-Alawi, A. I., Abdulmohsen, M., Al-Malki, F. M., and Mehrotra, A. 2019. "Investigating the barriers to change management in public sector educational institutions." *International Journal of Educational Management* vol.33. no. 1: 112-148.

Ana, A. 2020. "Trends in Expert System Development: A Practicum Content Analysis in Vocational Education for Over Grow Pandemic Learning Problems. "*Indonesian Journal of Science and Technology* vol.5, no. 2: 246–260.

Azmy, S. N. M. S., Abdullah, N. H., and Hadi Ayub, S. 2016. "Language and Aspiration of the Students on Global Outlook: a Review Based on Malaysia Education Development Plan (2013-2025)." *International Journal of Applied Linguistics and English Literature* vol.5, no. 6: 240-244.

Bernama. 2020. *Communication access is available throughout the period of movement control orders.* http://www.astroawani.com/berita-malaysia/akses-komunikasi-tersedia-sepanjang-tempoh-perintah-kawalan-pergerakan-234239. Astroawani.com. 19 March 2020.

Cosner, S. 2014. "Cultivating collaborative data practices as a schoolwide improvement strategy: A phase-based model of school leadership supports." *Journal of School Leadership* vol.24, no. 4 : 691-724.

Davis, G. 2019. *Exploring the Strategies Executive Leaders Need to Reduce Intergenerational Friction in a Business Organization.* Doctoral dissertation Colorado: Technical University.

Dolhan, H., and Ishak, N. 2017. "National education policy: Education development master plan–charting the future." *Revista Panamericana De Pedagogía. Saberes Y Quehaceres Del Pedagogo* vol.15, no. 2017: 13-32.

Doyle, A. 2020. *Definitions, skills and examples of workplace flexibility.* https://ms.chalized.com/definisi-kemahiran-dan-contoh-fleksibiliti-tempat-kerja/, retrieved on July 1, 2020.

Drucker, P F. 2017. *Human Prosperity in a Changing World.* Peter Drucker challenge 2017. The future economic man. PDC 2017.

Drucker, P. F. 2007. *Management challenges for the 21st century.* Routledge.

Hall, G. E. and Hord, S. M. 2014. *Implementing Change: Patterns, Principles and Potholes.* Edisi ke-4. Upper Saddle River, New Jersey: Pearson.

Hallinger, P. 2018. "Bringing context out of the shadows of leadership." *Educational management administration & leadership* vol.46, no. 1: 5-24.

Harris, A., Jones, M. and Huffman, J. B. 2017. *Teachers Leading Educational Reform: The Power of Professional Learning Communities*. New York: Routledge.

Helmi, Akhtar., and Ilhamie A. G. A. 2017. "Effective leadership communication." *Jurnal Syariah* vol.25, no. 3: 531-562.

Kahn, M. J., Maurer, R., Wartman, S. A., and Sachs, B. P. 2014. "A case for change: disruption in academic medicine." *Academic Medicine* vol.89, no. 9: 1216-1219.

Kapur, R. 2018. *Barriers to Effective Communication.* https://www.researchgate.net/publication/323794732_Barriers_to_Effective_Communication/citation/download.

Kemp, S 2019. *Global Digital Report.* https://wearesocial.com/global-digital-report-2019.

Kilber, J., Barclay, A., and Ohmer, D. 2014."Seven tips for managing Generation Y." *Journal of Management Policy and Practice* vol.15, no. 4: 80-91.

Mansaray, H. E. 2019. "The Role of Leadership Style in Organisational Change Management: A Literature Review." *Journal of Human Resource Management* vol.7, no. 1: 18-31.

Maryanti, R., Hufad, A., Sunardi., Nandiyanto, A. B. D., and Al-Obaidi, S. M. 2020. "Understanding COVID-19 particle contagion through aerosol droplets for students with special needs." *Journal of Engineering Science and Technology* vol.15, no.3:1909-1920.

Mulyanti, B., Purnama, W., and Parwinanto, R. E. 2020. "Distance Learning in Vocational High Schools during the COVID-19 Pandemic in West Java Province, Indonesia." *Indonesian Journal of Science and Technology* vol.5, no. 2: 271–282.

Naseri, H. (2019). "The Role of the Adventurer Manager in Order To Coordinate the Mind, Creativity and Change Management." *International Journal for Modern Trends in Science and Technology* vol.04, no.09: 35-40.

Ng, K. Y., Ang, S., and Chan, K. Y. 2008. "Personality and leader effectiveness: A moderated mediation model of leadership self-efficacy, job demands, and job autonomy." *Journal of Applied Psychology* vol.93, no. 4; 733-743.

Penton, S., and Pettersson, F. 2019. *Factors affecting managerial willingness to change: A case study on change management when implementing new digital technology.* Sweden: Stockholm.

Rodriguez, A., and Rodriguez, Y. 2015. "Metaphors for today's leadership: VUCA world, millennial and 'cloud leaders'." *Journal Management Development* vol.34, no. 7 : 854–866.

Yukl, G. 2013. *Leadership in organizations.* Harlow. England: Pearson Education Limited.

In: COVID-19 ISBN: 978-1-53618-903-2
Editors: A. B. D. Nandiyanto et al.

Chapter 17

NEW NORMS IN THE WORLD OF EDUCATION: THINK OUT OF THE BOX FROM MALAYSIAN SCHOOL ADMINISTRATOR'S PERSPECTIVE DURING PANDEMIC

***Nazeri Mohammad*[1,*] *and Arshad Jais*[2]**
[1]Department of International Education Cooperation and Relation, National Institute of Educational Management and Leadership, Genting Highlands, Malaysia
[2]Kuching Science School, Sarawak, Malaysia

ABSTRACT

Online education is a hot topic that is widely concerned in various countries today. However, the education of our children and youth has to continue because staying idle is contrary to the constitutional foundation

---

* Corresponding Author's Email: nazeri@ipgmksm.edu.my.

of civil societies. Online pedagogy is starting to nourish. In becoming a new normal, online, or digital teaching is a viable alternative to conventional face-to-face teaching and learning. In the era of mobile internet, countries around the world have made various effective attempts at online education, but online education is more of a supplement to school education, and large-scale normal online education lacks cases. The method of learning however largely depends on students' motivation; the motivation must come from students themselves. Beyond participating in the creation of norms, students must be given regular opportunities to interact with the norms through self-reflection, peer and class assessment, and discussion. The sudden and unpredictable nature of the COVID-19 crisis and its effect on work and enterprises call for a rethink of our way of life. Successful people in the coming decades need to be able to understand this interrelatedness and navigate across boundaries to leverage their differences and work in a globally collaborative way. Undeniably, there is an overall reevaluation of the significance and nature or everyone's work. The truth is, teaching online is not easy, but it can be done and can be rewarding. Increasing numbers of people are using their time during the Movement Control Order to build new skillsets, with an upsurge in enrolments in online learning. Therefore, the steps taken by our government must be supported to break the chain of transmission quickly while maintaining the competence of our students.

Keywords: Malaysian School Administrator's Perspective, new norms, pandemic, the world of education

1. Introduction

Coronavirus disease (COVID-19) has brought the world to a standstill but it has also helped pinpoint weaknesses in the education sector and presented opportunities for new norms and changes to kick in. None can predict the true impact of the pandemic on the global economy, but at this pivotal moment, there are clear choices to be made (Bringle et al. 2016b; Heimans and Timms 2014). To accomplish this condition, school administrators should support executive leadership and share the burden while maintaining appropriate separation from management. The way in which school administrators do their work at this time will be a critical factor in an organization's ability to emerge from the current crisis and push forward into a new era of economic recovery and opportunity for the benefit of all stakeholders (Al-Alawi et al. 2019; Cavazotte et al. 2013; Hallinger 2018).

Digital learning will continue to be a crucial part of post-Movement Control Order (MCO) education. Besides making improvements on internet accessibility and ICT facilities, the current exam-centric, the fast-paced education system needs to change (Pursel et al. 2016; Schankin et al. 2016; Zhou et al. 2020). E-learning tools provide educators and students with access to resources they could not have had otherwise, no matter their status or location (Helm et al. 2015). This has become painfully evident during the MCO. The current system's definition of success is narrow and based mainly on grades rather than outcome attainment as well as competency and character building. Economically, every additional MCO day will have a damaging impact. Making a bad situation worse, global oil prices slumped to new lows because of the COVID-19 pandemic. This makes it even more difficult for Malaysia to jump-start its economy while being mindful of fiscal prudence. Therefore, it is now more crucial than ever to think out-of-the-box to bolster the government's resources to fund its post-COVID-19 economic recovery (Husnu et al. 2016; Azmy et al. 2016).

2. Think Out of the Box

COVID-19 is a pandemic that illustrates how globally interconnected we are there is no longer such a thing as isolated issues and actions. The post-COVID-19 realm requires different ways of thinking and organizing the world. Educators across the world are experiencing new possibilities to do things differently and with greater flexibility resulting in potential benefits in accessibility to education for students across the world (Bringle 2016a; Rodriguez and Rodriguez 2015).

In Malaysia, the system is there, but there are things that can be done to make it better (Dolhan and Ishak 2017). Thinking outside the box may best be summarised by the assertion 'When you think outside the box, the box goes away'. Rethink the scheduling of classes in line with remote learning. Thinking outside the box is not easy since it involves leaving the psychological comfort zone, becoming open to new ways of seeing the world, and being willing to explore (Naseri 2019). In this ever-changing global environment, young people require resilience and adaptability skills that are proving to be essential to navigating effectively through this pandemic. So, if that is the worst outcome, what should institutions do to prevent that? Understanding how to learn involves deeper skills than mastery of study skills. Emotional intelligence, emotional health, and an understanding of the learning process are clearly related. We might conclude, therefore, that a good learner is able to think outside the box, and that since teachers are, by definition, also learners, those good teachers are out-of-the-box thinkers (Davis 2019; Stapa and Mohammad 2019).

Outside of marshaling all their resources to provide students without internet connectivity the support they need to teach and learn online, there are a few principles to follow. First, wherever possible, create active learning experiences ones in which there is synchronous communication, required class sessions, frequent opportunities for students to answer questions and defend answers, debate their peers, tackle problems, and the like (Zhou et al. 2020). Zoom might be suitable technologies for that, but schools should also investigate using an active learning platform. Second, remember that online learning is not about putting the class front and center like the MOOCs did. That means that teaching certain concepts might not be best accomplished through lecture capture technologies, but instead by showing a multimedia clip, something from Khan Academy, a brief simulation, by letting students teach each other (Khan et al. 2014).

3. New Norms in the World of Education

Norms are the agreements we make with each other. They represent community goals, and as such, all classroom members should be given the opportunity to contribute to their creation. Norms exist to be used by students, thus students must be able to define and explain them (Penton and Pettersson 2019; Philips et al. 2017). Additionally, choosing a few norms promote student familiarity and ownership of the norms. The community must be empowered and parents and teachers must rally together to build a strong support system amid this crisis (Schankin et al. 2016). The parents play a role in educating children when they are at home (Maryanti et al. 2020). This includes providing a conducive environment for learning and keeping distractions at bay. Parents must get their priorities right and they must be committed. The teachers and schools need strategies to ensure that learning outcomes are achieved (Pursel et al. 2016). Children need support when using online platforms. Parents and guardians need pedagogical competencies in assisting their children with online lessons as well. However, we are optimistic that things will fall into place eventually (Naseri 2019). Schools must maintain clear and constant communication with parents. A guide for parents who have to multitask between remote work, household responsibilities, and helping their children with school work, is needed. Parents and guardians can also build their own support system via chat and social media groups to exchange ideas and experiences (Hashim et al. 2020). We need a video library with content developed according to the national syllabus and curriculum, and accessible via digital devices. Rethink the scheduling of classes in line with remote learning. Physical attendance is only for teachers and students to touch base (Schankin et al. 2016). This method of learning however largely depends on students' motivation; the motivation must come from students themselves. Unfortunately, it will inadvertently filter those who want to learn and those who are less interested. Classrooms are made smaller to make it easier for teachers to get to know and engage with the students and parents (Bringle et al. 2016b).

These risk-control decisions have led millions of students into temporary homeschooling situations, especially in some of the most heavily impacted countries, like China, South Korea, Italy, and Iran. These changes have certainly caused a degree of inconvenience, but they have also prompted new examples of educational innovation. Although it is too early to judge how reactions to COVID-19 affect education systems around the world, there are signs suggesting that it could have a lasting impact on the trajectory of learning innovation and digitization. While school closures seem to present a logical solution to enforcing social distancing within communities, prolonged closures tend to have a disproportionately negative impact on the most vulnerable students. What we are learning from COVID-19, similar to what we have seen in previous pandemics, is that preparedness is crucial (Sangsawang 2020). While different scenarios exist, several of them assume that the COVID-19 spread will happen in waves, which means the process of addressing it should be cyclical.

4. Education Nudged and Pushed to Change Could Lead to Surprising Innovations

The COVID-19 pandemic has brought about a dramatic interruption in the way we do schooling across the globe. The slow pace of change in academic institutions globally is lamentable, with centuries-old, lecture-based approaches to teaching, entrenched institutional biases, and outmoded classrooms. However, COVID-19 has become a catalyst for educational institutions worldwide to search for innovative solutions in a relatively short period of time. In just the past few weeks, we have seen learning consortiums and coalitions taking shape, with diverse stakeholders including governments, publishers, education professionals, technology providers, and telecom network operators coming together to utilize digital platforms as a temporary solution to the crisis. In emerging countries where education has predominantly been provided by the government, this could become a prevalent and consequential trend to future education (Rodriguez and Rodriguez 2015).

5. The Digital Divide Could Widen

Most schools in affected areas are finding stop-gap solutions to continue teaching, but the quality of learning is heavily dependent on the level and quality of digital access. After all, only around 60% of the globe's population is online. Moreover, the less affluent and digitally savvy individual families are, the further their students are left behind. When classes transition online, these children lose out because of the cost of digital devices and data plans. Unless access costs decrease and quality of access increase in all countries, the gap in education quality, and thus socioeconomic equality will be further exacerbated (Bringle et al. 2016b).

The digital divide could become more extreme if educational access is dictated by access to the latest technologies (Firmansyah and Rahmawati 2018). Nobody thinks this is the way online education should be done. When students have expectations of face-to-face training, if the substitute for an emergency is proposed as interaction through a forum or a platform with limitations, satisfaction levels drop, because there is an apparent gap in those expectations, and students may prefer to postpone their course and wait for normal service to resume (Helms et al. 2015). If the substitution is carried out with a tool rich in interaction, this happens less often. Although e-learning from home is unavoidable in the current situation, the students are not able to focus as much as they can in a classroom. One of the ways e-learning has tried to mimic the social aspects of a classroom is with tools like message boards, Facebook groups, and yes, sometimes chatbots (Harisriani and Danuwijaya 2019). They give students the sense they are not just staring at an empty message board, but they are talking with real people about their homework (Kahn et al. 2014).

However, the pandemic is also an opportunity to remind ourselves of the skills students need in this unpredictable world such as informed decision making, creative problem solving, and perhaps above all, adaptability. The rapid spread of COVID-19 has demonstrated the importance of building resilience to face various threats, from pandemic disease to extremist violence to climate insecurity, and even, yes, rapid technological change. In our view as long as there is strict adherence to the safety guidelines and standard operating procedure (SOP), limiting the number of students to a class should not be an issue. Teaching and learning through online platforms must be strengthened as e-learning is the future of education (Ana 2020). The clear opportunity that has come out of this period is to press the "reset" button and we see areas where one can rebuild by recalibrating the mindset. The first thing that we need to do is upskill and reskill ourselves more intensively.

CONCLUSION

The COVID-19 pandemic will likely continue presenting challenges beyond those that come up in the course of routine virtual education. Even if this viral spread subsides, or a vaccination becomes readily available, the shift from online classes back to in-person learning may create disruptions of its own adjusting back to higher standards of accountability, weaning off of phone-checking habits, and transferring comments back to hard copies instead of digital notes. Hopefully, these experiences will serve as preparation for future challenges that come with the next epidemic, pandemic, and other disasters.

REFERENCES

Al-Alawi, A. I., Abdulmohsen, M., Al-Malki, F. M. and Mehrotra, A. 2019. "Investigating the barriers to change management in public sector educational institutions". *International Journal of Educational Management,* vol. 33, no. 1: 112 - 148.

Ana, A. 2020. "Trends in Expert System Development: A Practicum Content Analysis in Vocational Education for Over Grow Pandemic Learning Problems". *Indonesian Journal of Science and Technology,* vol. 5. no. 2; 71 - 85.

Azmy, S. N. M. S., Abdullah, N. H. and Hadi Ayub, S. 2016. "Language and Aspiration of the Students on Global Outlook: A Review Based on Malaysia Education Development Plan (2013 - 2025)". *International Journal of Applied Linguistics and English Literature,* vol. 5, no. 6, 240 - 244.

Bringle, R. G., Reeb, R. N., Brown, M. A. and Ruiz, A. I. 2016a. *Service learning in psychology: Enhancing undergraduate education for the public good.* Washington, DC: American Psychological Association.

Bringle, R. G., Ruiz, A. I., Brown, M. A. and Reeb, R. N. 2016b. "Enhancing the psychology curriculum through service learning". *Psychology Learning and Teaching,* vol. 15, no. 3: 294 - 309.

Cavazotte, F., Moreno, V. and Bernardo, J. 2013. "Transformational leaders and work performance: The mediating roles of identification and self-efficacy". *BAR-Brazilian Administration Review,* vol. 1, no. 4: 490 - 512.

Davis, G. 2019. *Exploring the Strategies Executive Leaders Need to Reduce Intergenerational Friction in a Business Organization.* Doctoral dissertation, Colorado Technical University.

Firmansyah, D. B. and Rahmawati, R. S. 2018. "Use of Multimedia-Based Teaching Media in Kanji Learning". *JAPANEDU: Jurnal Pendidikan dan Pengajaran Bahasa Jepang,* vol. 3. no. 1: 1 - 10.

Hallinger, P. 2018. "Bringing context out of the shadows of leadership". *Educational management administration and leadership,* vol. 46, no. 1, 5 - 24.

Haristiani, N. and Danuwijaya, A. A. 2019. "Gengobot: A chatbot-based grammar application on mobile instant messaging as language learning medium". *Journal of Engineering Science and Technology,* vol. 14, no. 6: 3158 - 3173.

Hashim, S., Masek, A., Abdullah, N. S., Paimin, A. N. and Muda, W. H. N. W. 2020. "Students' Intention to Share Information via Social Media: A Case Study of COVID-19 Pandemic". *Indonesian Journal of Science and Technology,* vol. 5, no. 2: 236 - 245.

Heimans, J. and Timms, H. 2014. "Understanding "new power". *Harvard Business Review,* vol. 92, no. 12: 48 - 56.

Helms, M. M., Rutti, R. M., Hervani, A. A., LaBonte, J. and Sarkarat, S. 2015. "Implementing and Evaluating Online Service Learning Projects". *Journal of Education for Busines,* vol. 90, no. 2015: 369 - 378.

Hunsu, N. J., Adesope, O. and Bayly, D. J. 2016. "A meta-analysis of the effects of audience response systems (clickerbased technologies) on cognition and affect". *Computers and Education,* vol. 94, no. 2016: 102 - 119.

Kahn, M. J., Maurer, R., Wartman, S. A. and Sachs, B. P. 2014. "A case for change: disruption in academic medicine". *Academic Medicine,* vol. 89, no. 9: 1216 - 1219.

Maryanti, R., Hufad, A., Sunardi, Nandiyanto, A. B. D. and Al-Obaidi, S. M. 2020. "Understanding COVID-19 particle contagion through aerosol droplets for students with special needs". *Journal of Engineering Science and Technology,* vol. 15, no. 3:1909 - 1920.

Naseri, H. 2019. "The Role of the Adventurer Manager in Order to Coordinate the Mind, Creativity and Change Management". *International Journal for Modern Trends in Science and Technology,* vol. 04, no. 09: 35 - 40.

Penton, S. and Pettersson, F. 2019. *Factors affecting managerial willingness to change: A case study on change management when implementing new digital technology*. https://www.diva-portal.org/smash/record.jsf?pid=diva2%3A1327286&dswid=-1922.

Phillips, L. A., Marron, J. K., Baltzer, C., Kichline, C., Filoon, L. and Whitley, C. 2017. *Overcoming Barriers to Service Learning in Higher Education*. Service Learning: Perspectives, Goals and Outcomes, Nova Science Publishers, Inc.

Pursel, B. K., Zhang, L., Jablokow, K. W., Choi, G. W. and Velegol, D. 2016. "Understanding MOOC students: Motivations and behaviours indicative of MOOC completion". *Journal of Computer Assisted Learning,* vol. 32, no. 3: 202 - 217.

Rodriguez, A. and Rodriguez, Y. 2015. "Metaphors for today's leadership: VUCA world, millennial and 'cloud leaders'". *Journal Management Development,* vol. 34, no. 7: 54 - 866.

Sangsawang, T. 2020. "An Instructional Design for Online Learning in Vocational Education according to a Self-Regulated Learning Framework for Problem Solving during the CoViD-19 Crisis". *Indonesian Journal of Science and Technology,* vol. 5, no. 2, 283 - 298.

Schankin, A., Bergmann, K., Schubert, A.-L. and Hagemann, D. 2016. "The allocation of attention in change detection and change blindness". *Journal of Psychophysiology,* vol. 31, no. 13: 94 - 106.

Stapa, M. A. and Mohammad, N. 2019. "The Use of Addie Model for Designing Blended Learning Application at Vocational Colleges in Malaysia. Asia-Pacific J.". *Inf. Technol. Multimed.,* vol. 8, no. 1: 49 - 62.

Zhou, L., Wu, Shanshan Zhou, M. and Li, F. 2020. 'School's Out, But Class' On', The Largest Online Education in the World Today: Taking China's Practical Exploration during the COVID-19 Epidemic Prevention and Control as an Example (April 15, 2020). *Best Evid. Chin. Edu.,* vol. 4, no. 2: 501 - 519.

In: COVID-19 ISBN: 978-1-53618-903-2
Editors: A. B. D. Nandiyanto et al.

Chapter 18

THE IMPACT OF COVID-19 ON THE INDONESIAN ECONOMY

Amir Machmud*

Departemen Pedidikan Ekonomi,
Fakultas Pendidikan Ekonomi Dan Bisnis,
Universitas Pendidikan Indonesia, Bandung, Jawa Barat, Indonesia

ABSTRACT

This study aimed to analyze the impact of corona virus disease 2019 (COVID-19) pandemic on the Indonesian economy. The study used a descriptive qualitative method, with the main study data taken from several articles published in several mass media and journals. The results of the study showed that the COVID-19 pandemic had a significant impact on the Indonesian economy, which in turn predicted Indonesia's economic growth in two scenarios: 2.3% (heavy) and minus 0.4% (very heavy). The implication of this finding is that the Indonesian government should prepare various post-pandemic COVID-19 policies both related to fiscal and monetary fields.

---

* Corresponding Author's Email: amir@upi.edu.

Keywords: COVID-19, economy, economic growth, pandemic

1. INTRODUCTION

World Health Organization (WHO) announced on 11 March 2020 regarding the change in the status of corona virus disease 2019 (COVID-19) to a pandemic. This is because of a significant increase in the number of case reports and the number of deaths from COVID-19 in whole part in the world (De Groot-Mijnes et al., 2005; Word Health Organization 2020). This pandemic has made a substantial impact on all the economic sectors. It is already widely-known that before developing into a pandemic, this virus was initially discovered in Wuhan City, Hubei Province, China in December 2019.

COVID-19 is a type of corona virus. This virus comes from animals or we use the term zoonotic (Maryanti et al., 2020a). This virus is very dangerous because it can infect the human body and result in death. This virus enters the human body through the nose and mouth (Maryanti et al., 2020b). This virus infects organs in the human body such as the digestive organs, liver, and lungs. People with COVID-19 usually experience symptoms of shortness of breath and fever. This virus is transmitted through droplets either directly or indirectly. The very small size of the virus results in the virus being easily transmitted and infecting the human body.

The number of confirmed COVID-19 cases from 22 January to 31 March 2020 experienced a significant surge (Ana 2020; Anggraeni et al., 2020). The number of case reports worldwide was 802,639 with a total of 39,014 deaths and a total of 172,319 patients recovered (Huang et al., 2020; Zhu et al., 2020; Li et al., 2020: Machmud and Minghat 2020).

The COVID-19 pandemic caused problems in various aspects in life. The COVID-19 pandemic also has an impact on economic, social, educational and public welfare aspects. In the economic aspect, it is possible to have inflation due to price increases (Machmud and Minghat 2020). In the educational aspect, it creates new problems for teachers and parents in the learning process for children. There are several conditions for children that do not allow distance learning (Maryanti et al., 2020b; Mulyanti 2020). Economic factors, infrastructure, and student abilities are the main factors in educational problems.

This study analyzed the impact of COVID-19 on Indonesian economy. The study was motivated by a decline in the level of consumption and investment that led to the economy as a whole. The call for physical distancing, working from home (WFH), studying from home (SFH), worshiping at home, and the prohibition of activities has caused the economic wheel to be almost stagnant. This study used a qualitative descriptive method by describing the phenomena that occurred due to the impact of the COVID-19 on the Indonesian economy. The source of the study referred to several articles published in several mass media and journals.

2. The Impact of COVID-19 on the Indonesian Economy

The impact of the COVID-19 pandemic on the economy is shown by the potential for shocks in the demand and supply of goods and services (Binder, 2020). From the supply side, the policy of physical distancing, social distancing, working from home, and staying at home caused a decline in the production activities in addition to the difficulties in the distribution of goods, while the demand side experienced a significant increase due to panic buying in meeting basic needs (Leung, Lam and Cheng 2020). This condition resulted in an increase in the prices of goods on the market (inflation). Indeed, it would ultimately reduce the purchasing power of the people, resulting in losses to producers which could result in high unemployment (Machmud and Minghat 2020; Weitzman 1982). Another economic impact is that the exchange rate of the Indonesian rupiah (IDR) against the US dollar (USD) has penetrated almost 1 USD = 17.000 IDR. This condition will have an impact on rising prices for imported goods, which incidentally still has a substantial number of goods needed by the people coming from imports. This condition is not surprising that there will lead to an economic crisis (Phelps 1968).

The Indonesian Central Statistics Agency (BPS) reported that the number of foreign tourist arrivals (tourists) recorded was 885,067 in February 2019. It decreased by 30.42% compared to the previous month and 28.85% compared to the same period in 2019. The decline in the number of foreign tourists is inseparable from the regional quarantine policy (lockdown) conducted by many countries in the world. A very significant decrease came from Chinese and Hong Kong tourists either year-on-year or month-to-month. The decline reached 94% from China and Hong Kong, down by 93.16% year on year, from February 2019 to February 2020 (Sugihamretha 2020).

Other impacts also affected the Indonesian capital market. While on the country's stock exchange, the Composite Stock Price Index (CSPI) on the trading day as of 7 April 2020 was corrected by 0.69% to 4,778.64 IDR. The transaction value on the Indonesia Stock Exchange (IDX) reached 9.6 trillion IDR with a record net sell of 527.65 billion IDR in the regular and non-regular markets. This condition shows that during the first quarter of 2020, CSPI recorded a decline of almost 28%. The most severe selling occurred in March 2020 which collapsed to value of 16.76%. Even on last 24 March 2020, the Jakarta Composite Index touched 3,911,716 IDR, the lowest level since August 2019 (Silalahi and Ginting 2020).

During the COVID-19 pandemic, the Indonesian government announced additional spending and financing for the 2020 state budget for handling COVID-19, amounting to 405.1 trillion IDR with allocations for social protection for 110 trillion IDR, health by 75 trillion IDR, tax incentives and stimulus for People's Business Credit (KUR) of 70.1 trillion IDR, as well as for financing the national economic recovery program of 150 trillion IDR, including credit restructuring and guarantees as well as SMEs and business financing to maintain economic resilience and recovery (Astuti and Mahardhika 2020).

As a further step to strengthen monetary and financial market stability together with Bank Indonesia, the Coordinating Ministry for Economic

Affairs, the Ministry of Finance, the Financial Services Authority (OJK) and the Deposit Insurance Corporation (LPS) have made a policy mix in order to strengthen economic stimulus in accordance with the authority of BI in the Government Regulation in lieu of the Act Law (Perpu) No. 1 Year 2020 dated 31 March 2020 concerning State Financial Policy and Financial System Stability for Handling the COVID-19 pandemic and/or in the context of dealing with threats that endangered the national economy and/or financial system stability signed by President Jokowi, The policy mix is at least as follows:

1. Reducing BI 7-Day Reverse Repo Rate (BI7DDR) policy rates in February and March by 25 bps;
2. Increasing the intensity of triple intervention in the spot market, Domestic Non Delivery Forward (DNDF), and purchasing loan letter (SBN) in the secondary market;
3. Reducing the minimum mandatory giro (GWM) of conventional commercial bank foreign exchanges from 8 to 4%;
4. Extending the SBN repo tenor and auction every day to strengthen the easing of rupiah liquidity and increase the frequency of FX Swap auctions to every day to ensure adequate liquidity;
5. Extending the underlying DNDF transaction types so that they can hedge the ownership of ownership Rupiah in Indonesia;
6. Reducing Rupiah GWM by 50 bps for banks conducting export-import activities, financing to SMEs and/or other priority sectors;
7. Loosening the provisions of Macroprudential Intermediation Ratio (RIM); and
8. Providing hygienic money, reducing costs Payment System in Indonesia (SKNBI), the establishment of a 0% QR Code Indonesian Standard (QRIS) *Merchant Discount Rate* (MDR) for micro business merchants, and supports the distribution of non-cash funds for government programs such as the Hope Family Program (PKH) and Non-Cash Food Aid (BNPT) Social Assistance Program, the Workers Card Program, and the Smart Indonesia Card (Masudin et al., 2020).

Based on the above conditions, the overall COVID-19 pandemic has negatively influenced Indonesia's economic growth. Sri Mulyani Indrawati, Indonesia Minister of Finance, predicted two possible scenarios that occurred on Indonesia's economic growth as the impact of the COVID-19 pandemic, namely heavy and very heavy.

In a severe scenario, GDP is predicted to grow 2.3%, while this year's very scenario of economic growth could be minus 0.4%. This condition caused a significant decline in economic activities and has the potential to put pressure on financial institutions because credit cannot be paid while companies have experienced difficulties from revenues (Phan et al., 2020).

To deal with these conditions, the Indonesian government must have prepared various policies after the COVID-19 pandemic, which are both related to fiscal and monetary aspects. Quoting Ibn Khaldun's model of the father of Islamic economics, to maintain economic stability, it is possible to apply the Sharia Socio-Economic Dynamics Model (Affandi and Astuti 2013; Chapra 1999; Chapra 2008). The formulation of this model has eight important elements:

1. Government power (al-mulk) cannot be realized except by the implementation of Sharia;
2. Sharia cannot be implemented except by government (al-mulk);
3. The government cannot obtain power except from the people (ar-rijal);
4. Society cannot be supported except by wealth (al-mal);
5. Wealth cannot be obtained except from development (al-'imarah);
6. Development cannot be achieved except through justice (al-'adl);
7. Justice is a benchmark (al-mizan) that God will evaluate in His people; and
8. The government is charged with the responsibility to realize justice.

In the effort to recover Indonesia's economy, variables such as government, society, and law have important roles in bringing about the welfare of society. The economic recovery of a country will be realized depending on the strengths and weaknesses of the political authorities that they succeed in realizing.

CONCLUSION

The results of the study showed that the COVID-19 pandemic had a significant impact on the Indonesian economy, which in turn predicted Indonesia's economic growth in two scenarios: 2.3% (heavy) and minus 0.4% (very heavy). This finding implies that the Indonesian government should prepare various post-pandemic COVID-19 policies both related to fiscal and monetary fields. This research is still in the stage of descriptive analysis related to the impact of the coronavirus on the global economy. Further other research can look at the impact of the coronavirus pandemic on society which is more focused on the conditions and behaviors that occur in society.

REFERENCES

Affandi, A., and Astuti, D. P. 2013. "Dynamic model of Ibn Khaldun theory on poverty." *Humanomics* vol. 29, no. 2: 136-160.

Ana, A. 2020. "Trends in Expert System Development: A Practicum Content Analysis in Vocational Education for Over Grow Pandemic Learning Problems. " *Indonesian Journal of Science and Technology* vol. 5, no. 2: 246-260.

Anggraeni, S., Maulidina, A., Dewi, M. W, Rahmadianti, S., Rizky, Y. P. C., Arinalhaq, Z. F., Usdiyana, D., Nandiyanto, A. B. D., and Al-Obaidi, A. S. M. 2020. "The Deployment of Drones in Sending Drugs and Patient Blood Samples COVID-19." *Indonesian Journal of Science and Technology* vol. 5, no. 2: 193-200.

Astuti, P. B., and Mahardhika, A. S. 2020. "COVID-19: How does it impact to the Indonesian economy?." *Jurnal Inovasi Ekonomi* 5, no. 2. http://202.52.52.22/index.php/JIKO/article/view/11751.

Binder, C. 2020. "Coronavirus fears and macroeconomic expectations." *Review of Economics and Statistics*, no. 2020 (May): 1-27. https:// doi/abs/10.1162/rest_a_00931.

Chapra, M. U. 1999. "Socioeconomic and political dynamics in Ibn Khaldun's thought." *American Journal of Islamic Social Sciences* vol. 16, no. 4: 1-7.

Chapra, M. U. 2008. "Ibn Khaldun's theory of development: Does it help explain the low performance of the present-day Muslim world?." *The Journal of Socio-Economics* vol. 37, no. 2: 836-863.

De Groot-Mijnes, J. D., Van Dun, J. M., Van Der Most, R. G., and De Groot, R. J. 2005. "Natural history of a recurrent feline coronavirus infection and the role of cellular immunity in survival and disease." *Journal of virology* vol. 79, no. 2: 1036-1044.

Huang, C., Wang, Y., Li, X., Ren, L., Zhao, J., Hu, Y., Zhang, L., Fan, G., Xu, J., Gu, X., Cheng, Z., Yu, T., Xia., Z., Wei, Y., Wu, W., Xie X., Yin, W., Li, H., and Cao, B., 2020. "Clinical features of patients infected with 2019 novel coronavirus in Wuhan, China." *The lancet* vol. 395, no. 10223: 497-506.

Leung, C. C., Lam, T. H., and Cheng, K. K. 2020. "Mass masking in the COVID-19 epidemic: people need guidance." *Lancet*, 395(10228):945.

Li, Q., Guan, X., Wu, P., Wang, X., Zhou, L., Tong, Y., Xing, X. Zhou, L., Tong, Y., Ren, R., Leung, K. S. M., Lau E. H. Y., Wong, J. Y., and Xiang, N. 2020." Early transmission dynamics in Wuhan, China, of novel coronavirus–infected pneumonia." *New England Journal of Medicine* vol. 382, no. 12 (March): 1199-1207.

Machmud, A., and Minghat, A. D. B. 2020. "The Price Dynamics of Hand Sanitizers for COVID-19 in Indonesia: Exponential and Cobweb Forms." *Indonesian Journal of Science and Technology* vol. 5, no. 2: 1-9.

Maryanti, R., Hufad, A., Sunardi, Nandiyanto, A. B. D., Manullang, T. I. B. 2020b. "Understanding Coronavirus (COVID-19) as a Small Particle to Students with Special Needs." *Horizon* vol. 2, no. 1: 121-130.

Maryanti, R., Hufad, A., Sunardi., Nandiyanto, A. B. D., and Al-Obaidi, S. M. 2020a. "Understanding COVID-19 particle contagion through aerosol droplets for students with special needs." *Journal of Engineering Science and Technology* vol. 15, no. 3:1909-1920.

Masudin, M., Amsal, A., Lisnawati, L., Nasrul, N. and Hafid, F. 2020. "Admission of New Students through Joint Selection (SIMAMA) of the Health Polytechnic of the Ministry of Health, Palu during the COVID-19 Pandemic." *Poltekita: Jurnal Ilmu Kesehatan* vol. 14, no. 1: 1-10.

Mulyanti, B., Purnama, W., and Parwinanto, R. E. 2020. "Distance Learning in Vocational High Schools during the COVID-19 Pandemic in West Java Province, Indonesia." *Indonesian Journal of Science & Technology* vol. 5, 271-282.

Phelps, E. S. 1968. "Money-wage dynamics and labor-market equilibrium." *Journal of political economy* vol. 76, no. 4 (Part 2): 678-711.

Silalahi, D. E. and Ginting, R. R. 2020. "The Government of Indonesia's Fiscal Policy Strategy to Manage State Revenue and Expenditure in the Face of the Covid-19 Pandemic." *Jesya (Jurnal Ekonomi & Ekonomi Syariah)* vol. 3, no. 2, 156-167.

Sugihamretha, I. D. G. 2020. "Policy Response: Mitigating the Impact of the Covid-19 Outbreak in the Tourism Sector." *The Indonesian Journal of Development Planning* vol. 4, no. 2: 191-206.

Weitzman, M. L. 1982. "Increasing returns and the foundations of unemployment theory." *The Economic Journal 92,* no. 368: 787-804.

World Health Organization. 2020. *Laboratory testing for coronavirus disease 2019 (COVID-19) in suspected human cases: interim guidance,* 2 March 2020 (No. WHO/COVID-19/laboratory/2020.4). World Health Organization.

Zhu, N., Zhang, D., Wang, W, Li, X., Bo Yang., Song, J., Zhao, X, Huang, B., Shi, W., Lu, R., Niu, P, Zhan, F., Ma, X., Wang, D., Xu, D., Wu, G., George F. Gao., and Wenjie Tan. 2020. "A novel coronavirus from patients with pneumonia in China, 2019." *New England Journal of Medicine* vol. 382. no. 8(February): 727-733.

In: COVID-19 ISBN: 978-1-53618-903-2
Editors: A. B. D. Nandiyanto et al.

Chapter 19

THE GLOBAL IMPACTS OF COVID-19: RISK AND CRISIS MANAGEMENT IN AFFECTED COMPANY

***Eddy Soeryanto Soegoto*[1] *and Senny Luckyardi*[2]**
[1]Faculty of Economics, Universitas Komputer Indonesia,
Bandung, Jawa Barat, Indonesia
[2]Faculty of Postgraduate, Universitas Komputer Indonesia,
Bandung, Jawa Barat, Indonesia

ABSTRACT

The economic decline becomes the most severe phenomenon that hit the world besides the medical impact of the coronavirus outbreak. Southeast Asia countries as the middle-income countries require a better strategy to successfully respond to Coronavirus Disease 2019 (COVID-19) pandemic. Moreover, the highly uncertain condition makes it difficult for the affected companies' management in decision and policy-making. Therefore, this chapter aimed to develop better risk and a crisis management as the right response towards rapid and sudden change in crisis situation. In particular, it suggests ways that decision makers can adjust their company management for dealing with the extreme condition.

The chapter explored risk and crisis management of some management experts using descriptive analysis, literature review, and qualitative technique. The chapter resulted in risk and crisis management strategies for reducing losses but at the same time providing protection for their employee considering people's safety is second to none. The way of how companies react will bring big impacts to control the economic downturn in the middle of a global recession that now seems inevitable.

Keywords: pandemics, risk and crisis management, companies, South East Asia

1. INTRODUCTION

The emergence of Coronavirus Disease 2019 (COVID-19) pandemic causes large-scale mortality and morbidity, trade and travel networks disruption, as well as stimulating civil unrest (Di Marco et al. 2020). This is not the first time when global pandemic led the world economy to devastation. The SARS outbreak in 2003, the H1N1 pandemic in 2009, and the West African Ebola outbreak from 2013 to 2016 each have caused economic damages by more than US$ 10 billion. The current outbreak of COVID-19 once again hit the world with the huge socio-economic impact caused by international travel restriction and the quarantining of people in almost all affected countries. The considerable crisis hit almost all companies, especially in the field of tourism such as hotels, resorts, restaurants, and airlines. The disruption of supply chains also incredibly affected food, medicines, and the manufactured products industry. The economic impact is estimated to be higher than the US $150 billion (Smith et al. 2019). On the focus as company management and from the point of view of a manager, COVID-19 that is spreading human suffering in economics has brought uncertainty conditions in all affected companies (Machmud and Minghat 2020). This extraordinary condition pushed them to provide risk analysis and risk management in order to minimize the financial and psychological loss.

Southeast Asia which is occupied by most of the middle-income countries and developing countries must prepare the appropriate strategy since the crises is predicted to be worse than the developed countries. Loayza and Pennings (2020) in their research stated that the developing countries can be more severely affected by economic crises besides mass unemployment and business closures. Its ripple effects can produce a set of other crises which are financial, sectoral, balance-of-payments, and debt crises. Furthermore, this extreme pandemic may cause a humanitarian crisis such as worsening poverty, a dire decline of basic social services in education, health, safety, and stimulating social conflict, violence, and crime (Loayza and Pennings 2020). There are 11 affected countries in South East Asia namely: Singapore, Indonesia, Philippines, Malaysia, Thailand, Vietnam, Brunei Darussalam, Cambodia, Myanmar, Laos, and Timor Leste (Sirkeci and Yucesahin 2020). The updated data on 20 April, 2020 showed that the high number of cases is suffered by Singapore, while the highest mortality number in South Asia is suffered by Indonesia (World Health Organization 2020). Even though the crisis caused by the pandemic is global, the response to anticipate the impact is local. However, different countries show different approaches in responses as well as different companies react differently toward the resulting crisis.

Extreme efforts are needed in an extreme situation. Companies need to know the risks that might occur and what risk mitigation strategies can be applied to overcome the risks. Managerial implications need to be taken from the risk analysis to make a better effect on the company (Giannakis and Papadopoulos 2016). There are several studies concerning risk analysis where the researchers predict and measure the loss caused by the COVID-19 pandemic. A research confirmed that today, Composite Stock Price Index (IHSG) significantly decreased and lost almost 50% from the initial value on December 2019 (Utari, 2015). Asian Development Bank in its research estimated a global impact of US$77 to US$347 billion (or 0.1% to 0.4% of global GDP) (Dayrit and Mendoza, 2020). In line with this, the Center for Economic Policy and Research stated that COVID-19 hit many factories in Asia, especially in China, Japan, the Republic of Korea, and Singapore. Collectively, the United States, China, Japan, Germany, UK, France, and

Italy account for 60% of the global economy, 65% of global manufacturing, and 41% of global manufactured exports (Maliszewska et al. 2020). The World Health Organization (WHO) researchers predicted that East Asia and Pacific (EAP) will suffer the biggest GDP losses countries due to their relatively deep integration through trade and direct impact on tourism, as an example Cambodia (3.20%), Singapore (2.10%), China (2.30%), Thailand (3%), Vietnam (2.70%), and Malaysia (2.10%) (Mendoza, 2020). However, the paper describing risk management from the point of view of practitioners; in this terms company management; is required to broaden insight in building better risk management. It is crucial for all companies' management to have sufficient knowledge concerning risk and crisis management including taking preventive action, predicting upcoming uncertainty, building adjustment, and developing adaptation ability to survive in the long run.

This chapter attempts to develop better risk management as the right response toward rapid and sudden change. In particular, it suggests ways that the decision-makers can adjust company management for dealing with extreme condition. The chapter used descriptive analysis, literature study, and qualitative method in order to present a well-described subject.

2. What Is the Risk? And How It Can Be Different from the Crisis?

In summary, the risk is anything that negatively impacts the achievement of objectives as measured by their likelihood and impact. Risk can be defined as the actual deviation from the expected yield (Gollier 2018). The definition of risk is emphasized on the negative impact of achieving goals, although the exact definition is still growing. The definition of risk is still debatable considering the fact that well-measured and well-managed risk can increase innovation and greater opportunity to achieve goals (positive impact). On the other hand, the terms of crisis refer to dangerous situations that have a huge impact on everyone which can be caused by several factors such as the plague, natural disaster, technology, bad management, terrorism, war, and scarcity (Tong and Zhang 2020), whereas crisis management can be interpreted as a process that addresses organizations with a major event that threatens to harm the organization, stakeholders, or the general public. There are three elements that are most common for defining crises: threats to the organization, elements of surprise, and short time decisions. Unlike risk management, which involves assessing potential threats and finding the best way to avoid threats, crisis management deals more with threats that have already occurred.

The crisis which is assessed through the business perspective is a situation that leads to greater intensity of the problem, disruption of daily business running, affecting the image of the company, interfering company's overall work system, affecting community social pattern. In facing the crisis, the government has the authority to intervene. In facing the risk, the company has its authority to solve the problem. The common thing from risk and crisis that is both cases may trigger companies in conducting transformation and building resilience through the hard conditions. In a good response, both conditions may become a catalyst for companies to get better and survive in the long run (Martin et al. 2017).

3. Types of Risk versus Types of Crisis

Risks can be classified differently depending on which segment of business operations they are related to. Risks are divided into two categories: internal and external risks (Salamai et al. 2019). Business risks that occur within the business activities in the companies are called internal business risks and including the following external business risks which are sources that are outside the company such as the COVID-19 pandemic. The size of risk can be predicted from the data released by WHO regarding the decline in GDP and export illustrated in Figure 1.

Figure 1 shows the decreasing of GDP that is predicted to be experienced by several countries in East Asia Pacific (EAP) released by the

World Health Organization (WHO). Global GDP is expected to decrease by 2.10%, while developing and high-income countries' GDP is expected to decrease by 2.50 and 1.90%, respectively. Moreover, exports at a global level are expected to decrease by 2.50%. China is predicted to suffer a decrease in production across all sectors and goods as well as showing a reduction in exports of 3.70%. Vietnam shows a decrease in its total exports by only 1% because Vietnam fills the gap left by the decrease in Chinese exports. China is the most affected country in the East Asia and Pacific region in terms of export declines, followed by Laos (3.60%), Cambodia (3.90%), and Singapore (4.40%) (Barua 2020a).

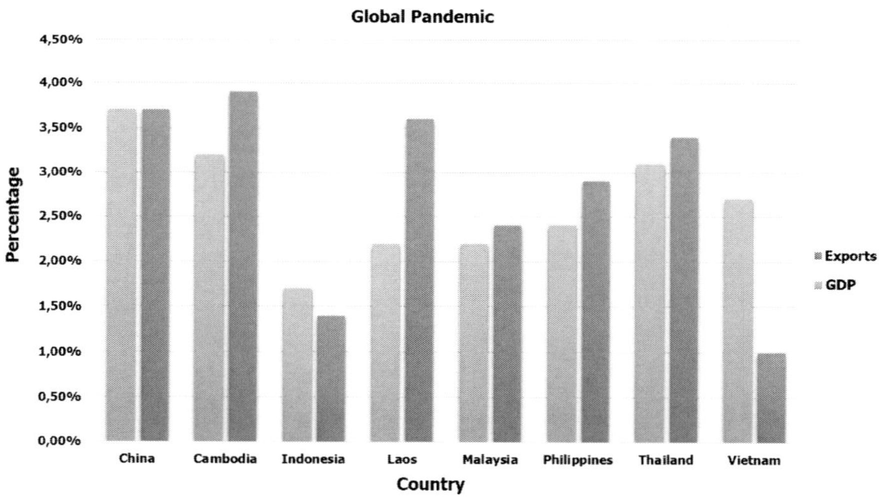

Figure 1. GDP and export implication of global pandemic scenario for EAP countries (% deviation from the benchmark (World Health Organization 2020).

People quarantined in almost every affected area have disrupted the supply chain due to the underutilization of labor and capital. Moreover, with an increase in its trade costs, the import costs for the rest of the world turns into a decline in global exports. The decline will lead to an economic crisis. Company management needs to have good knowledge concerning the stages of the crisis, which are divided into several stages, namely prodromal or symptoms of the crisis, acute, chronic, and healing (Bundy et al. 2017).

At the stage of Prodromal or Symptoms of Crisis, all events or signals of the crisis have begun to appear but the company continues to carry out activities as usual. If the company cannot catch this signal by not implementing crisis management, it will have a big impact on the next stage. As an example, when a company hears that coronavirus had spread in various countries but Indonesia has not yet had an impact, then this is a signal for the company to prepare a strategy if the virus enters Indonesia so that at the next stage, the company can survive.

At the acute stage, the crisis is not so obvious but has begun to be felt slowly by the company. At this stage, the term "point of no return" also means the company has no chance to re-improve the situation if the signal in the prodromal process is not heeded by doing good crisis management. For example, when the government firstly found the COVID-19 cases in Indonesia, the company continued to run the company as usual and prepared scenarios for alternative work such as working from home.

At this chronic stage, government intervention has emerged and affected the entire business process as a whole because the company has had an impact on the crisis. It is at this stage that the company implements a strategic policy so that the business can continue working. As an example, when Jakarta or Indonesia is on the lockdown, it can affect overall business activities such as supply chains and also export or import activities.

The last stage of the crisis is the healing stage. The company will begin to improve and reorganize the workings and structure of human resources. However, at this time, the company also began to adapt to all conditions if the company experienced a crisis that was quite long (Barro 1991).

4. Three Assumptions on Risk and Crisis Management Planning

4.1. Quick Recovery Assumption

In a quick recovery assumption, we assume that the COVID-19 pandemic will be overcome before the end of this year. Community transmissions in East Asia and Europe are brought under control. Consumer confidence also starts to return, even in the setting of sustained transmission, due to lower case fatality ratio, case-growth slowdown, and promising treatment options. Aviation, tourism, and hospitality sectors back to normal as countries lift travel bans (Maliazewaka et al. 2020). In this assumption, companies must design strategies by identifying crisis threats and opportunities. Companies must also be able to analyze the company's SWOT in facing a crisis as well as made a long-term strategy preparation. In this situation, a manager should translate theoretical planning into reality and practicing the responses with appropriate personnel and other resources. For this condition, management should involve senior members who have sufficient experience and knowledge to design risk and crisis management planning. After those who familiar with the situation conducting an analysis, companies need to implement strategic programs in dealing with crises.

4.2. Slow Down Recovery Assumption

A slowdown recovery assumption has been indicated with the transmission case in East Asia and the Middle East, while transmission in Europe is still growing (Maliazewaka et al. 2020). Consumer confidence also remains decrease. Demand recovery depends on the evolution of disease; some sectors (e.g., consumer goods) recover faster. It is too early to predict when the COVID-19 will be resolved. This also causes the vagueness of many companies about their priorities at the end of this pandemic. This is not surprising as it is difficult to predict what position the company will be in or what resources will be available in this assumption. The impact on business continuity is likely to be severe in a slow-down recovery assumption. However, in this condition, communication management and trust are very important in building resilience to a “shocking” impact. Communication management between governments, non-governmental organizations, media, and telecommunications in times of crisis should be well-maintained to make problem mapping easier.

4.3. Pessimistic (Recession) Assumption

The pessimistic assumption is indicated with the expansion of disease to other parts of the world, including confirmed transmissions in the rest of North America, Africa, and India. Consumer confidence remains low, and air-travel restrictions remain in place until late 2020 (Maliazewaka et al. 2020). During the time when we were writing this chapter, the pandemic has not reached its peak yet. The researchers predict the second phase of COVID-19. The worse assumption should be made to make companies well-prepared with this ongoing crisis.

The following are the suggested steps as risk and crisis management in all assumptions, especially in the worst condition.

5. Maintaining Good Communication

The COVID-19 crisis has stimulating civil unrest and labor demonstration. Communication by those who oversee the situation is often critical. Maintaining good communication also means protecting employees. This pandemic has been disturbing either mentally or economically. Therefore, good communication can stimulate resilience toward the worst assumption of the COVID-19 crisis. Since the pandemic tremendously changes the way of work and the way of life, then giving support to employees becomes more crucial. Report and socialization of new policy must be conveyed by those who have good communication skills. Leaders and top management should communicate their policy continuously to the employees.

6. Create a Special Team

Companies should create a special team to handle the crisis. The team is assigned to monitor the physical health and psychological condition of the employees. Companies should provide online consultation and counseling services to reduce the stress of the employees. The team should update information related to the socio-economic conditions, report to the CEO, and inform the employees. Supply chain monitoring should also become their work priority as well as the sales number. The information must be transferred to a related division for forecasting risk and designing a good response. This team should design specific daily, weekly, and monthly targets by continuing adjustment to recent conditions. They must define priority in the effort to overcome the crisis, determine the most valuable people in the company, and make sure the liquidity of the company.

7. Supply Chain Management

Company management is suggested to find the second supplier. This step aims to find suppliers of raw materials with a closer location. This step has a positive side of greater long-term supply chain resilience. Safety stock and recalculate raw material inventory is also an effort that can help to maintain the supply chain. This step aims to consider the resilience of ready raw material stock for production to deal with the fluctuations in demand in times of crisis.

8. Customer Management

This pandemic has caused a downturn in direct sales (face-to-face method). The company management must adjust their method to maintain customer loyalty. Online sales obviously have become a new trend in the pandemic era (Dirgantari et al. 2020) Stay at home as social distancing jargon means that people are purchasing products from home. This must stimulate every company to make digital transformation and strengthen digital infrastructure.

9. Change the Risk into Opportunity

Several companies have changed their production to product mask, medical equipment, and many more to find opportunity in the middle of the crisis. Of course, this cannot be conducted by all companies. Creating some innovations in sales and promotions also become crucial needs for companies to survive against the crisis.

10. Growth is Replaced with Survival Strategies

Several business sectors are predicted to experience the worst impact of a pandemic. In these sectors, survival strategies should be well-planned to replace growth strategies. The rapid response should be managed to allocate company resources in the effort to overcome the crisis overall rather than just increasing sales targets. Below is some analysis of business continuity in the most affected sectors:

11. Tourism

Travel restrictions have been widely applied to minimize the spreading of COVID-19. Travel restriction is defined as government order to stay at home and prohibition to move to other jurisdictions and closure of international borders. The exception of travel restriction is made for permanent residents and essential services. Meanwhile, the closure of international border is not enforced for returning nationals and permanent residents/visa holders (Wilson et al. 2020). The tourism industry contributes around 10.3% of global gross domestic product and generates roughly one in four of the world's new jobs over the past five years. Travel restriction in such an extreme manner in almost all territories around the world would result in more than 100 million job losses this year. Asia is suffering the biggest job losses in this sector; with a total of 60 million job losses; compare to other continents (UNWTO 2020). Short- and long-term survival strategies show the organization's capacity to respond to a crisis.

The tourism product is included in the service which is intangible. It is also complex since it consists of numerous different service providers and organizations. Hotel service, transportation companies, restaurants, tourism destination management/private sector, media, local community, and government/public sector are engaged in the tourism image. These service providers should contribute to the creation of favorable images for the fast recovery of the tourism sector. However, the safety aspect is the most important for the customer to visit tourism after the pandemic. In addition, the investment in human resource management in responding and managing crises has become a major risk mitigation issue for organizations in the tourism sector. Thus, resources investment in HRM initiatives involving to change corporate culture to deal effectively with crisis situations benefit organizations in both ethical and business perspectives (Mitroff 2004; Pforr and Hosie 2008). The holistic approach should be created by involving all stakeholders. The media has a role to deliver correct and consistent information and support image rejuvenation. The government should take an action in determination of tax incentives, special import provision to stimulate foreign investment, tax relief, extended credit to businesses, increased funding. The private sector should focus on marketing and promotions and the best way to handling customers. The local community has the role to inform tourists about the situation and security advice at the destination (Martents et al. 2016).

12. PROPERTIES

The decrease in economic growth and purchasing power due to pandemic has a tremendous impact on the decline of demands in the properties sector. The other impact of the crisis was the fund withdrawing by the investors, and temporarily discontinuation of distributing credit from the bank to the property sector. As the survival strategy, the property companies should shift their marketing target to Suburban areas since the demand in this area may increase due to businesses relocating from areas that have been quarantined. The strategy will keep the fixed costs for businesses holding leases at the same number, even in the face of declining occupancy and declining revenue (Sikich and Gear 2018).

13. UTILITIES (ELECTRIC, GAS AND OTHER INFRASTRUCTURE POWER SUPPLIES)

The great track record as a provider of critical infrastructure in the pandemic makes the utility company to be responsive to emergency situation. The global pandemic could stimulate the permanent destabilization of the power and utility sector. The high loss of workforce has led to respond ability decreasing in the maintenance. Furthermore, the inability to meet demands resulting in the prices increasing for energy and related products. The high demand for information systems to operate facilities and pipelines creates security vulnerabilities for this industry (Sikich and Geary 2018). The information system should develop to create clean and efficient energy. Although, during the pandemic, the domestic electricity consumption increased because most people were staying at home. On the other hand, the pandemic has pursued the rapid growth of renewable energy. Hence, the focus of recovery strategy in this sector should be focused on the security of energy supply and creates innovation in renewable energy (Wang et al. 2020).

14. COMMUNICATIONS INDUSTRY (VOICE, DATA AND OTHER INFORMATION SYSTEMS)

Work from home becomes the most popular word during the pandemic. Through technology, people are enabled to work remotely and at the same time also enable greater information exchange. Economists predict that fixed costs remain unchanged regardless of demand in this sector (Sikich and Geary 2018). The high demand for this sector should be answered with a high investment in the skillful personnel. Human resource management should create a good system to prevent the loss of skilled workforce since it creates potential system vulnerabilities

15. Banking and Finance

The disruption of worldwide economy is experiencing by the banking and finance sector. However, severe outbreaks are not new for countries in Asia. The COVID-19 outbreak was often likened to the SARS epidemic in 2003, which hit mainland China, Hong Kong, and Singapore very hard, and plunged each country's economy into a recession that makes the local government better equipped to deal with a similar crisis. Major economies in Asia have learned from past crises and built strong financial balances to reduce their economies in the face of external shocks. Governments in the Asian region are also learning quickly from China's response to the outbreak. In addition, companies in Asia also have stronger cash positions. Asian and Western markets show that more Asian companies have a net cash position, which means they have the ability to reinvest in the business and potentially gain market share (Bloom et al. 2005).

16. Transportation

The transportation sector has become the worst devastated caused by the pandemic of COVID-19. The travel restriction, quarantine of thousand people worldwide, flight restrictions, lack of workforce, inability to ship goods to markets has made this sector experience the tremendous impact that hard to be recovered (Barua 2020). This pandemic makes people even more reluctant to switch to using public transportation because of the high concern over the transmission of COVID-19 in public spaces. We need greater efforts to get out of the crisis situation that arises in the transportation sector. The government policy to give the secure feeling to the people to use transportation is urgently needed. This effort must be supported by the discipline culture of citizens and the management of public transportation company.

CONCLUSION

This paper has presented three assumptions in risk and crisis management in the COVID-19 outbreak that might evolve. Pandemic risks may largely jeopardize the market position and financial position of affected companies in South East Asia. Even more, South East Asia which is occupied by developing countries will suffer more economic destruction compared to developed countries. Pandemic is global, but the response is local. The way of how companies react will bring big impacts to control the economic downturn in the middle of a global recession that now seems inevitable. The company management cannot merely think about the plannable or plan for the unthinkable, but they must learn to think about business continuity planning in the unplannable situation such as pandemic of COVID-19.

REFERENCES

Barro, R. J. 1991. "Economic Growth in a Cross-Section of Countries." *The Quarterly Journal of Economics* vol. 106, no.2:. 407-443.

Barua, S. 2020a. "*Understanding Coronanomics: The economic implications of the coronavirus (COVID-19) pandemic*." Available at SSRN 3566477. https://dx.doi.org/10.2139/ssrn.3566477.

Barua, S. 2020. "*COVID-19 pandemic and world trade: Some analytical notes*." Available at SSRN 3577627. https://papers.ssrn.com/sol3/papers.cfm?abstract_id=3577627.

Bloom, E., De Wit, V., and Carangal-San Jose, M. J. 2005. *Potential economic impact of an avian flu pandemic on Asia.* https://www.think-asia.org/handle/11540/2165.

Bundy, J., Pfarrer, M. D., Short, C. E., and Coombs, W. T. 2017. "Crises and crisis management: Integration, interpretation, and research development." *Journal of Management* vol.43, no 6:1661-1692.

Dayrit, Manuel, and Ronald U. Mendoza. "*Social cohesion vs COVID-19.*" Available at SSRN 3555152 (2020). https://dx.doi.org/10.2139/ssrn.3555152.

Di Marco, M., Baker, M. L., Daszak, P., De Barro, P., Eskew, E. A., Godde, C. M., and Karesh, W. B. 2020. "Opinion: Sustainable development must account for pandemic risk." *Proceedings of the National Academy of Sciences* vol.117, no.8: 3888-3892.

Dirgantari, P. D., Hidayat, Y.M., Mahphoth, M. H., and Nugraheni, R. 2020. "Level of Use and Satisfaction of E-Commerce Customers in Covid-19 Pandemic Period: An Information System Success Model (ISSM) Approach." *Indonesian Journal of Science and Technology* vol.5, no. 2: 261–270.

Giannakis, M., and Papadopoulos, T. 2016. "Supply chain sustainability: A risk management approach." *International Journal of Production Economics* vol.171, no.2016: 455-470.

Gollier, C. 2018. "*The economics of risk and uncertainty.*" Edgartonline: Edward Elgar Publishing Limited.

Loayza, N. V., and Pennings, S. 2020. "*Macroeconomic Policy in the Time of COVID-19: A Primer for Developing Countries.*" https://elibrary.worldbank.org/doi/abs/10.1596/33540.

Machmud, A., and Minghat, A. D. B. 2020. The Price Dynamics of Hand Sanitizers for COVID-19 in Indonesia: Exponential and Cobweb Forms. *Indonesian Journal of Science & Technology* vol.5, no. 2: 176 - 184.

Maliszewska, M., Mattoo, A., and Van Der Mensbrugghe, D. 2020. The Potential Impact of COVID-19 on GDP and Trade: A Preliminary Assessment. *World Bank Policy Research Working Paper*, (9211). https://elibrary.worldbank.org/doi/abs/10.1596/1813-9450-9211.

Martens, H. M., Feldesz, K., and Merten, P. 2016. "Crisis management in tourism–a literature-based approach on the proactive prediction of a crisis and the implementation of prevention measures." *Athens Journal of Tourism* vol.3, no. 2: 89-101.

Martin, H., Durr, D., Smith, M., Finke, R., and Cherry, A. 2017. "Analysis of GMO food products companies: financial risks and opportunities in the global agriculture industry." *African Journal of Economic and Sustainable Development* vol.6, no. 1: 1-17.

Mitroff, I. I. 2004. "*Crisis Leadership: Planning for the Unthinkable*." Wiley, 2004.

Pforr, C and Hosie, J.P. 2008. "Crisis Management in Tourism. Preparing for Recovery." *Journal of Travel and Tourism Marketing* vol.23, no. 2: 249-264.

Salamai, A., Hussain, O. K., Saberi, M., Chang, E., and Hussain, F. K. 2019. "Highlighting the importance of considering the impacts of both external and internal risk factors on operational parameters to improve Supply Chain Risk Management." *IEEE Access* vol.7, no. 2019: 49297-49315.

Sikich, and Geary W. 2018. "*Potential Economic Consequences of a Pandemic.*" Logical: Management system.

Sirkeci, I., and Yucesahin, M. M. (2020). "Coronavirus and Migration: Analysis of Human Mobility and the Spread of Covid-19." *Migration Letters* vol.17, no.2: 379-398.

Smith, K. M., Machalaba, C. C., Seifman, R., Feferholtz, Y., and Karesh, W. B. 2019." Infectious disease and economics: The case for considering multi-sectoral impacts." *One Health* vol. 7, no. 2019 (June): 100080- 100090.

Tong, X., and Zhang, H. 2020. "A Comprehensive Analytical Framework for Risks, Disasters and Crises." In *China's Emergency Management*, no.2020(July): 3-40. https://link.springer.com/chapter/10.1007/978-981-13-9140-8_1.

United Nations World Tourism Organization. 2020. *Impact Assessment of the COVID-19 Outbreak on International Tourism.* UNWTO

Worldwide. https://www.unwto.org/impact-assessment-of-the-covid-19-outbreak-on-international-tourism.

Utari, R. 2015. "*Designing a Supply Chain Risk Mitigation Strategy at Pt Atlas Copco Nusantara Using the House of Risk Method*." Doctoral dissertation: Institut Teknologi Sepuluh Nopember.

Wang, B., Yang, Z., Xuan, J., and Jiao, K. 2020. "Crises and opportunities in terms of energy and AI technologies during the COVID-19 pandemic." *Energy and AI*. https://www.ncbi.nlm.nih.gov/pmc/articles/PMC7273151/

Wilson, N., Barnard, L. T., and Baker, M. 2020. "*Rationale for border control interventions and optionsto prevent or delay the arrival of Covid-19 in New Zealand: Final commissioned report for theNew Zealand Ministry of Health.*" Ministry of Health.

In: COVID-19
Editors: A. B. D. Nandiyanto et al.
ISBN: 978-1-53618-903-2

Chapter 20

CONSUMER PURCHASING PATTERNS IN RESPONSE TO COVID-19 PANDEMIC IN INDONESIA

Puspo Dewi Dirgantari[1,*], Yusuf Murtadlo Hidayat[1], Rury Nugraheni[1] and Mohd Halim Mahphoth[2]

[1]Business Education, Faculty of Economics and Business Education, Universitas Pendidikan Indonesia, Bandung, Jawa Barat, Indonesia

[2]Faculty of Business and Management, Universiti Technologi MARA Cawangan, Melaka, Malaysia

ABSTRACT

As the coronavirus disease 2019 (COVID-19) crisis continues around the world, consumer behavior on purchasing pattern has started to change. The outbreak of the COVID-19 has a major impact not only in the health sector but also on the economy, including on economic activities relating to the process of purchasing goods or services. The condition of the COVID-19 pandemic followed by the adoption of social distancing led to

* Corresponding Author's Email: puspodewi@.upi.edu.

consumer new behavior in determining purchasing patterns or purchasing decisions. This chapter investigated whether consumers purchase decisions are changing or not during the pandemic. This study used the literature study with secondary data support. It was found that consumers are shifting to online and digital shopping decisions through online media to reduced-contact channels. The results of the study are expected to be a reference for related parties, especially for suggesting some decision in the policy makers and government.

Keywords: buying decision, purchasing patterns, pandemic

1. Introduction

The world concern very well about the coronavirus 2019 (COVID-19) outbreak that occurred. The reality of this new pandemic surprised the world. Based on the Chinese National Health Commission until 12 a.m. on 4 February 2020, this pandemic has caused 20,471 people to be infected in China (including Hong Kong, Macao and 150 Taiwanese) and the Chinese National Health Commission has also confirmed that there are 23 countries outside China that have infected, including Indonesia (Wyplosz 2020; Dirgantari 2020). The positive number of COVID-19 in Indonesia has now reached five thousand cases as of 18 April 2020 with a death rate due to positive COVID-19 of 9.13%. As many as 8.68% of the number of people who are positive COVID-19 has recovered (This data was submitted by the Government Spokesperson for Handling COVID-19, Achmad Yurianto (Kompas 2020).

The increasing number of positive COVID-19 has affected many sectors such as tourism, aviation, health, mass media, government, e-commerce, social media, and entertainment media. The government has also made a policy to carry out all activities at home such as studying, working, and worshiping. So far, there have been 10 regions that have implemented Large-Scale Social Restrictions (known as PSBB) as an effort to break the spread of COVID-19. This is certainly increasingly limiting community activities outside the home, in which usually we can shop directly to markets or supermarket and nowadays people must shop Online. Indeed, this is easier and faster, and this does not have to gather with people (Kompas 2020).

During the COVID-19 pandemic, business competition was very fierce, reflected by the number of companies that sought to capture market share and new markets through a variety of ways and innovations displayed in the products or services they produced (Velavan et al., 2020). Companies must be able to determine the right marketing strategy so that the business can survive and the main objectives of the company can be achieved.

Several factors are the reason for a company to get its own place in the hearts of the community. For example, company must consider how a company sets competitive prices, conduct effective promotions, shape the image and build a good corporate reputation in the eyes of consumers, as well as good and satisfying quality of products. They also need to find ways to get their old customers back with a new mindset from the traditional mindset to the online mindset.

In most countries, customers adapt to make transactions, access Products, and services that are minimal in contact and digitally based (El Zowalaty et al., 2020). When consumers are restricted in shopping, they find and adopt newer ways to shop through technology. In countries badly affected by COVID-19, consumers begin to hoard food and other important items, and isolate themselves from the crowd. Thus, patterns in shopping change, and they adopt newer ways to shop through e- commerce (Buana 2020).

In this situation, people who were previously reluctant to shop online are now setting up online accounts on various e-commerce platforms, experiencing a completely new customer journey. Once they feel comfortable shopping online, they might never go back to their old ways. e-commerce has undermined offline retailing for a long time, but this pandemic has accelerated the trend (Bakhtiar 2020). The government also began to look at the e-commerce sector as one solution to overcome the tax deficit due to the economic slowdown. E-commerce has actually been able to attract many consumers in Indonesia before the COVID-19 outbreak. E-commerce is also one of the main drivers of making Indonesia the country with the largest digital economic value in Southeast Asia reaching $ 40 billion in 2019 and it is predicted to increase to $ 130 billion by 2025. With more retail shops and consumers forced to turn to e-commerce, its growth can be increased and even further (Corbitt, Thanasankit and Yi 2013).

E-commerce or online shop, provides a variety of products needed by the community ranging from household needs, electronics, clothing, and others. They also provide various kinds of conveniences to consumers and various other promotions such as discounts, cashback, and other bonuses (Foster 2016). Various kinds of offers provided by this online shop certainly attract consumers to shop. With the closure of physical stores, brands are increasingly pivoting to a direct-to-consumer (D2C) business model. D2C brands have a simplified proposition that cuts out retailers – selling directly to consumers through mobile and digital channels. They can meet household needs easily and quickly. They still follow the rules applied without going out of the house, but the goods will arrive safely and securely with an online shop. The convenience provided in shopping is expected to help government programs to "stay at home" (Lucas et al., 2020; Dirgantari et al., 2020).

The use of various e-commerce services continues to increase, based on research conducted by similar web shows an increase of 2.05% in e-commerce in Indonesia within 28 days and will continue to increase as consumers spend more time to stay at home (SimiliarWeb 2020).

Thus, the purpose of this study was to find out how people's buying patterns were during the COVID-19 pandemic outbreak. The results of this study are expected to provide information about businesses in selecting and determining strategies that can influence purchasing decisions with businesses able to survive in increasingly competitive competition during the COVID-19 pandemic outbreak.

2. Method

This research was a descriptive research with a literature study approach by finding references and theories, which were obtained as a research path for the study of literature serve as the basic foundation and the main tool for research practice in the middle of the field. The results of this study used to identify consumer buying patterns through changes in consumer behaviour in making purchasing decisions and strategies, so that companies could survive in increasingly fierce business competition during the COVID-19 pandemic outbreak.

3. Results and Discussion

According to Kotler, a purchasing decision is a problem-solving process that consists of an analysis of needs and desires, information search, assessment of the source of selection for purchasing alternatives, purchasing decisions, and behaviour after purchase. In general, making a decision is the selection of actions from two or more alternative choices. Of the various factors that influence consumers in buying a product or service, consumers usually always consider the quality, price, and products that have been previously identified (Said et al., 2020).

The purchase decision process includes five stages. These stages are

1. being aware of needs;
2. searching for information;
3. evaluating product alternatives;
4. making a purchase decision; and
5. post-purchase behaviour.

The buying process starts long before the actual purchase. Marketers need to focus on the entire buying process, instead of focusing on the purchase decision alone (Kotler and Armstrong 2018). The consumer decision-making process begins with them realizing their needs and insatiable desires. Then, the consumer will realize the difference between his actual status (as a case) and the ideal needs they want to meet through several social and psychological aspects. These needs are what motivate and stimulate them to make decisions (Mullins et al., 2011; Mullins et al., 2008).

The importance of purchasing decisions appear, especially for shopping commodities. Risks that are a consequence of this decision are (Lahindah and Siahaan 2018):

1. functional risk: the product does not perform its function as expected;
2. financial risk: the product does not match (or is the same) as the price paid;
3. social risk: the product may endanger others;
4. psychological risk: products can affect (or influence) consumer from their consumers;
5. time risk: product failure can cause a loss of opportunity to be satisfied from consuming other alternative products.

To find out how and when consumers begin to show behavioural changes in making purchasing decisions, we conducted a study of shopper behaviour during the beginning of the pandemic in China and extended to other countries that were also affected. Current reports monitored a growing trend in the consumer environment when news of COVID-19 reached the public sphere and found that consumers went through six stages of knowledge based on their awareness of COVID-19 that spread in their communities (Velavan et al., 2020):

a. proactive health-minded buying: increasing interest in having a product that has a relationship in maintaining welfare or health.
b. Reactive health management: prioritizing products in an effort to prevent infection.
c. Panty preparation: increasing in product purchases that have a long-term shelf life and increase store visits.
d. Quarantined living preparation: increasing online shopping, decreased store visits and signs of supply chain irregularities.
e. Restricted living: increasing in prices due to limited availability and hinder the fulfilment of online needs.

f. Living a new normal: increasing health awareness when returning to their activities.

The literature on purchasing decisions explains that many factors influence purchasing decisions. Some factors that influence purchasing decisions include price, products and services (Basu et al., 1995). Consumers are willing to sacrifice their money to buy certain products if the product is able to meet their expectations (Parasuraman and Berry 1991). The evaluation of a product or service based on several considerations is only determined based on its external appearance, such as brand, price, or packaging, which directly or indirectly will affect the decision-making process (Zeithaml 1988).The price, promotion, and reputation of the company have a great influence on the customer in influencing the formation of a buying decision. It was explained that the more competitive the price given by the seller, the greater the purchasing decisions made by the customer. Likewise, with promotions, the more intensive and attractive promotions that are held will increase the probability of consumer decisions to buy them and a good assessment of the company is also one of the factors that can influence the formation of purchasing decisions. This is because consumers will always look for companies that provide a specification in accordance with what this is expected by consumers (Ayu 2019). Buying decisions made by potential buyers are not always direct purchasing decisions only but also pending purchase decisions. One of the reasons is that funds are not yet available for purchase (Kim et al., 2008; Anggraeni et al., 2020). When prospective buyers have an interest in a particular product and already have a trust in the seller's account in question, then they will give a 'mark' on the seller's account or product.

CONCLUSION

COVID-19 pandemic give opportunity to evaluate consumers lifestyle choices. The purchasing decisions helped to contribute to the food, electronics, clothing and other industries which were sluggish because of the closure of shopping centres and the borders of social activities. There are also negative risks that must be faced by consumers during this pandemic, namely functional risk, financial risk, social risk, psychological risk, and time risk. They are also triggered by security problems, loss of payment checks, accumulation of bills, and uncertainty the store. Thus, companies should pay more attention to prices and set a competitive price in addition to the quality of services in accordance with the wishes of consumers, update their customer personas and communication strategy, and giving maximum quality of product and good performance.

References

Anggraeni, S., Maulidina, A., Dewi, M.W, Rahmadianti, S., Rizky, Y. P. C., Arinalhaq, Z. F., Usdiyana, D., Nandiyanto, A. B. D., and Al-Obaidi, A. S. M. 2020. "The Deployment of Drones in Sending Drugs and Patient Blood Samples COVID-19." *Indonesian Journal of Science and Technology* 5, no. 2: 193–200.

Ayu, A. D. 2019. *Actualization of Social Justice Values in Buying and Selling Activities in Lawang Traditional Market, Malang Regency.* SKRIPSI Jurusan Pendidikan Pancasila dan Kewarganegaraan-Fakultas Ilmu Sosial: Universitas Malang.

Bakhtiari, K. 2020. *How Will The Pandemic Change Consumer Behaviour.* https://www.forbes.com/sites/kianbakhtiari/2020/05/18/ how-will-the-pandemic-change-consumer-behavior/#3fb398cf66f6.

Basu, Swasta, D. H., and Irawan. 1995. *Modern Marketing Management.* Libert: Yogyakarta.

Buana, D. R. 2020. "Analysis of Indonesian Society Behavior in Facing the Corona Virus Pandemic (Covid-19) and Tips for Maintaining Mental Welfare." *SALAM: Jurnal Sosial dan Budaya Syar-i* 7: no.3, 1-10.

Corbitt, B. J., Thanasankit, T., and Yi, H. 2003) "Trust and e-commerce: a study of consumer perceptions." *Electronic commerce research and applications*, 2(3):203-215.

Dirgantari, P. D., Hidayat, Y. M., Mahphoth, M. H., and Nugraheni, R. 2020. "Level of Use and Satisfaction of E-Commerce Customers in Covid-19 Pandemic Period: An Information System Success Model (ISSM) Approach." *Indonesian Journal of Science and Technology* vol.5, no.2: 86-95.

El Zowalaty, M. E., and Jarhult, J. D. 2020. "From SARS to COVID-19: A previously unknown SARS-CoV-2 virus of pandemic potential infecting humans–Call for a One Health approach." *One Helath vol.9*, no. 2020 (June):100124-100134.

Foster, B. 2016. "Impact of Brand Image on Purchasing Decision on Mineral Water Product "Amidis"(Case Study on Bintang Trading Company)." *American Research Journal of Humanities and Social Sciences vol.2*, no. 2016: 1-11.

Kim, D.J., Ferrin, D.L. and Rao, H.R., 2008. "A trust-based consumer decision-making model in electronic commerce: The role of trust, perceived risk, and their antecedents." *Decision support systems vol.44, no. 2*: 544-564.

Kompas. 2020. "Data Covid-19 di Indonesia." *Kompas.com,* April 18, 2020. [COVID-19 data in Indonesia]. *Kompas.com,* April 18, 2020. https://www.kompas.com/covid-19.

Kotler, P., and Armstrong, G. 2018. *Principles of Marketing. Pearson Education*. http://library.wbi.ac.id/repository/212.pdf.

Lahindah, L., and Siahaan, R. 2018. "The Influence of Product Innovation and Service Quality to Buying Decision and the Impact to Repeat Buying at Progo Road Bandung." *The Asian Journal of Technology Management vol.11. No.2*: 118-124.

Lucas, B., Elliot, B., and Landman, T. 2020. *Online Information Search During COVID-19*. arXiv preprint arXiv:2004.07183. https://arxiv.org/abs/2004.07183.

Mullins, C. D., Obeidat, N. A., Cuffel, B. J., Naradzay, J., and Loebel, A. D. 2008. "Risk of discontinuation of atypical antipsychotic agents in the treatment of schizophrenia." *Schizophrenia Research vol.98. no.1:* 8-15.

Mullins, R. F., Dewald, A. D., Streb, L. M., Wang, K., Kuehn, M. H., and Stone, E. M. 2011. "Elevated membrane attack complex in human choroid with high risk complement factor H genotypes." *Experimental eye research vol.93, no.4*: 565-567.

Parasuraman, A., and Berry, L. L. 1991. *Marketing services: competing through quality.* Simon and Schuster: New York. e-book.

Said, S., Kamase, J., Ella, H., Rachman, A., and Dunggio, T. 2020. "Big data and content marketing on purchase decisions online in Indonesia." *American Journal of Economics and Business Management vol.3, no.1*: 168-177.

Velavan, T. P., and Meyer, C. G. 2020. "The COVID-19 epidemic." *Trop. Med. Int. Health 25, no. 3*: 278-280.

Wyplosz, C. 2020. *The good thing about coronavirus.* (No.Article).https://repository.graduateinstitute.ch/record/298221.

Zeithaml, V. A., Berry, L. L., and Parasuraman, A. 1988. "SERVQUAL: a multiple-item scale for measuring consumer perceptions of service quality." *Journal of Retailing vol.64, no.1*: 12-40.

In: COVID-19
Editors: A. B. D. Nandiyanto et al.
ISBN: 978-1-53618-903-2

Chapter 21

ANALYSIS OF THE APPLICATION OF THE MOBILE VENDING MACHINE AS A DISTRIBUTION TOOL FOR COVID-19 BASIC PROTECTIVE ASSISTANCE FOR THE INDONESIAN SOCIETY

Bachrul Tias[1], Cahyanisa Alifa Pramesti[1], Cuk Khim[1], Muhammad Shofwan Qobus[1], Salma Salsabila[1], Sri Anggraeni[1,*], Dian Usdiyana[1] and Asnul Dahar Minghat[2]

[1]Fakultas Pendidikan Ilmu Pengetahuan Alam,
Universitas Pendidikan Indonesia, Bandung, Jawa Barat, Indonesia
[2]Razak Faculty of Technology and Informatics,
Universiti Teknologi Malaysia, Skudai, Johor, Malaysia

[*] Corresponding Author's Email: anggraeni_said.upi.edu.

Abstract

The world is currently experiencing extraordinary event after coronavirus disease 2019 (COVID-19) first appeared in Wuhan, Hubei Province, China. This event is declared as a pandemic because it spread widely throughout the world including Indonesia. Indonesia has a *Work From Home* (WFH) system that is assumed ineffective because there are still many people who are unable to stop going to their office. They have economic limitations, so they also find it difficult to get personal protective equipment to avoid being exposed by the COVID 19 viruses. This study used qualitative analysis with data obtained from online questionnaires. The data obtained states that the Vending Machine Mobile is considered effective in solving problems. The Vendible has related to the difficulties of the public to access personal protective equipment to avoid being exposed to the COVID 19.

Keywords: basic personal protective equipment, COVID-19, Indonesia, Vendbile

1. Introduction

Currently the world is experiencing extraordinary event after the Novel Coronavirus Disease (COVID-19) was declared as a pandemic by World Health Organization (WHO) on 30 January 2020. This virus was first discovered in Wuhan, Hubei Province, China in December 2019 and spread very quickly throughout China (Zheng et al., 2020; Putra and Abidin, 2020). In Indonesia, people infected on Nov 2019, and COVID-19 were first discovered on 2 March 2020 (CNN Indonesia, 2020a; Anggraeni et al., 2020). Based on the data obtained from Worldometers, the spread of this case takes place so quickly. On 19 April 2020, there were 6,248 cases in Indonesia, 535 of them died (CNN Indonesia, 2020b).

COVID-19 is an infectious disease caused by a newly discovered coronavirus. The COVID-19 virus spreads in the form of small droplets that are usually released by people who have been infected while sneezing or coughing (Rawan and Triwidiastuti, 2000). These droplets generally will not move but fall to the ground or a surface within a few seconds. This is the reason social distancing or physical distancing effectively prevents its spread (Sauer, 2020).

This virus spreads in the form of droplets released by the infected people (Maryanti et al., 2020). This virus will not move but fall to the surface. Social distancing or physical distancing is effective in preventing the spread of this virus. However, social distancing or physical distancing affects various aspects such as economic, social, and environmental aspects. Moreover, Indonesia is still a developing country whose economy is not as good as developed countries. In implementing the *Work From Home* (WFH) system, our society has difficulties because there are still many people who have to work to provide needs for their family.

Previous researches on COVID-19 stated that using masks or face masks during religious rituals to prevent the spread of the virus (Dong et al., 2020) are a must, and a tool or website to track COVID-19 cases in real time (Liputan 6, 2020) are needed. These two studies are different from our researches on Mobile Vending Machines (Vendbile) which can help distribute tools to prevent the spread of COVID-19 such as masks, hand sanitizers, and hand washs in areas that need these items throughout Indonesia.

This research answered some of the problem formulations including the socialization on the importance of COVID-19 prevention tools and systems to the society, how Vendbile works to the society, and how important Vendbile is for Indonesian. We conducted this research based on the apprehension we experienced because there are still many people who find it difficult to get tools such as masks and hand sanitizers to prevent COVID-19.

2. Vending Machine Mobile

Vendbile is one of the many ideas of transportation equipment that helps the government in distributing COVID-19 prevention tools (medicines, masks, hand wash, and hand sanitizer) using vending machines on an open truck. Illustration of a Mobile Vending Machine is presented in Figure 1.

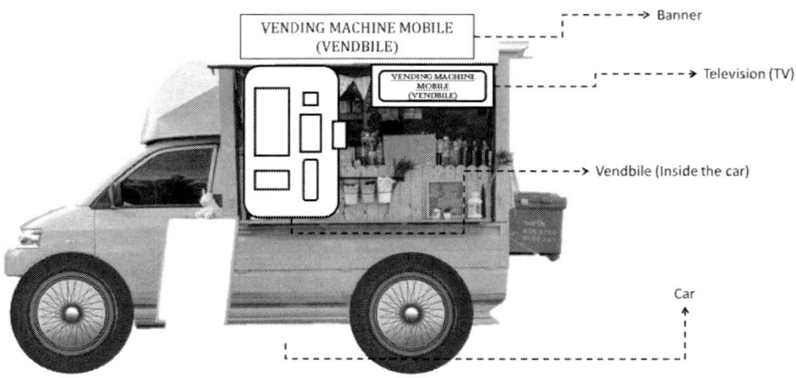

Figure 1. Illustration of the Mobile Vending Machine design as a distribution tool for COVID-19 basic protective aid.

The distribution equipment proposed is presented in Figure 2. The tool is designed in three angles view namely, the front, left and right side, and backside as shown in Figure 2(a), 2(b), and 2(c), respectively. Figure 2(d) shows the media used to explain the usage procedure of this aid distribution tool.

This tool is an automatic machine but it needs a driver, however, the driver still has to maintain physical distancing. Therefore, Vendbile is equipped with a guide written on the banners and small TVs in order to help people to know how to use it. People need to bring their identity cards, before using Vendbile apply hand sanitizer, scan the identity card, choose the desired items, and after getting the items, they applied hand sanitizer again.

3. RESEARCH METHOD

The research method used was a qualitative research method. Qualitative research methods emphasize data trends (Syandri and Akbar, 2020). This research took place during April 2020. The method in this study was a quantitative method with qualitative analysis and a questionnaire-based research method distributed online. After the information collected from a number of samples, information processed and analyzed qualitatively.

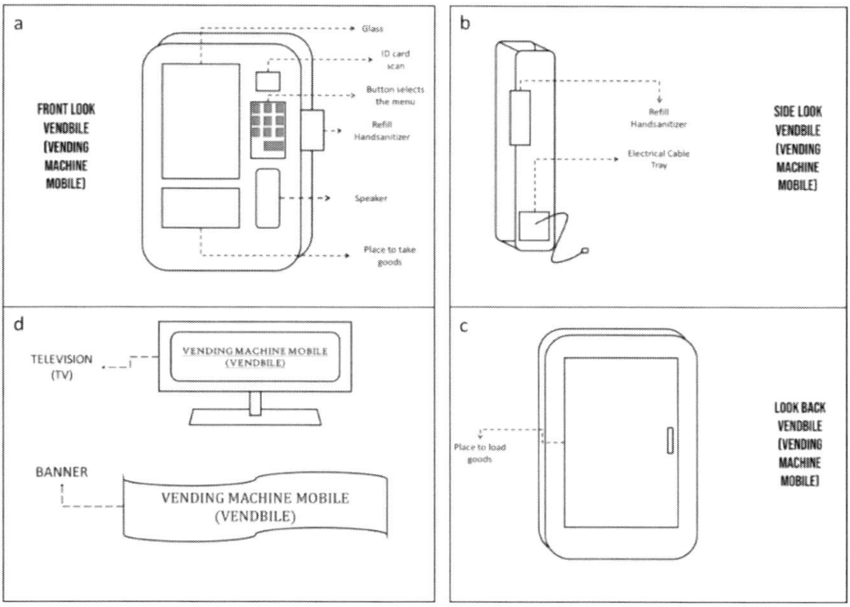

Figure 2. The visual appearance of the Mobile Vending Machine as a distribution tool for COVID-19 basic protective. Figures (a), (b), (c), and (d) respectively are the design of the device design from the front, side, back, and appearance of the media for the procedure to use the tool.

4. RESULTS AND DISCUSSION

This questionnaire form divided into two parts, the first part was the identity of the respondents, and the second part was related to the Vendbile. The second part consisted of 23 questions with one final question regarding suggestions and input for the further development of the Mobile Vending Machine in order to fit in with the COVID-19 prevention assistance standard (medicines, masks, and hand wash or hand sanitizer).

There were 180 respondents that answered the questionnaire which was distributed through social media.

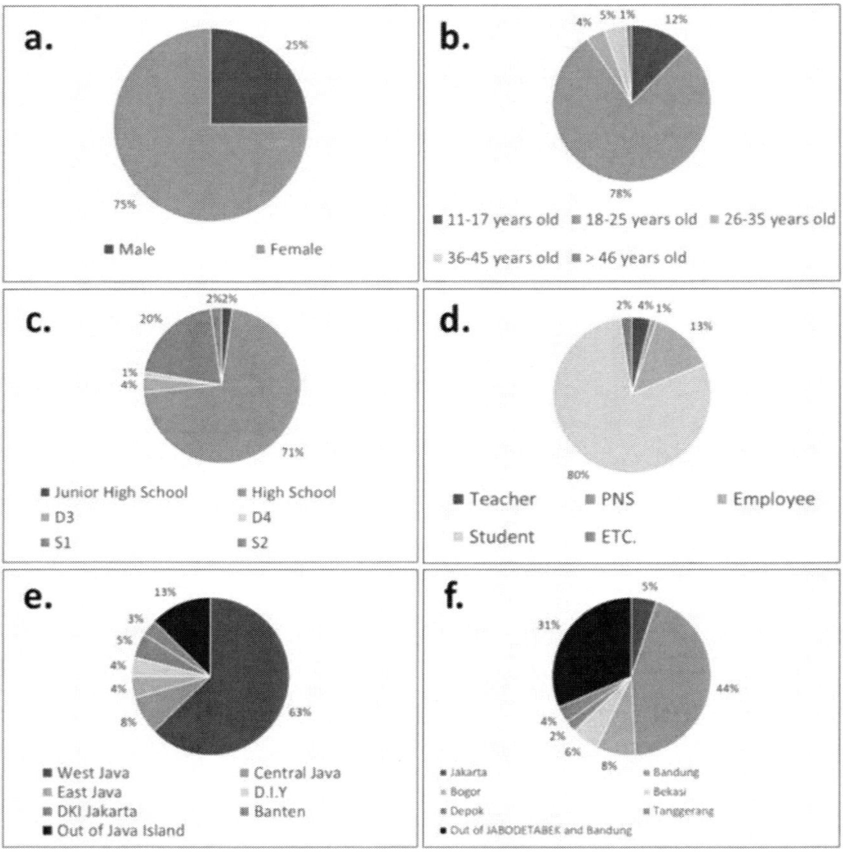

Figure 3. Identity of the 180 respondents.

Research showed that 75% of the respondents were female (Figure 3(a)). The most dominant respondents' age range is between 18-25 years (Figure 3(b)).

Most of the respondents' education level is a senior high school, followed by undergraduate and the rest were spread fairly evenly among the levels of junior high school education, diploma, and master degree (Figure 3(c)). The majority of respondents worked as students (Figure 3(d)). The majority of respondents residing in West Java and many of them are from the city of Bandung, while other respondents came from various regions outside West Java, from Central Java, DKI Jakarta, and the rest were scattered in various regions in Indonesia (Figure 3(e) and 3(f)).

On the question of how the situation and condition in the environment around the respondent during the COVID-19 pandemic, the majority of people answered that it was in good situation and condition (Figure 4(a)).

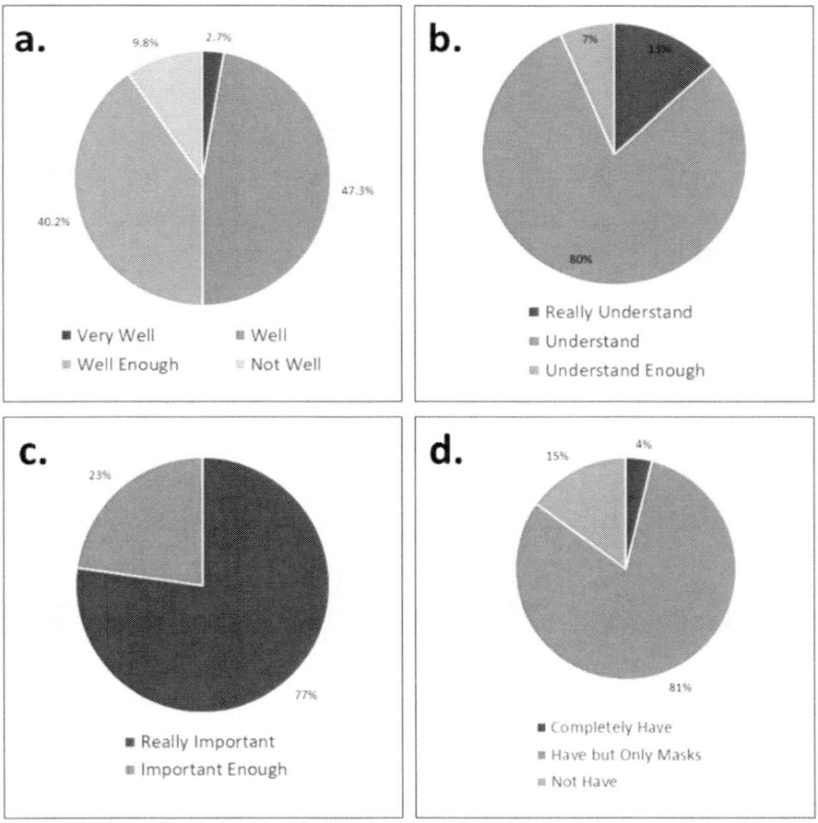

Figure 4. Public opinion about the situation and conditions in the surrounding environment (a), understanding the prevention procedures and protective equipment from COVID-19 (b), public opinion about the importance of standard protective equipment (c), and ownership of standard protective equipment that reaches all groups according to the society (d).

Respondents who answered, mostly came from West Java, especially from the city of Bandung. The next question is about the respondents' understanding of the COVID-19 prevention procedure and the tools used. The majority of people understood it (Figure 4(b)). The result showed that the readiness and outreach based on information and messages disseminated by the government and the society have almost reached to all groups. The result of the next question is presented in Figure 4(c). Respondents' opinions about the importance of standard protective equipment such as masks and gloves indicated that society has understood and considered this situation was important as well as the prevention of COVID-19. Out of 180 respondents, 138 respondents considered that the standard protective equipment was very important. Continuing from the discussion of the previous questions, it can be concluded that Indonesian people have had awareness in terms of basic prevention through the importance of using protective equipment such as mask and glove.

Furthermore, the results in Figure 4(d) shows that majority of people (81%) only have masks as standard Personal Protective Equipment (PPE). This shows that the distribution of protective equipment was not evenly needed for the general public, especially those who live in West Java. Many factors could affect this, one of which is the limited access to transportation as a result the distribution only happens in certain areas.

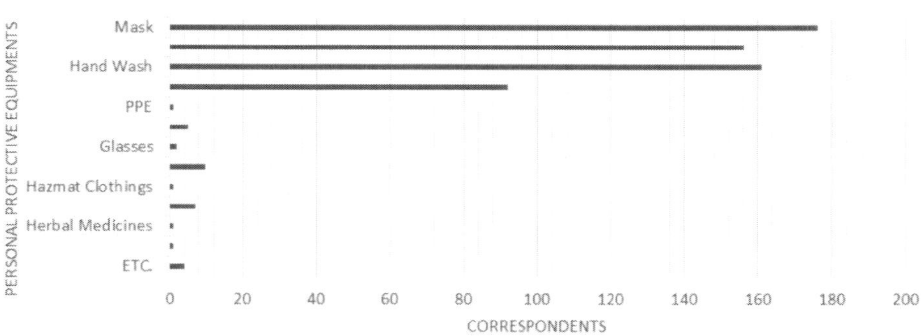

Figure 5. Graph of the most important personal protective equipment for the society.

Meanwhile, people's understanding of personal protective equipment produces data as shown in Figure 5, 176 respondents chose mask as the most important equipment. Some respondents also added other things that were also important such as disinfectant, glasses, hazmat clothing, vitamins, herbal medicine, and jacket. Based on the response, we concluded that the society has already known items to prevent the spread of COVID-19.

In Figure 6(a), 88% of the respondents had difficulties in obtaining protective equipment.

In Figure 6(b), the information to be taken is the availability of PPE around society. 37% of respondents lived close to a place where information about personal protective equipment to prevent COVID-19 transmission could be accessed. The status of the PPE distribution showed that respondents still felt that the distribution had the Barrier, as shown in Figure 6(c). Then in Figure 6(d), survey results showed that the majority of respondents, did not feel the distribution costs to the society burdensome but the rest felt the government was burdening them with the costs.

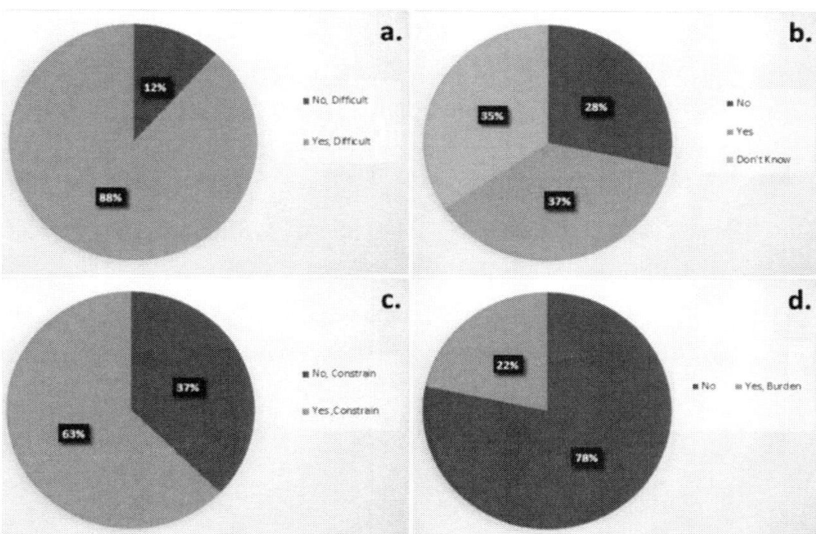

Figure 6. Difficulties of the society in obtaining personal protective equipment (a), availability of personal protective equipment in the environment around the society (b), public opinion regarding the obstacles in the distribution of aid equipment (c), and regarding the imposition of transportation costs for assistance (d).

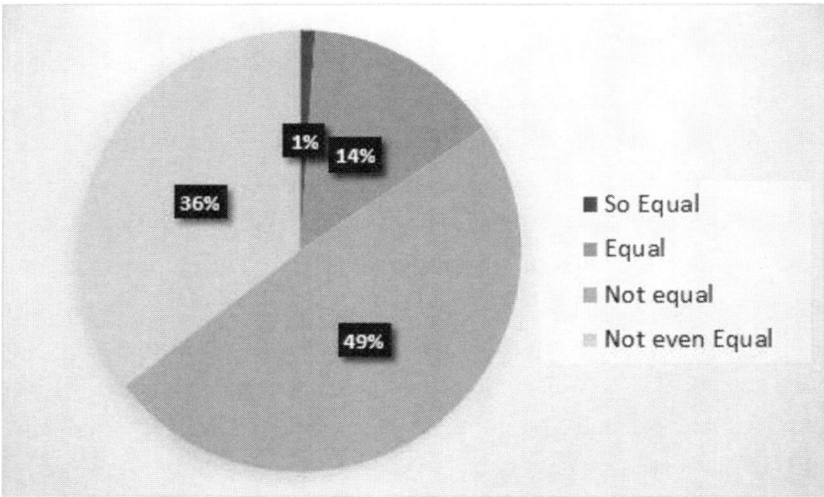

Figure 7. Equitable distribution level of personal protective aid equipment from COVID-19.

In Figure 7, 49% of the respondents stated that there was still a lack of equalization of the prevention tools. It could be concluded that the majority of respondents still felt unsatisfied with the distribution and that there was still uneven distribution.

In Figure 8(a), we obtained the results of the data that the society gave full support to if an attempt was made to provide the PPE distribution tools. It could be concluded that society really needed a tool to distribute PPE so that the tool would be easily accessed by society without having to wait for a long time. In Figure 8(b), the respondents would put the people who needed it first. Hospitals that received PPE assistance well were government-owned hospitals, while private hospitals still had difficulties in getting PPE assistance. In urban areas, private hospitals still found it was very difficult to get PPE and also in rural areas (World Health Organization, 2020).

In Figure 9, data collection is related to the idea of developing a Mobile Vending Machine to help distribute the personal protection and prevention tools of COVID-19.

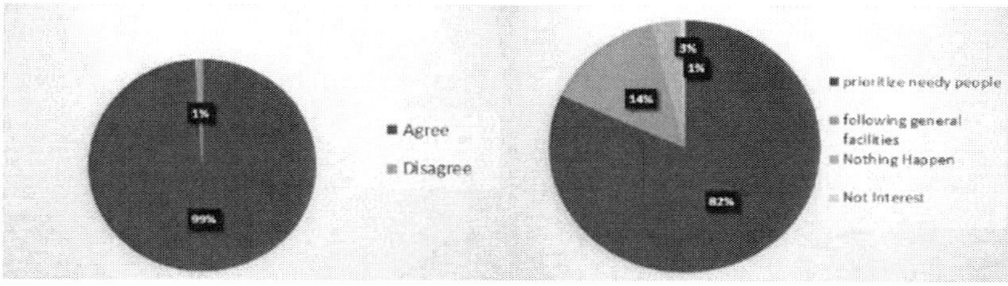

Figure 8. Respondents regarding the planned provision of aid distribution tools (Vendbile) and their impact on the distribution of distribution to the society (a) and the respondents' opinions in using Vendbile if it has been realized (b).

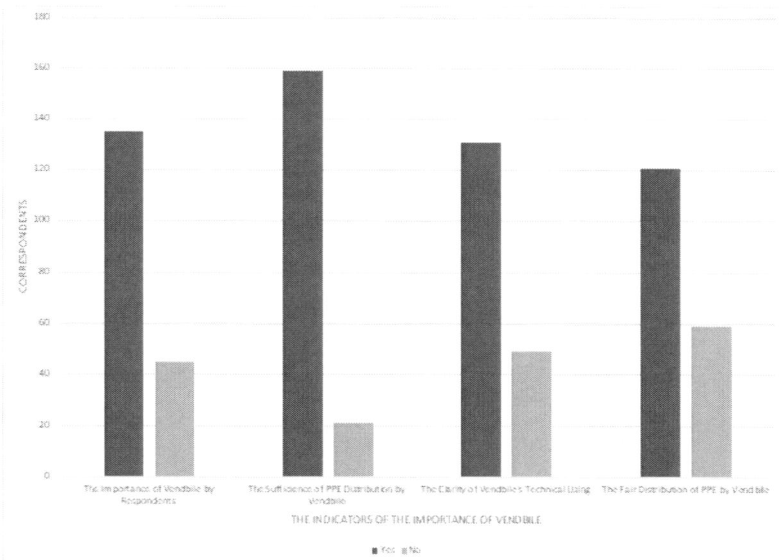

Figure 9. Graph the importance of Vendbile to the society.

Vendbile is important for respondents. According to respondents, these tools were sufficient to help the distribution evenly. The technical and procedures for using Vendbile according to respondents were quite clear. For respondents, Vendbile could be a good idea in the distribution of personal protective equipment. This shows that this idea received a positive response from society.

The next question was about Vendbile license to operate around society settlements. As a result, the majority of people responded that it should be based on the situation and conditions in the areas where it operates.

Furthermore, regarding the availability of respondents to become volunteers who participated in supplying Vendbile stock, the majority of people answered that they were not willing to participate. The next question is about the availability of the society to participate in socializing Vendbile to the surrounding environment. It shows that the majority of people answered that they were willing to participate. It means that society is willing to participate in socializing Vendbile in order to help the neighborhood to get sufficient information about Vendbile.

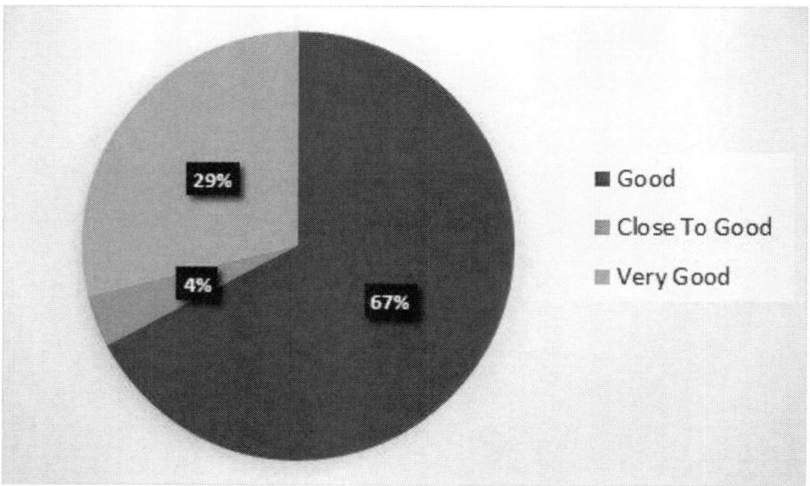

Figure 10. Vendbile breakthrough for the society.

On questions related to the existence of Vendbile in their areas regularly that can increase the number of vehicles on the road and add a little pollution in the environment, the majority answered it depended on the situation and conditions.

This shows that it would be wise if we operate Vendbile based on the situation and conditions of the areas. Furthermore, according to the respondents, the right and effective time for Vendbile to operate was in the morning. This shows that the operation of Vendbile will be more precise and effective in the morning because most people do not have many activities in the morning so, if the Vendbile would operate in the morning it can make the distribution even.

In Figure 10, the majority of people answered that Vendbile was very good. This shows that Vendbile can be useful to help the society especially on the equal distribution of COVID-19 prevention tools, especially in the red zone and in the underdeveloped, remote, and outermost regions in Indonesia. Quoted from CNN Indonesia, East Nusa Tenggara Province, for example, requires 17 million liters of disinfectant containing chlorine, while, at present, South Sumatra needs 250 million ordinary masks and DI Yogyakarta Province still lacks 3.2 million PPE (CNN Indonesia, 2020; Worldometers, 2020).

Conclusion

From this study, we can conclude that currently the society is experiencing difficulties in obtaining COVID-19 standard prevention tools. This problem is caused by hoarding the standard prevention tools conducted by some people. Then, based on the respondents' answers, Vendbile is a good and effective breakthrough to assist the government in distributing prevention tools in order to make it more equitable. However, the operations must be based on the current situation and conditions in society.

Acknowledgment

We acknowledged Program Bangdos, Universitas Pendidikan Indonesia for supporting this study.

References

Anggraeni, S., Maulidina, A., Dewi, M. W, Rahmadianti, S., Rizky, Y. P. C., Arinalhaq, Z. F., Usdiyana, D., Nandiyanto, A. B. D. and Al-Obaidi, A. S. M. 2020. "The Deployment of Drones in Sending Drugs and

Patient Blood Samples COVID-19". *Indonesian Journal of Science and Technology,* vol. 5, no. 2: 193 - 200.

CNN Indonesia. 2020a. "Darurat Corona, Tito Akui Masih Ada Daerah Kekurangan APD". CNNIndonesia.com. April 8, 2020. [Corona emergency, Tito admits there are still areas that lack PPE]. *CNN Indonesia.* April 8, 2020. https://www.cnnindonesia.com/nasional/20200408095145-20-491503/darurat-corona-tito-akui-masih-ada-daerah-kekurangan-apd.

CNN Indonesia. 2020b. "Jokowi Umumkan Dua WNI Positif Corona di Indonesia" ["Jokowi Announces Two Positive Corona Indonesian Citizens"]. *CNNIndonesia.com.* March 2, 2020. https://www.cnnindonesia.com/nasional/20200302111534-20-479660/jokowi-umumkan-dua-wni-positif-corona-di-indonesia.

Dong, E., Du, H. and Gardner, L. 2020. "An interactive web-based dashboard to track COVID-19 in real time". *The Lancet Infectious Diseases,* vol. 20, no. 5: 533 - 534.

Liputan 6. 2020. *IDI Sebut Distribusi APD ke Daerah Terkendala Birokrasi.* Liputan6.com. April 8, 2020. *IDI Called the Distribution of PPE to Bureaucratic Constrained Areas.* https://www.liputan6.com/news/read/4231040/idi-sebut-distribusi-apd-ke-daerah-terkendala-birokrasi.

Maryanti, R., Hufad, A., Sunardi, Nandiyanto, A. B. D. and Al-Obaidi, S. M. 2020. "Understanding COVID-19 particle contagion through aerosol droplets for students with special needs". *Journal of Engineering Science and Technology,* vol. 15, no. 3:1909 - 1920.

Putra, Z. A. and Abidin, S. A. Z. 2020. "Application of SEIR Model in COVID-19 and the Effect of Lockdown on Reducing the Number of Active Cases". *Indonesian Journal of Science and Technology,* vol. 5, no. 2: 185 - 192.

Rawan, P. and Triwidiastuti, S. E. 2000. *Pengantar Metode Penelitian.* [*Introduction to Research Methods*]. Retrieved from Repository UC: http://repository.ut.ac.id/4195/1/MMPI5202-M1.pdf.

Sauer, L. M. 2020. *What Is Coronavirus?* Hopkins Medicine. https://www.hopkinsmedicine.org/health/conditions-and-diseases/coronavirus.

Syandri and Akbar, F. 2020. "Penggunaan Masker Penutup Wajah Saat Salat Sebagai Langkah Pencegahan Wabah Coronavirus Covid-19" ["The Use of a Face Mask during Prayer as a Prevention Step for the Coronavirus Covid-19 Outbreak"]. *SALAM: Jurnal Sosial dan Budaya Syar-I,* vol. 7, no. 3: 261 - 268.

World Health Organization. 2020. *Coronavirus*. WHO Worldwide. https://www.who.int/health-topics/coronavirus#tab=tab_1.

Worldometers. 2020. *Corona viruse cases in Indonesia*. Worldometer: https://www.worldometers.info/coronavirus/country/indonesia/.

Zheng, Y. Y., Ma, Y. T., Zhang, J. Y. and Xie, X. 2020. "COVID-19 and the cardiovascular system". *Nature Reviews Cardiology,* vol. 17, no. 5: 259 - 260.

In: COVID-19 ISBN: 978-1-53618-903-2
Editors: A. B. D. Nandiyanto et al.

Chapter 22

HEALTH TRUCK MOBILE COMMUNITY HEALTH SERVICES FOR COVID-19

Anjani Nurfitriana[1,*], Dea Puspha Annisa[1], Fitria Faizah Hilman[1], Sri Anggraeni[1], Dian Usdiyana[1] and Asnul Dahar Minghat[2]

[1]Fakultas Pendidikan Ilmu Pengetahuan Alam, Universitas Pendidikan Indonesia, Bandung, Jawa Barat, Indonesia

[2]Razak Faculty of Technology and Informatics, Universiti Teknologi Malaysia, Malaysia

ABSTRACT

Coronavirus disease 2019 (COVID-19) is an infectious disease caused by a new type of coronavirus namely severe acute respiratory syndrome coronavirus 2 (SARS-CoV-2). The disease has spread to 118 countries and infected 119,179 people on Feb 2020. Indonesia is currently affected by the COVID-19 outbreak. This has an impact on the economic, social, and educational systems. In these conditions, the transportation system also needs attention. The distribution of drugs and rapid test equipment to rural

* Corresponding Author' Email: anggraeni@upi.edu.

areas during the pandemic is a serious barrier. The number of areas that still lack of health facilities has caused lower health care for the community, including the current handling of COVID-19, such as the rapid test tool in every public health center in Indonesia. One solution that can be provided from this problem is the provision of Health Truck to help provide health services to deal with COVID-19, especially rapid tests on areas where health facilities are lacking. The rapid test tools available on this Health Truck can at least help in handling COVID-19, so that the provision of health services in remote areas can be overcome.

Keywords: COVID-19, disease, coronavirus, transportation, health, rapid test

1. Introduction

The new type of coronavirus has started to become a concern of the world community after on January 20, 2020, health authorities in Wuhan City, Hubei Province, China, said three people died in Wuhan after suffering from pneumonia caused by the virus (Febrian 2020; Razon 2020). The disease is caused by a new type of coronavirus namely severe acute respiratory syndrome coronavirus 2 (SARS-CoV-2) and the disease is named corona virus disease 2019 (COVID-19) by world health organization (WHO) (World Health Organization 2020).

Coronavirus is a large family of viruses that cause diseases ranging from mild to severe symptoms. Common signs and symptoms of coronavirus infection include symptoms of acute respiratory disorders such as fever, coughing, and shortness of breath. In severe cases, it can cause pneumonia, acute respiratory syndrome, kidney failure, and even death (Maryanti et al., 2020). The clinical signs and symptoms reported are mostly fever, with some cases having difficulty breathing, and X-rays show extensive pneumonia infiltrates in both lungs (Kementerian Kesehatan Republik Indonesia 2017).

In March 2020, Indonesia began to be affected by this disease and after World Health Organization (WHO) declared this disease a global pandemic. At present, 18 April 2020, 5923 people have been positively identified as having COVID-19, 520 people have died, and 607 people have successfully recovered (Halim 2020). The Health Service recognizes the lack of COVID-19 treatment facilities in all regions of Indonesia to closely monitor people from exposure to the SARS-Cov-2 virus. One of them is the lack of supervision regarding public health itself (Nugraha 2020). Therefore, in the midst of the COVID-19 pandemic, Faculty of Mathematics and Science Education at the Indonesian University of Education students are developing ideas related to transportation systems that are relevant for conducting health surveillance in areas with minimal health facilities. The proposed idea is a health care transportation media that can maintain and control public health during the COVID-19 pandemic, especially for conducting rapid tests. Rapid test is an initial screening method to detect antibodies, namely IgM and IgG, which are produced by the body to fight coronavirus (Nareza 2020). These antibodies will be formed by the body when expose to coronavirus. The rapid test system used is a door to door system, so that it can prevent people from crowding in large numbers in one place simultaneously.

This idea still requires data to support it. So, we conduct research through online media. The confidentiality of personal data sent is guaranteed and processed for this research purpose only. Transportation media are provided to help the community, especially during the emergency COVID-19 pandemic, which is in an area with limited health facilities.

2. METHOD

The method used was a descriptive method using a questionnaire. The questionnaire was designed in such a way and then distributed randomly through online media to various regions in Indonesia. The collected data used as the source of information needed to develop ideas about the health care transportation media that can maintain and control public health during the COVID-19 pandemic. The data was processed by analyzing each question.

3. Results and Discussion

There were 221 participants participated on the online media questionnaire about the idea of the Health Truck to maintain and control public health, specifically to carry out a rapid test. The data shows various ages for both women (71%) and men (29%), from various backgrounds such as students, civil servants, entrepreneurs, teachers, and housewives.

Table 1. The number of participants in various regions

No.	Residential area	Number of Participants
1	West Jakarta	3
2	East Jakarta	3
3	South Jakarta	0
4	North Jakarta	0
5	Central Jakarta	0
6	Bogor City	6
7	Depok City	7
8	Cimahi City	12
9	Bandung	24
10	Tanggerang City	0
11	South Tanggerang City	0
12	Serang City	0
13	Cilegon City	2
14	Surakarta City	0
15	Cirebon City	2
16	Bogor Regency	25
17	Bekasi Regency	2
18	Bandung Regency	17
19	Subang Regency	40
20	Karawang Regency	1
21	Purwakarta Regency	2
22	Pandeglang Regency	0
23	Tanggerang Regency	3
24	Other Areas	72

Based on Table 1, most participants were from the areas of West Jakarta, East Jakarta, Bogor City, Depok City, Cimahi City, Bandung City, Subang Regency. Meanwhile, participants were from other regions, such as Kutai Kartanegara Regency, Garut Regency. In this context, we only choose five regions with the most participants to be discussed, which are Cimahi City, Bandung, Bogor Regency, Bandung Regency, and Subang Regency.

Most of the participants were well aware of the dangers, symptoms, and prevention of COVID-19. Some participants chose to have their health checked into various health services while others choose to stay at home or do self-isolation and then had their observation after symptoms worsen (Putra and Abidin, 2020). In accordance with the circular letter submitted by the Indonesian government, if you experience some symptoms that indicate COVID-19 and people must stay at home to isolate themselves. In addition, people who appear to be healthy or fine are still encouraged to continue to take various precautions to reduce the spread of COVID-19 (Jogloabang 2020).

Based on Figure 1, participants who need a rapid test are those live in Cimahi and Bandung cities that are red zone area, as shown in Figures 1(a) and 1(b) require a rapid test, but they do not make this much of a problem because they assume that their area has already had adequate health facilities in handling COVID-19. Meanwhile, Subang Regency, Bandung Regency, and Bogor Regency which are shown in Figures 1(c), 1(d), and 1(e) are areas with a high percentage of needs regarding the handling of COVID-19, especially for rapid tests. This may be due to various factors, for example, in Subang Regency has a very large number of People under monitoring, but is also limited to the procurement of rapid test equipment (Firmansyah 2020). Therefore, people really need this health facility.

Most of the participants (46.15%) stated that there were closest health services that could conduct COVID-19 tests, there were also participants (22.18%) who said there were no health services in their area, and the rest (31.67%) were participants who still doubted the existence of facilities in the area.

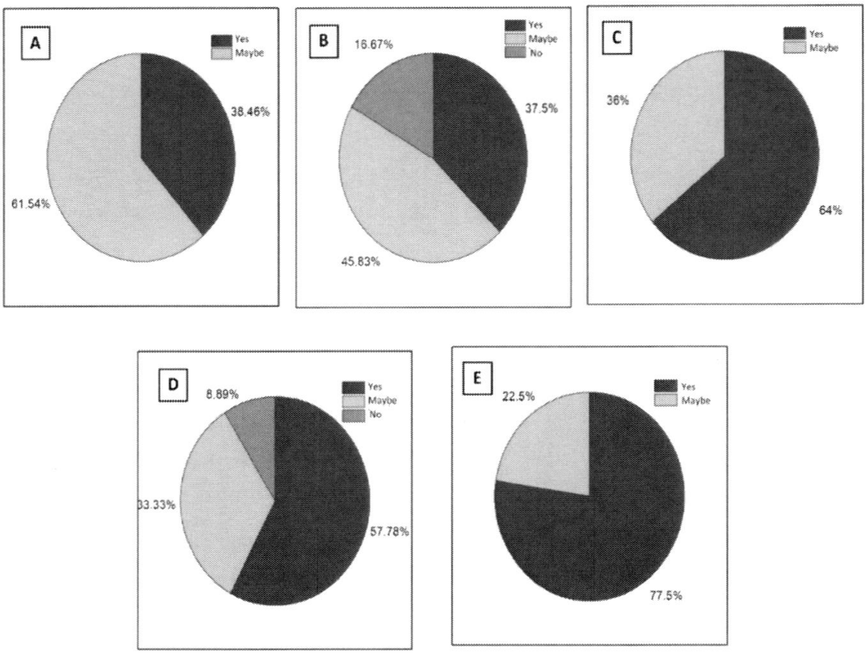

Figure 1. (a) Participants who need rapid tests in Cimahi City, (b) Participants who need rapid tests in Bandung, (c) Participants who need rapid tests in Bogor Regency, (d) Participants who need rapid tests in Bandung Regency, and (e) Participants who need a rapid test in Subang Regency.

Based on the data obtained, the health services available in the participant area were mostly clinics, puskesmas, and hospitals. However, the procurement of COVID-19 tests at clinics and puskesmas was limited due to limited health facilities or a limited number of rapid test equipment. As many as 50.23% of participants stated that the community might experience difficulties in handling health, 32.58% of other participants responded that they did not experience any difficulties at all, and only 17.19% of participants stated that they experienced difficulties in handling health. In fact, not all health services can handle problems related to COVID-19. One solution that can be provided from this problem is a health care transportation media that can maintain and control public health during the COVID-19 pandemic. Furthermore, in handling COVID-19, about 91.4% of participants needed special transportation to help with health management and control, then, only about 8.5% did not need it.

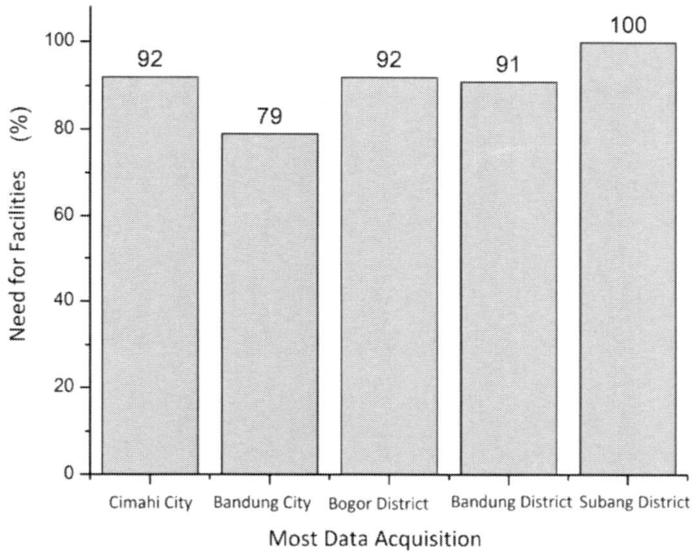

Figure 2. Distribution of needs for health facilities in various regions.

Figure 2 shows the data distribution of the needs of health facilities in various regions of Indonesia. Cimahi City, Bandung City, Bogor Regency, Bandung Regency, and Subang Regency are the regions with the highest number of participants. Based on Figure 2, Subang Regency is the area that most needs health facilities. Then, followed by Cimahi City, Bandung Regency, and Bogor Regency which are the COVID-19 red zone areas.

Therefore, to overcome the problem of limited health services, we propose ideas to participants regarding transportation media, namely Health Truck. Health Truck is a health care transportation media that can maintain and control public health during the COVID-19 pandemic. In the Health Truck, there are several health services, especially rapid tests needed by the community during a pandemic like this. In this Health Truck idea, we pay attention to various health service protocols, both for patients and medical personnel, provided by the government based on World Health Organization technical guidelines (World Health Organization 2020).

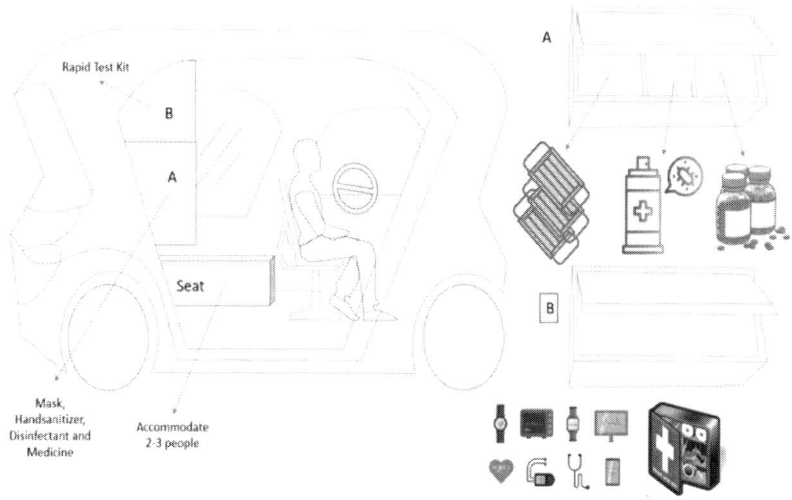

Figure 3. Health Truck Design.

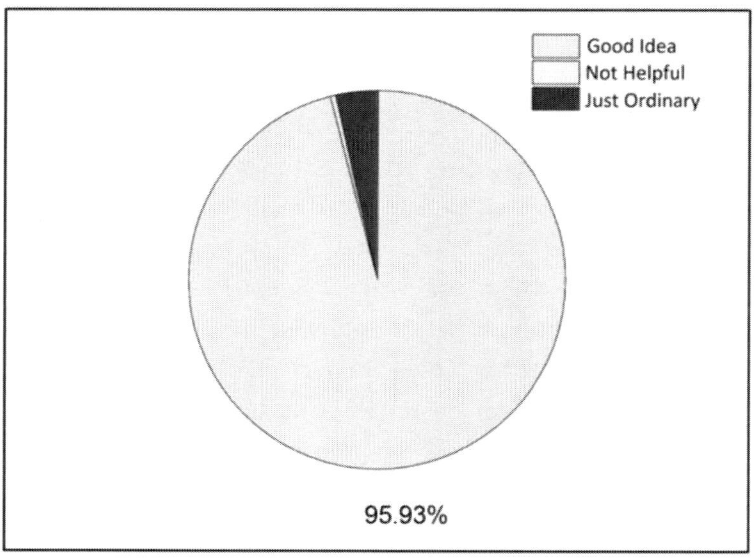

Figure 4. Participants who support the idea of Health Truck.

The shape of or designated Health Truck as can be seen in Figure 3, is a medium-sized car that has a futuristic look with various health facilities and personal protective equipment inside. The shape of the Health Truck is deliberately designed smaller than a truck so it can be driven on narrow roads.

Figure 4 shows the data of participants who supported our ideas. After the participants learned about the purpose and function of this Health Truck, most of the participants were very supportive of our ideas and hoped that this would be the solution to the existing health service problems. Even after the end of the epidemic, this transportation can continuously be used, especially in remote areas that lack health facilities.

If this transportation media was built, most of the participants think that they would participate to take the test as long as it is free of charge. According to the participants, the Health Truck was also effective in preventing transmission of COVID-19, participants also stated that many areas or regions would need this Health Truck.

Based on the results of the questionnaire, participants revealed that there were still many needs of the community in the prevention of COVID-19 such as masks, hand sanitizers, disinfectants, Personal Protective Equipment (PPE), rapid tests and swab tests. The swab or RTPCR test results are more accurate than the rapid test. Therefore, swab test or RTPCR is important to ensure whether someone infected by the COVID-19 (Majni 2020).

Conclusion

Based on the method we carried out on 221 participants, it can be concluded that the majority of the community needs additional facilities to deal with the COVID-19 pandemic. Through our ideas in the form of Health Truck, it is expected that it can support the community in facing the COVID-19 pandemic.

Acknowledgment

We acknowledged Program Bangdos, Universitas Pendidikan Indonesia for supporting this study.

References

Febrian, A. A. 2020. "Asal Mula dan Penyebaran Virus Corona dari Wuhan ke Seluruh Dunia" ["The Origin and Spread of the Corona Virus from Wuhan to Around the World"]. *IDN Times Bali*. April 17, 2020. https://bali.idntimes.com/health/medical/ denny-adhietya/asal-muasal-dan-perjalanan-virus-corona-dari-wuhan-ke-seluruh-dunia-regional-bali.

Firmanysah, D. 2020. "Jalani Rapid Test, 13 Warga Subang Terindikasi Corona." ["Take a Rapid Test, 13 Subang residents are indicated by Corona"] *Detik.com*. March 17, 2020. https://news.detik.com/berita-jawa-barat/d-4973110/jalani-rapid-test-13-warga-subang-terindikasi-corona.

Halim, D. 2020. UPDATE: "Kini Ada 5.923 Kasus Covid-19 di Indonesia, Bertambah 407 ["Now There are 5,923 Covid-19 Cases in Indonesia, Up 407"]." *Kompas.com*. March 24, 2020. https://nasional.kompas.com/read/2020/03/24/15442831/update-kini-ada-686-kasus-covid-19-di-indonesia-bertambah-107-pasien? page=all.

Indonesia. Kementerian Kesehatan Republik Indonesia. 2020. *Pedoman Kesiapsiagaan Menghadapi Corona Virus Disease (COVID-19).* [*Corona Virus Disease (COVID-19 Preparation Guidelines*]. https://www.persi.or.id/images/2020/data/pedoman_kesiapsiagaan_covid19.pdf.

Jogloabang. 2020. "SE HK.02.01/MENKES/202/2020 tentang Protokoler Isolasi Diri Sendiri dalam Penanganan COVID-19." ["SE HK.02.01/MENKES/202/2020 concerning Self-Isolation Protocol in Handling COVID-19"] *Jogloabang.com*. March 17, 2020. https://www.jogloabang. com/kesehatan/se-hk0201menkes2022020-protokol-isolasi-diri-sendiri-penanganan-corona-virus-disease.

Majni, F. A. 2020. "Mengenal Rapid Test dan Swab Test." ["Knowing Rapid Test and Swab Test"] *Media Indonesia.com*. April 15, 2020. https://mediaindonesia.com/ read/detail/304226-mengenal-rapid-test-dan-swab-test.

Maryanti, R., Hufad, A., Sunardi., Nandiyanto, A. B. D., and Al-Obaidi, S. M. 2020. "Understanding COVID-19 particle contagion through aerosol droplets for students with special needs." *Journal of Engineering Science and Technology* vol.15, no.3:1909-1920.

Nareza, M. 2020. "Kenali Apa Itu Rapid Test untuk Virus Corona" ["Recognizing Rapid Test for the Coronavirus"]. *Alodokter.com*. April 17, 2020. https://www.alodokter. com/kenali-apa-itu-rapid-test-untuk-virus-corona.

Nugraha, A. 2020. "Dinkes Jabar Akui Fasilitas untuk Penanganan COVID-19 Masih Kurang" ["West Java Health Office Admits Facilities for Handling COVID-19 Are Still Lacking"]. *Liputan6.com*. March 10, 2020. https://www.liputan6.com/ health/read/4198171/dinkes-jabar-akui-fasilitas-untuk-penanganan-covid-19-masih-kurang.

Putra, Z. A., and Abidin, S. A. Z. 2020. "Application of SEIR Model in COVID-19 and The Effect of Lockdown on Reducing The Number of Active Cases." *Indonesian Journal of Science and Technology* vol.5, no.2: 185 - 192.

Razon, B. C. 2020. "COVID 19: Impetus for "Community Spirits" among Filipinos." *Indonesian Journal of Science and Technology* vol.5, no.2: 201-208.

World Health Organization (WHO). 2020. Naming the coronavirus disease (COVID-19) and the virus that causes it. *WHO Worldwide*. https://www.who.int/emergencies/diseases/novel-coronavirus-2019/technical-guidance/naming-the-coronavirus-disease-(covid-2019)-and-the-virus-that-causes-it.

World Health Organization. 2020. Materi Komunikasi Risiko COVID-19 untuk Fasilitas Pelayanan Kesehatan. *WHO Worldwide*. [COVID-19 Risk Communication Material for Health Care Facilities]. *WHO Worldwide*. https://www.who.int/docs/defaultsource/searo/indonesia/covid19/riskcommunicationforhealthcarefacility.pdf?sfvrsn=9207787a_2.

In: COVID-19 ISBN: 978-1-53618-903-2
Editors: A. B. D. Nandiyanto et al.

Chapter 23

Automatic Slit for Delivering Food Aid to Workers and Medical Personnel in Motorized Vehicles

Ghina Mufidah[1], Thyta Medina Salsabila Erlangga[1], Hasna Nadaa Fida Karima[1], Fitria Felashopa[1], Sri Anggraeni[1,*] and Asnul Dahar Minghat[2]

[1]Fakultas Pendidikan Ilmu Pengetahuan Alam, Universitas Pendidikan Indonesia, Bandung, Jawa Barat, Indonesia

[2]Razak Faculty of Technology and Informatics, Universiti Teknologi Malaysia, Skudai, Johor, Malaysia

Abstract

Since the coronavirus disease 2019 (COVID-19) pandemic began to spread in Indonesia, the government has implemented several policies. Implementing physical distancing and encouraging workers to work at

* Corresponding Author's Email: anggraeni_said@upi.edu.

home and encouraging students to study at home are among those policies. Although this policy has been made, workers including medical personnel still have to work outside. COVID-19 has also impacted the workers' income and as a result, they find it difficult to meet their daily needs. Therefore, we designed an automatic box on a vehicle to distribute food aid to medical personnel and workers who do not work from home using the Drive-thru system. This drive-thru system was chosen because it is easy and supports government efforts in implementing physical distancing.

Keywords: drive-thru, automatic box, COVID-19, food transportation

1. Introduction

Coronavirus disease 2019 (COVID-19) is a disease that causes respiratory infections (Maryanti et al., 2020). This virus is a large family of coronavirus discovered after Middle East Respiratory Syndrome (MERS) and Severe Acute Respiratory Syndrome (SARS) (World Health Organization 2020; Anggraeni et al. 2020). This outbreak started in December 2019 in Wuhan, China, until it spread throughout the world and arrived in Indonesia in early March 2020 (Azanella 2020). The existence of this outbreak affects several aspects, one of which is the distribution of logistical needs. These are in line with government policies that require a reduction in outdoor activities. Most people have to work at home, but some still have working outside as the spread of COVID-19 continues to increase. Workers are losing their incomes and having difficulty meeting their daily needs (Putra and Abidin 2020).

Coronavirus affects those who make a living as private employees, laborers, and in particular workers in the informal sector. Many companies have laid off employees without pay. Although inofficial workers continue to sell their products, their income decreases due to limited community activities (Indraini 2020). Online drivers are affected by this policy as well as they lose up to 70% of their daily income. Besides supporting the family at home, they also need to pay for other needs, one of which is lunch (Media Indonesia 2020).

Another problem that arises is a large number of medical workers who are exhausted and need food aid to meet their food needs. Medical personnel in Banten claimed that the workload was getting heavier. The shift scheduled for four turns, and medical personnel who has the third shift scheduled, from 05:00 p.m. until 1:00 a.m., do not to get food (Lesmana 2020). As known, the safety of medical personnel is not only a matter of the quality and sufficiency of Personal Protective Equipment (PPE) but also of the food to sustain the stamina. The medical personnel has to give a balanced diet and sufficient vitamins to secure their immune system (SeRiau 2020).

With this idea, there is a need to evolve ideas related to the appropriate transportation network to support the government's efforts to reduce the spread of COVID-19 by adopting the concepts of physical distance, yet to accommodate the food needs of those who are unable to work from home including medical personnel. The ideas that can be executed. Our proposed idea is to build automatic cars and motorbikes transportation.

In this case, the drive-thru systems in Indonesia has conducted by the One-stop Administration Services Office. Indonesian's drive-thru system is efficient to use and has received a strong response from society (Wardani and Rumiyatun 2017). Another innovation using the drive-thru system is the rapid test in Bogor city. Besides, Bogor city, Indonesia Ministry of Communication and Information also held COVID-19 RAPID test for media workers and employees. This action is part of an attempt to break the sequence of coronavirus spread. So, there is a need to develop the ideas related to the appropriate transportation network to support the government's efforts to reduce the spread of COVID-19 reffering to the effectiveness of using drive thru in the previous case. RAPID Test are carried out with the drive-thru system in order to avoid crowds and conform to the coronavirus prevention protocol on physical distancing (Kontan 2020). The drive-thru system is used to prevent greater transmission (Kosasih 2020). Many countries still continue to use the drive-thru system during the increased spread of COVID-19 one of which is Spain. Spain ranks second with the number of positive patients reaching more than 136 thousand and deaths exceeding 13,341 as per Tuesday on 7 April 2020. Facing a growing number of deaths, Spain began to apply the drive-thru system for funerals (LPPM

UM 2020). It inspired us to create concepts following the drive-through system.

2. AUTOMATIC CAR BOX AND MOTOR

Using a drive-thru system to distribute food to people who cannot work from home starting from the middle to lower class workers and medical personnel is a breakthrough. This mode of transport supports the physical distancing efforts being implemented by the government during the COVID-19 pandemic. The designed automatic car box and motorcycle box is used to distribute free food to people who cannot work from home and to medical personnel. Workers or motorists who will distribute the food aids do not need physical contact with the recipients, because they could take the food themselves through the gap/window box.

In general, the difference between a drive-thru system using a motorcycle and a car is on the target customers. The motorbike box is used for small-scale deliveries to homes/residential areas, while car automatic box is used for larger scales such as for medical workers, or people who cannot work from home as seen in Figure 1. The automatic box can be used both for motorbikes and cars. As for motorbikes, the box is placed on the back, fitted with an inner layer that can keep food fresh and is resistant to cold and hot heat. In addition, the box is spacious in order to maintain food condition. The food is put in the package from the back of the box, as shown in Figures 1(a) and 1(b). The rationale for using a motorcycle is to make things easier for the courier to reach densely populated areas. The courier must also follow the protocol in compliance with government guidelines, such as the use of helmets and other protective equipment. Figure 1(c). shows a box in a car. The idea of a car is very much like a motorcycle case, except the scale is greater and could carry more food. The courier will press the button to open the window. People can directly take food through without having physical contact with the courier. The food is hygienic because it is placed in another room. As soon as the food is taken, the new food box will appear automatically.

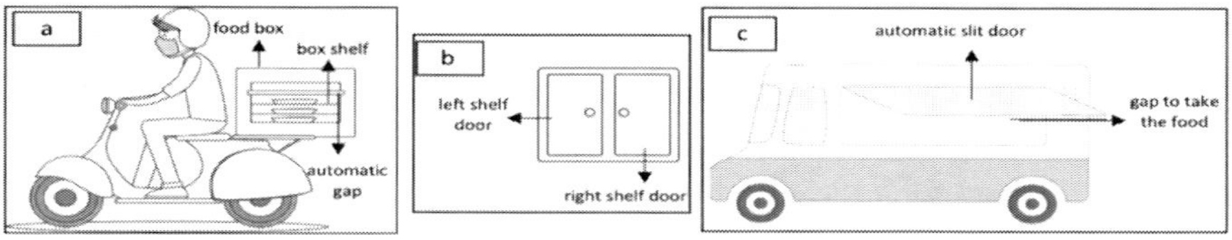

Figure 1. Automatic Drive thru box illustration. Figures (a), (b), and (c) respectively are automatic box illustration drawings on the motor from the "side" direction, from the "back" , and automatic box illustration drawings on the car from the "side" direction.

Knowing that there is a large number of medical personnel who are exhausted and the declining income of people who cannot work from home, then this idea is created in order to help people who cannot work from home by distributing food aids for them. The food is free of charge. We believe that this idea requires feedback and suggestions so the concept would be more effective and efficient. As a result, we conducted an online survey using the Google form targeted at various categories of people.

3. METHOD

The study was conducted online using the Google form on 17 April 2020 from 09:00 a.m. to 15.15 p.m. Forms made in questionnaires and distributed to different groups of people. The questionnaire consisted of questions relating to identity age, educational background, occupation, and the area of residence. It also had questions that matched the data needed to support this concept, as well as a comment section where the respondents could write recommendations.

4. RESULTS AND DISCUSSION

Questionnaire forms distributed through social media and 101 responded to it. Most respondents were in the age range of 16 - 25 years old. In the last education-related questions, more than half of the respondents were high school and undergraduate students. Knowing the respondent's education level was needed to predict their maturity in responding to the questionnaire given. Furthermore, most of the respondents were students, some of the respondents worked as civil servants, employees, and entrepreneurs. On questions related to residential areas, dominant respondents lived in West Java spreading from the city of Bandung, Cianjur regency, Bandung regency, Bekasi regency, Bogor regency, Majalengka regency, Subang regency, Cimahi city, Cirebon city, West Bandung regency, Sukabumi regency, Bekasi city, Bogor city, and Depok city. The respondents also came from outside West Java and Java.

There were 21 questions related to the data needed in developing the concept. On the final question, participants could write suggestions. On questions related to the condition and situation in their area, some respondents responded that the conditions and situation got better because the number of COVID-19 positive patients was less than in other regions. However, there were also respondents who felt that conditions and situations in their area worse because a number of COVID-19 positive patients were rising and many who lived in the Red Zone area still went working, because they had to support their families. On questions related to whether or not many communities around the area could not work from home, we found out that quite a lot of people could not work from home because they were still in the Green Zone area so they still felt safe.

We also found out that there were still quite a lot of people around the respondents who could not work from home such as online motorcycle taxi riders. Respondents' answers related to the question of whether or not the respondents knew about food aids from the government, half of the respondents had already known that the government provided food aids to the community.

On questions related to the equal distribution of food aids organized by the government, most respondents responded that food aids were not evenly distributed. That means not everyone who needed food aids was entitled to receive them.

The next question related to the need for food aids for people who cannot work from home and medical personnel, many respondents stated that food aids for them were needed because the salary that someone earns cannot be measured precisely. It means there were many who earned incomes but worried about what food to bring home for the family. Furthermore, on the question related to whether or not people who could not work from home and medical personnel found it difficult to get food aids, almost half of the respondents stated that food aids were difficult to get, but there were also people who did not know about the difficulty that medical personnel and people who cannot work from home experience in getting the food assistance.

For the question of what assistance needed by people who could not work from home and medical personnel, it was found that the majority of respondents thought they needed personal protective equipment (PPE), masks, and hand sanitizers as seen in Figure 2. We analyzed that people who cannot work from home and medical personnel needed these items because this pandemic requires everyone to be hygienic and clean to protect them from the invisible germs and viruses.

In the beginning, there was a panic buying phenomenon and some people hoarded these items. It can be concluded that this has caused difficulties for people to get PPE, masks, and hand sanitizers during this pandemic.

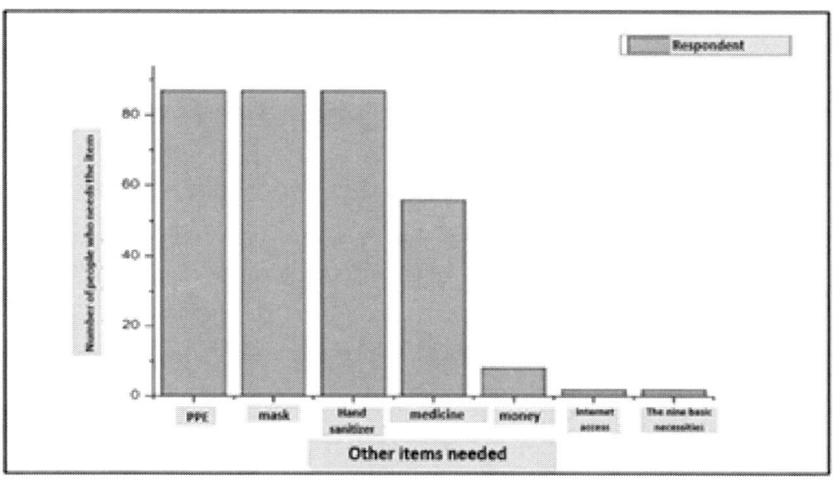

Figure 2. Data on basic needs besides food aids.

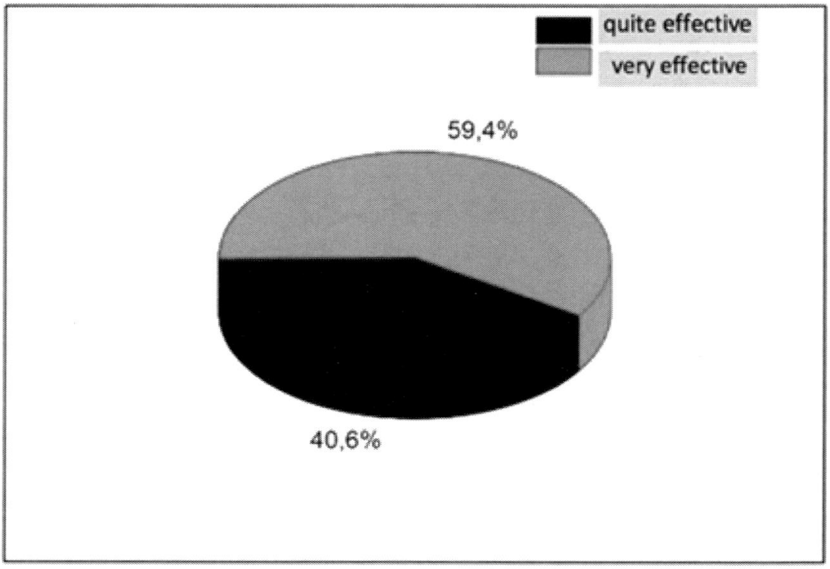

Figure 3. Data on the effectiveness of ideas to be realized by applying physical distancing.

The next question related to the ideas of whether our design could be considered effective in implementing physical distancing, most of the participants answered that it was quite effective and none of them answered ineffective (Figure 3). It can be concluded that this idea could become a breakthrough in implementing physical distancing if it is executed. This idea is considered quite effective because it is quite difficult for people to maintain physical distancing due to urgent needs such as buying basic necessities.

The respondents were then asked to answer whether the government's food aids were given to the right person, and in fact, more than half the number of respondents responded that the government's assistance had not been given to the person who was entitled to receive the aid. The next question, respondents were asked to state certain groups of people who need food aids rather than people who cannot work from homeworkers and medical personnel. Respondents gave suggestions that people who were entitled to receive food aids other than people who cannot work from homeworkers and medical workers were the poor, marginal people, people who had no income, middle-to-lower society, the elderly, traders, private employees, online motorcycle taxi riders, orphans, pedicab drivers, daily laborers, unemployed people, volunteers, workers laid off due to the COVID-19 pandemic, factory workers, farmers, homeless people, orphanages, tutors, beauty workers, homeworkers, overseas students, public transportation drivers, middle and lower workers, administrators at places of worship, and all Indonesian people who are certainly affected by the COVID-19 pandemic.

The next question was asked to the respondent regarding whether or not the respondent knew the difficulties of people who cannot work from home workers and medical personnel in getting food, most of the respondents considered it was not difficult for them to get food. Respondents were also asked to give advice, what staple foods were needed and almost all respondents responded that the staple foods needed were rice, vegetables, side dishes, and fruits. A small number of respondents suggested that other food aids needed also include milk, vitamins, canned foods, and snacks. The next question related to the development of this idea on its effectiveness using a motorcycle, more than half of respondents answered effectively considering this idea prioritizes the principle of physical distancing to break the chain of COVID-19 spread.

Then, the next question related to the costs required whether the production would spend an excessive amount of money, some respondents stated that this idea required quite an excessive amount of money. Moreover, this idea is suspected to cause new problems because there may be a gap between recipients and non-recipients, so respondents are asked to comment on it. Most of the respondents agreed that there would be a gap between recipients and non-recipients, but some respondents believed that if this idea would be implemented in a respectful and equitable way then there would be no issue of social inequality between recipients and those who are not getting aid.

Furthermore, our design would be developed using bio solar as a fuel source. Almost all respondents thought it was possible to implement the use of bio solar, but there are also a small number of respondents who did not respond to this question. The respondents were also asked to address whether there might be hurdles to the distribution of food and to provide examples of what barriers could emerge. Respondents gave examples of obstacles that might occur, including distance, access to the area, road conditions, time, unequal distribution, corruption of food aid, food aid shortages, the goods capacity, physical contact, courier safety, and food delivery concerns exposed to COVID-19.

The last question was about the corruption of food aids which could have been found by respondents. More than half of the respondents had never seen any corruption in food aids committed by any individuals, but there were also respondents who often encountered corruption in food aids. The last data was the feedback where respondents could include ideas, feedback, and expectations that we could use to improve our design to be more effective and productive. The suggestions given by respondents include list of the eligible recipients, the impact on this idea to the community, fairness, and equity on the distribution, safety on the distribution, transparency on the distribution to prevent corruption, coordination with many parties, strict rules for couriers, and involve local community leaders.

CONCLUSION

Our idea is still possible to be implemented although it still needs to be re-examined since there are still many things that need to be considered and developed. This assistance is not only proposed for people who cannot work from homeworkers and medical personnel but is also needed for all people affected by the COVID-19 including middle-to-lower society as well as those who are unable to meet their daily needs. The community also hoped that the assistance provided would also include medical needs, financial assistance, and internet access for students and college students. The respondents also expect that this concept could be properly designed, fairly, on schedule, and uniformly implemented in order to reduce the issues or effects that might be created and would not create additional challenges for the community and would help the efforts of the government to socialize physical distancing.

ACKNOWLEDGMENT

We acknowledged Program Bangdos, Universitas Pendidikan Indonesia for supporting this study.

REFERENCES

Akurat. 2020. "The number of COVID-19 victims is booming, the Spanish government uses the Drive Thru burial technique". *Akurat news*, April 02, 2020. https://akurat.co/news/id-1074852-read-jumlah-korban-covid19-membludak-pemerintah-spanyol-gunakan-teknik-pemakaman-drive-thru.

Anggraeni, S., Maulidina, A., Dewi, M. W, Rahmadianti, S., Rizky, Y. P. C., Arinalhaq, Z. F., Usdiyana, D., Nandiyanto, A. B. D., Al-Obaidi, A. S. M. 2020. "The Deployment of Drones in Sending Drugs and Patient Blood Samples COVID-19". *Indonesian Journal of Science and Technology,* vol. 5, no. 2: 193 - 200.

Azanella, L. A. 2020. "Virus Corona: Penyebab, Gejala, Pencegahan, dan Kapan Harus Segera ke Dokter". ["Corona Virus: Causes, Symptoms, Prevention, and When to See a Doctor Immediately"]. *Kompas.com*, March 31, 2020. https:// www.kompas.com/tren/read/2020/03/31/162000665/virus-corona--penyebab-gejala-pencegahan-dan-kapan-harus-segera-ke-dokter?page=all.

Indraini, A. 2020. "Sedihnya Nasib Pekerja Harian yang Pendapatannya Seret Dibikin Corona" ["The sad fate of daily workers whose income is dragging is made by Corona"]. *Detik.com*, April 03, 2020. https://finance.detik.com/berita-ekonomi-bisnis/d-4963596/sedihnya-nasib-pekerja-harian-yang-pendapatannya-seret-dibikin-corona.

Kontan. 2020. "Kominfo Holds COVID-19 Rapid Test for Media Workers and Employees". *Kontan,* April 09, 2020. https://pressrelease.kontan.co.id/release/kominfo-gelar-rapid-test-covid-19-untuk-pekerja-media-dan-pegawai.

Kosasih. 2020. "Use the Drive Thru System, This is the Appearance of the Corona COVID-19 Test in Bogor". *Liputan6.com*, March 29, 2020. https://www.liputan6.com/otomotif/read/4213636/gunakan-sistem-drive-thru-ini-penampakan-tes-corona-covid-19-di-bogor.

Lesmana, A. S. 2020. "Corona Nurse Sincerity: Work Getting Heavier, Night Shif Cannot Eat". *Banten Suara*, March 26, 2020. https://banten.suara.com/read/2020/03/26/151135/keikhlasan-perawat-corona-kerja-makin-berat-shif-malam-tak-dapat-makan?page=all.

LP2M UM. 2018. *Panduan Pembuatan Book Chapter UM.* [*Guideline to make Book Chapter UM*]. http://lp2m.um.ac.id/panduan-pembuatan-msopen-book-chapter-um/.

Maryanti, R., Hufad, A., Sunardi., Nandiyanto, A. B. D. and Al-Obaidi, S. M. 2020. "Understanding COVID-19 particle contagion through aerosol droplets for students with special needs". *Journal of Engineering Science and Technology,* vol. 15, no. 3:1909 - 1920.

Media Indonesia. 2020. "Atasi Dampak Covid-19, Ojek Online Dapat Bantuan Makanan". *Media Indonesia*, April 02, 2020. [Overcoming the Impact of Covid-19, Online Ojek Get Food Aid]. *Media Indonesia*, April 02, 2020. https://mediaindonesia.com/read/detail/300850-atasi-dampak-covid-19-ojek-online-dapat-bantuan-makanan.

Putra, Z. A. and Abidin, S. A. Z. 2020. "Application of SEIR Model in COVID-19 and the Effect of Lockdown on Reducing the Number of Active Cases". *Indonesian Journal of Science and Technology,* vol. 5, no. 2:185 - 192.

SeRiau. 2020. "Medical personnel not only need PPE, but also adequate nutrition, Kartini: PPE is necessary but nutrition is also considered". *SeRiau,* March 31, 2020. http://seriau.com/mobile/detailberita/36517/parlemen/DRPD-Pekanbaru/tenaga-medis-tidak-hanya-butuh-apd-tapi-juga-gizi-yang-memadai--kartini--apd-perlu-tapi-gizi-di-perhatikan-juga-.

Wardani, K, D. and Rumiyatun. 2017. "The Influence of Taxpayer Knowledge, Taxpayer Awareness, Motor Vehicle Tax Sanctions, and the Samsat Drive Thru System on Motor Vehicle Taxpayer Compliance". *Jurnal Akuntansi,* vol. 5, no. 1: 15 - 24.

World Health Organization. 2020. *Q&A on coronaviruses (COVID-19).* https://www.who.int/bulletin/online_first/COVID-19/en/.

In: COVID-19 ISBN: 978-1-53618-903-2
Editors: A. B. D. Nandiyanto et al.

Chapter 24

MOBILE FOOD TRUCK TO ASSIST PEOPLE'S FOOD FULFILLMENT DURING THE COVID-19 PANDEMIC IN THE LARGE-SCALE SOCIAL RESTRICTIONS AREA

Wafa Raihanah Arwa[1], Muhammad Rayhan Fadillah[1], Nabila Nurul Anisa Az Zahra[1], Imam Imadudin[1], Sri Anggraeni[1] and Asnul Dahar Minghat[2]

[1]Fakultas Pendidikan Ilmu Pengetahuan Alam, Universitas Pendidikan Indonesia, Bandung, Jawa Barat, Indonesia

[2]Razak Faculty of Technology and Informatics, Universiti Teknologi Malaysia, Skudai, Johor, Malaysia

ABSTRACT

The health crisis is happening in the world today because the number of infected people with coronavirus disease 2019 (COVID-19) continues to grow day by day. This happens because the virus that infects the respiratory system spreads rapidly. COVID-19 is transmitted by a droplet of an infected person. The world currently applies a social distancing to prevent the transmission of the COVID-19, including Indonesia. However, social distancing has impacted the economy, especially on the food access problem. Therefore, we carried out research aimed at developing ideas related to transportation systems for food fulfillment during the COVID-19 pandemic, which is the provision of Mobile Food Trucks. This research conducted using a quantitative method with a technique method of a survey by filling out the questionnaire online through the Google form application. The survey was responded by 259 respondents from the provinces of Banten, Jakarta, and West Java. The results of this study indicate that society indeed has difficulty in fulfilling its basic food needs in the middle of the pandemic due to the implementation of social distancing. The basic food fulfillment facilities currently available also do not fully fulfill the needs of the community. Besides, the survey results also showed that the public responded well to the idea of this Mobile Food Truck.

Keywords: COVID-19, food truck, social distancing, transportation system

1. Introduction

A mysterious case of pneumonia has reported in Wuhan, China, at the end of December 2019. A few days later, the virus that caused this disease has been identified and called coronavirus novel. (Anggraeni et al. 2020; Mulyanti et al. 2020). Corona virus is a type of virus that originates from animals and can infect the human body. This virus is very dangerous because it can cause death (Maryanti et al. 2020). This virus enters the human body through the nose or mouth and is transmitted through droplets. Data shows 66% of patients are related to a seafood market in Wuhan, Hubei Province of China (Huang et al. 2020). Recently, World Health Organization (WHO) has named this disease as coronavirus disease 2019 (COVID-19) (Perhimpunan Dokter Paru Indonesia 2020; Razon 2020).

Indonesia is one of the countries with a high spread of COVID-19. Quoted from the JHU Research Center website, Indonesia is among the countries with the highest spread of the COVID-19 in Southeast Asia with 5,923 infected cases as of April 17, 2020 (Johns Hopkins Coronavirus

Resource Center 2020). The spread of the COVID-19 has led to many new policies made by the government. One of them is the regional quarantine policy which can help reduce the spread of the COVID-19. According to the European Centre for Disease Prevention and Control (ECDC), social distancing needs to be conducted because the COVID-19 is likely to spread through aerosols (Eurosurveillance Editorial Team 2020). Besides, social distancing is carried out to minimize the spread of the COVID-19 from infected to non-infected and aims to reduce the need for the health system. Besides, social distancing is the most effective treatment for those vulnerable to infection (Pfattheicher et al. 2020, Maryanti et al. 2020). According to WHO in the Interim guidance issued on March 19, 2020, quarantine during the initial outbreak can slow the peak of the epidemic (World Health Organization 2020).

In Indonesia, regional quarantine has been implemented in several regions. Especially for regions with a high number of infected cases, such as Jakarta and West Java provinces, which have implemented Large-Scale Social Restrictions (LSSR) system for their residents. LSSR which is carried out as a social distancing movement does have a positive impact, that is, reducing the mobility of the community or helping to carry out social distancing to reduce the possibility of the spread of the COVID-19. However, social distancing also has significant social and economic impacts (Dalton et al. 2020). The economy can become unstable amid this pandemic situation (Center for Food Safety and Applied Nutrition 2020). These things certainly happen because of the limitation of community activities, this is what then moved us to make a breakthrough in the transportation system during the COVID-19 pandemic to facilitate access for the community. The breakthrough that we made was supported by the state of the community during the COVID-19 pandemic which required to stay at home since activities outside the home were limited.

People certainly needs to fulfill their basic needs, especially food fulfillment. The current conditions are quite impossible for people to go out routinely to fulfill their food needs because markets are usually visited by many people. Therefore, U. S. Food and Drug Administration in their article entitled Food Safety and the COVID-19 stated that we must follow four key steps for food safety which are clean, separate, cook, and chill to prevent foodborne diseases (Center for Food Safety and Applied Nutrition 2020; Machmud and Minghat 2020). Referring to the conditions mentioned earlier, we are trying to make a breakthrough or a new idea in the transportation system that makes it easier for people to fulfill their food during the COVID-19 pandemic.

2. Idea Development

People need to fulfill their daily basic food needs; however, it is quite difficult to do during the COVID-19 pandemic. We developed a transportation idea during the COVID-19 pandemic named a Mobile Food Truck to assist people to provide food fulfillment during the COVID-19 pandemic in the LSSR areas in Indonesia. The idea of a Mobile Food Truck is the provision of transportation to help the implementation of social distancing where this truck will sell the needs of the basic food. This food truck will operate from house to house so that people can access food and also the foods are sold easily. This food truck operates from house to house in order to avoid direct contact with many people and minimize trading in the market. The basic foods sold are also obtained from market traders so

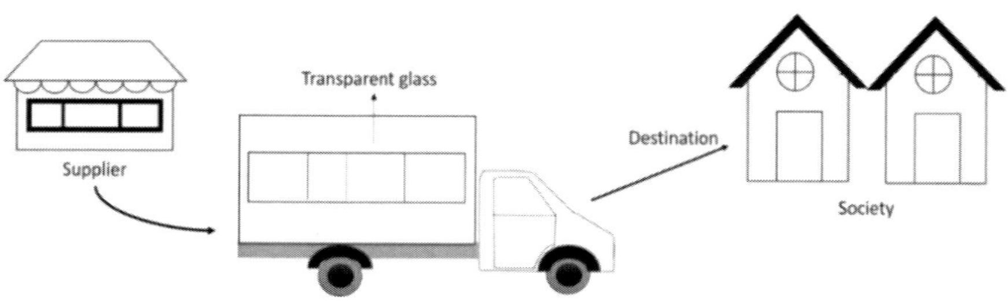

Figure 1. The illustration of Food Truck Idea.

that it can become a consideration for traders to participate in the success of LSSR. Basic foods that are sold in a food truck will not be touched directly by the buyer, the buyer only mentions items they want to buy and the seller will pick it up for the buyer. The buyer can also choose by pointing the desired items through the transparent glass on the Mobile Food Truck (Figure 1).

3. METHOD

We conducted a study on April 17, 2020, as a review to develop our ideas. We used quantitative data collection methods with a technique method of online surveys and questionnaire using the Google form application that contains several questions arranged according to the theme with several answer options. The data obtained then processed as a data source that could help in the development of our ideas. The questionnaire was distributed specifically in the provinces of Banten, Jakarta, and West Java in areas in the three provinces with a high COVID-19 case.

4. RESULT AND DISCUSSION

The total participants in this study using Google form were 259 participants, dominated by female participants. Participants who participated in filling this questionnaire were mostly in the age range of 16-20 years (see Figure 2(a)), and they are students. In addition, some participants were housewives and other occupations, as shown in Figure 3(b).

Most of the participants came from regions in Banten province, followed by participants from regions in West Java Province and participants from Jakarta Province. The distribution of participants' residence is presented in Figure 3. From the personal data filled in the questionnaire distributed via Google form, it could be concluded that most participants came from among students from the regions of Banten, Jakarta, and West Java Provinces.

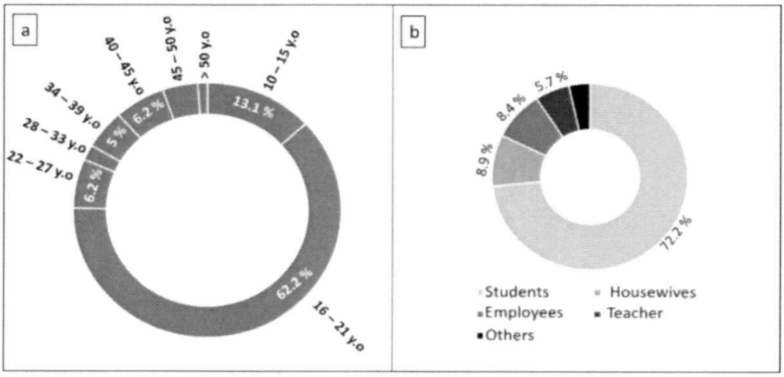

Figure 2. (a) Participants age and (b) participants status.

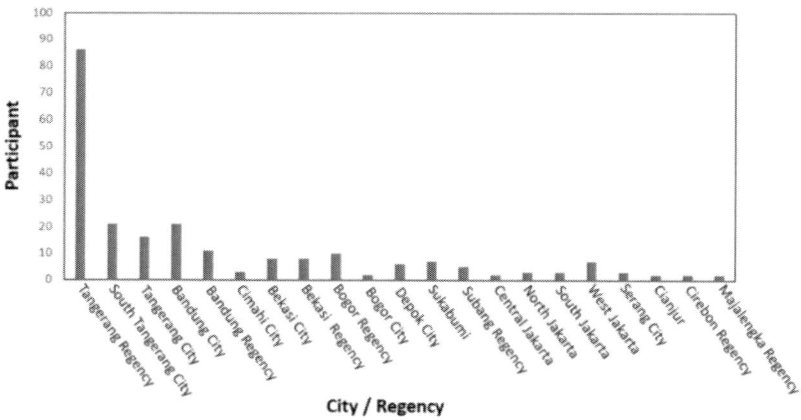

Figure 3. The Distribution of Participants Residence.

There were twenty questions asked to the participants relating to the COVID-19 pandemic which then led to the theme of our study. From the questions filled in by the participants, different results were obtained. Based on survey data, almost all of the participants have known and understood physical/social distancing. Survey results showed that participants were people from areas where LSSR implemented. From the data obtained it could be concluded that the average community residing in the area of the implementation of the LSSR has known and understood about physical/social distancing which is the key to the implementation of the LSSR itself.

In this survey, we presented questions related to our ideas which would later be able to support the development of our ideas. We included questions related to the fulfillment of basic food needs in participants' respective home areas during the COVID-19 pandemic. Survey data showed that most participants had no difficulty getting food during social distancing (see Figure 4(a)). The participants were the people who fulfilled their basic needs (mainly basic food needs) by going to markets and supermarkets. Then, although social distancing had been applied, most participants still went to the market occasionally, even some participants still routinely went to the market as shown in Figure 4(b).

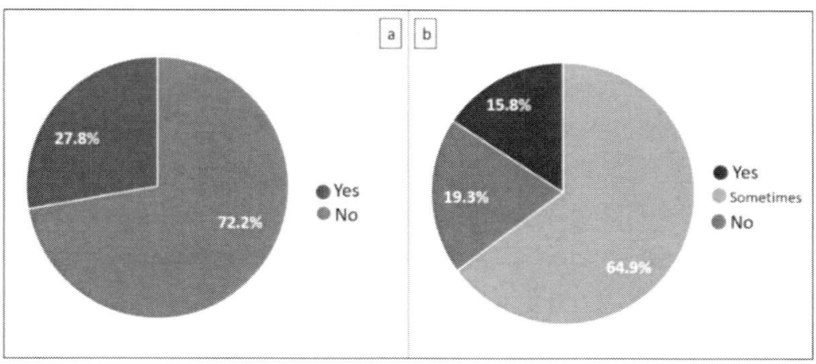

Figure 4. (a) Participants difficulties in fulfilling food and (b) intensity of participants going to the market.

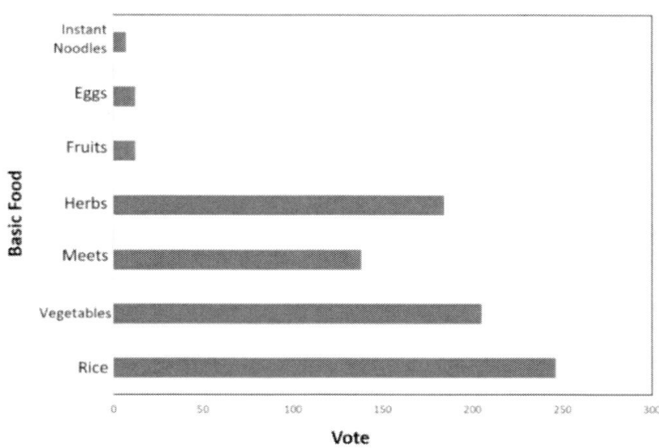

Figure 5. Participants basic food needs.

The types of the most needed basic food during the COVID-19 pandemic according to the survey results are presented in Figure 5. Participants could choose more than one option provided and rice was the most needed basic food according to the participants' choices, followed by vegetables, herbs, and other basic food needs.

Although many participants still went to the market, most participants admitted that there was fear of going to the market during this pandemic. Most participants also admitted that it was not conducive to go to the market in the middle of this pandemic. Almost all participants were concerned about physical contact with many people when they were going to the market. Participants were also worried about food conditions that were openly displayed in the markets and had direct contact with many people (see Figure 6(a)). The market situation in the residence of most participants has slightly reduced visitors although it was still categorized as a crowded condition. Besides, participants responded to some difficulties in meeting basic food needs during the COVID-19 pandemic. One of the main difficulties was because some traders closed their shops, which then led to difficulties in fulfilling other basic food needs encountered by participants. Therefore, it could be stated that the implementation of social distancing, or in general the implementation of the LSSR in the residence of the participants are related to one another. Other than that, there were other difficulty factors explained by the participants, i.e., the lack of public transportation, supplies that were running out (especially in stores), and some of the participants explained because of the fear of leaving their houses as shown in Figure 6(b).

Figure 7 shows the fulfillment of the basic foods of the participants if they did not go to the market. They mostly bought basic food needs at a shop near their homes. Besides, participants also chose delivery and waiting for peddlers as an option to fulfill other basic food needs. However, according to more than half of the participants, options such as food shops near houses and peddlers could not fulfill all the basic food needs of participants. Delivery options also could not fully help in fulfilling the participant's basic food needs, because according to the participant's explanation some shops did not have delivery services, making it difficult for participants to access.

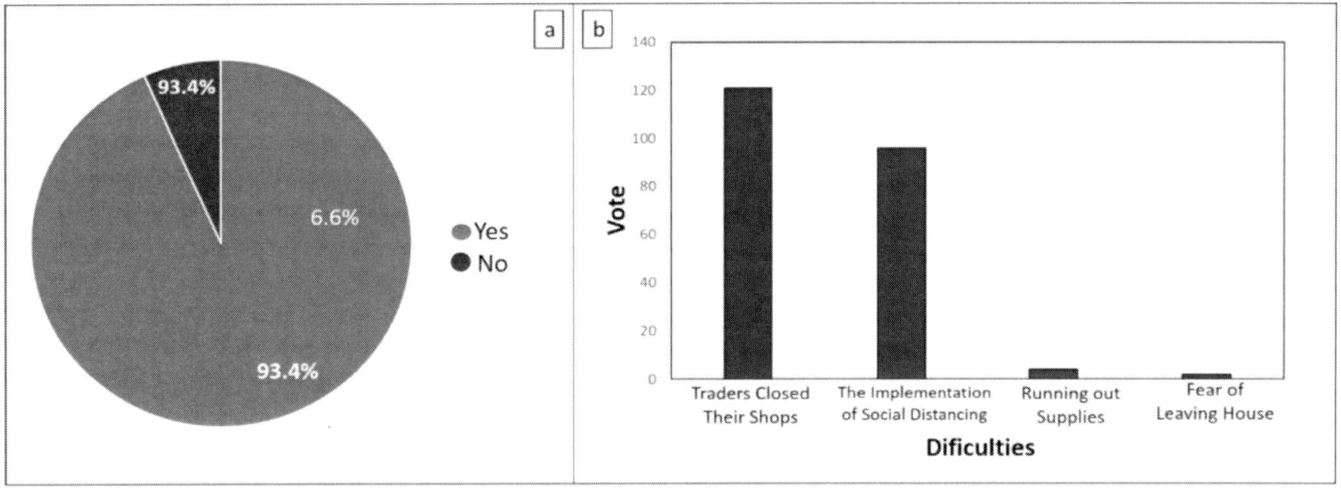

Figure 6. (a) Percentage of participants concerns about physical contact and (b) participants difficulties in the fulfillment of basic food.

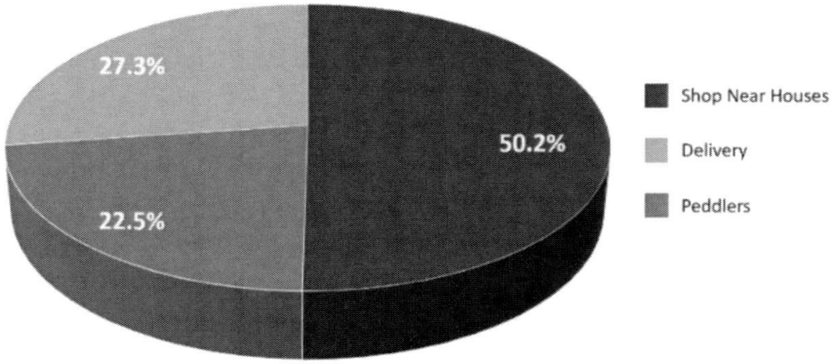

Figure 7. Sources of the food fulfillment if participants did not go to the market.

Some participants also explained that it was not uncommon for participants to have stored food supplies at home. However, afterward, the data was obtained that most participants felt worried that some of the stored food supplies were no longer fresh and would be stale and then wasted.

Delivery and peddlers were the options of the fulfillment of basic food needs during this pandemic that were mostly chosen by participants. The data obtained also showed that participants responded well that delivery and peddlers helped fulfill food during the COVID-19 pandemic. Some participants also responded related to peddlers, the intensity of peddlers in the participants' residence was reduced during this pandemic. Besides, from the survey data, it was found that most participants were worried about the food conditions that peddlers sold were openly displayed.

In this questionnaire, we included several questions that were directly related to the ideas we had in order to see the communities' response to our idea. The data obtained from these questions could later be used as suggestions/input. We presented our ideas related to the transportation system during this pandemic. Most of the participants responded well to our idea by assuming that this food truck idea could be a solution to reduce the difficulty of the community in accessing food during LSSR. Participants also responded that the most appropriate time for a food truck to operate in areas affected by LSSR was in the morning and operated three times a week.

Conclusion

From all the survey data obtained, it could be concluded that the community indeed experienced difficulties in fulfilling basic needs during this pandemic. The problem in fulfilling food at the current pandemic is due to the limitation of citizens' activities with the implementation of LSSR in some areas. Facilities to fulfill basic food needs such as peddlers, food shops close to community houses also have shortcomings, that is, not all basic food needs could be obtained from these facilities because the citizens usually buy more complete basic foods by going to the market. The community's concern to leave the house and the condition of food that is displayed openly is also a problem. Food that is left open is feared to be contaminated by COVID-19. Then, judging from the participants' situation and response, the idea of a Mobile Food Truck that transports basic food could be a solution to the fulfillment of the needs of the basic food of the community during the COVID-19 pandemic, mainly in the area where the LSSR is implemented.

Acknowledgments

Bangdos, Universitas Pendidikan Indonesia is acknowledged.

References

Anggraeni, S., Maulidina, A., Dewi, M. W., Rahmadianti, S., Rizky, Y. P. C., Arinalhaq, Z. F., Usdiyana, D., Nandiyanto, A. B. D., and Al-Obaidi, A. S. M. 2020. "The Deployment of Drones in Sending Drugs and Patient Blood Samples COVID-19." *Indonesian Journal of Science and Technology* vol. 5, no. 2: 193-200.

Center for Food Safety and Applied Nutrition. 2020. "Food Safety and the Coronavirus Disease 2019 (COVID-19)." www.fda.gov/food/food-safety-during-emergencies/food-safety-and-coronavirus-disease-2019-COVID-19.

Dalton, C., Corbett, S., and Katelaris, A. 2020. Dalton, Craig B., Stephen J. Corbett, and Anthea L. Katelaris. "Pre-emptive low cost social distancing and enhanced hygiene implemented before local COVID-19 transmission could decrease the number and severity of cases." *The Medical Journal of Australia* vol. 212, no. 10: 1-10.

Eurosurveillance Editorial Team. 2020. "Updated rapid risk assessment from ECDC on the novel coronavirus disease 2019 (COVID-19) pandemic: increased transmission in the EU/EEA and the UK." *Eurosurveillance* vol. 25, no. 10. doi: 10.2807/1560-7917.ES.2020.25.10.2003121.

Huang, C., Wang, Y., Li, X., Ren, L., Zhao, J., Hu, Y., Zhang, L., Fan, G., Xu, J., Gu, X., Cheng, Z., Yu, T., Xia., Z., Wei, Y.,Wu, W., Xie X., Yin, W., Li, H., and Cao, B. 2020. Clinical features of patients infected with 2019 novel coronavirus in Wuhan, China. *The Lancet* vol. 395, no 10223: 497-506.

Johns Hopkins Coronavirus Resource Center. 2020. *Johns Hopkins experts in global public health, infectious disease, and emergency preparedness have been at the forefront of the international response to COVID-19.* https://coronavirus.jhu.edu/map.html.

Machmud, A., and Minghat, A. D. B. 2020. "The Price Dynamics of Hand Sanitizers for COVID-19 in Indonesia: Exponential and Cobweb Forms. *Indonesian Journal of Science & Technology* vol. 5, no. 2: 176-184.

Maryanti, R, Hufad, A, Sunardi, Nandiyanto, A. B. D, Manullang, T. I. B. 2020. "Understanding Coronavirus (COVID-19) as a Small Particle to Students with Special Needs." *Horizon* vol. 2, no. 1: 121-130.

McKibbin, W. J., and Fernando, R. 2020. "The global macroeconomic impacts of COVID-19: Seven scenarios." Centre for Applied Macroeconomic Analysis vol. 19, no. 2020: 1-45.

Mulyanti, B., Purnama, W., and Parwinanto, R. E. 2020. "Distance Learning in Vocational High Schools during the COVID-19 Pandemic in West Java Province, Indonesia." *Indonesian Journal of Science and Technology* vol. 5, 271-282.

Perhimpunan Dokter Paru Indonesia. 2020. *Panduan Praktik Klinis: Pneumonia 2019-nCoV* [*Clinical Practice Guide: 2019-nCoV Pneumonia*]. PDPI: Jakarta. https://klikpdpi.com/bukupdpi/wp-content/uploads/2020/04/C-PPK-Pneumonia-COVID-19-dengan-komplikasi-3.pdf.

Pfattheicher, S., Nockur, L., Böhm, R., Sassenrath, C., and Petersen, M. B. 2020." The emotional path to action: Empathy promotes physical distancing during the COVID-19 pandemic." *Psyarxiv Preprint* vol. 3, no. 2020. https://psyarxiv.com/y2cg5/.

Razon, B. C. 2020. "COVID 19: Impetus for "Community Spirits" among Filipinos." *Indonesian Journal of Science and Technology* vol. 5, no. 2: 201-208.

World Health Organization. 2020. *Considerations for quarantine of individuals in the context of containment for coronavirus disease (COVID-19): interim guidance*, 19 March 2020. ttps://apps.who.int/iris/handle/10665/331497?localeattribute=ar&fbclid=IwAR10FZIeAe8pzRBvZNc8MJB9lnOtJvCLV5lZQmPC2pKBHKYyJbaXSxloIrA.

In: COVID-19 ISBN: 978-1-53618-903-2
Editors: A. B. D. Nandiyanto et al.

Chapter 25

MINI HELICOPTER AS DISINFECTANT SPRAYER (HYPOCHLOROUS ACID)

***Aulia Rachmah*[1], *Fauzia Utami Malik*[1], *Rully Ilham Pratama*[1], *Shalma Nurlatifah*[1], *Sri Anggraeni*[1] and *Asnul Dahar Minghat*[2]**

[1]Fakultas Pendidikan Matematika dan Ilmu Pengetahuan Alam, Universitas Pendidikan Indonesia, Bandung, Jawa Barat, Indonesia
[2]Razak Faculty of Technology and Informatics, Universiti Teknologi Malaysia, Skudai, Johor, Malaysia

ABSTRACT

This research was conducted as an effort to reduce the spread of coronavirus disease 2019 (COVID-19). One of the efforts here is in the form of an idea to spray disinfectant using a mini helicopter. The background of this research is from the fact that current prevention of COVID-19 the spread conducted is still considered to be less effective. Although the government has now appealed for social distancing, there are still many people who do not understand the urgency of social distancing so that the number of COVID-19 cases continues to grow. Spraying disinfectants is also very necessary to eliminate viruses that stick to objects and viruses that are still airborne. Researchers have an alternative idea to spray hypochlorous acid periodically using a mini helicopter. This research was conducted using a survey method with the help of google form media. Based on the survey results, the research subjects argued that social distancing and spraying disinfectants became effective ways to prevent the spread of COVID-19. More than half of the research subjects stated that the idea of developing a mini helicopter for spraying disinfectants is possible to prevent the spread of COVID-19. The priority area for spraying according to research subjects is the COVID-19 the red zone area.

Keywords: disinfectant, hypochlorus acid, mini helicopter, social distancing, the spread of COVID-19

1. Introduction

Coronavirus is a type of virus from the corona viridae family that can infect the respiratory system both humans and animals. This virus is more commonly found in animals. The coronavirus was first identified in the 1960s. It was named Corona because of its body structure that looked like a crown (Verizarie 2020). The disease caused due to being infected with this virus is called COVID-19 (Maryanti et al. 2020). Coronavirus can cause mild disturbances to the respiratory system, severe lung infections, also death. This virus can affect anyone, both infants, children, adults, the elderly, pregnant women, and nursing mothers. This virus was first discovered in Wuhan city, China, at the end of December 2019 (Anggraeni et al. 2020). The virus is transmitted very quickly and has spread to almost all countries, including Indonesia, in just a few months (Merry 2020; Hasyim et al. 2020).

In March 2020, in Depok, Indonesia, there were two people affected by this disease. Then the spread was so fast that on 18 April 2020 there were positive cases of 19,248 people, 535 people died and 631 people were cured. The initial prevention steps set by the government to encourage people to work, worship, and study at home (BBC News 2020). It was quite effective to reduce mass gatherings. The next step is using a mask when leaving the house, washing hands with flowing water, maintaining physical endurance, and spraying disinfectants (Kevin 2005). Disinfectant in the medical view is a compound to prevent infection by destroying or dissolving pathogenic microorganisms by being imposed on non-living tissue such as operating rooms, operating instruments/medical devices, etc. In another sense, it kills germs, bacteria, and also viruses by destroying or dissolving them. This disinfectant is used in non-living tissues, such as equipment/rooms that want to be sterilized so that the disinfectant is currently used to sterilize rooms or other facilities (Vembi 2020).

Disinfection is prevention of various types of dangerous organisms, both viruses, bacteria, and fungi that can cause disease transmission. Spraying disinfectant is done to the aforementioned (Fathiyah 2020). Spraying disinfectants is often used on a person's body and WHO (World Health Organization) says disinfectants are dangerous if sprayed on the human body (Achmad 2020). Disinfectants that are sprayed on the body automatically will have accumulated harmful particles that are inhaled and enter the respiratory tract, either from detergents or alcohol (Aris 2020).

We developed ideas related to the transportation system to reduce the spread of COVID-19 in regions in Indonesia using mini helicopters. This idea still requires data from the Indonesian people, so we distributed questionnaires about our ideas for research purposes. It is hoped that this idea can be developed and be able to assist Indonesian people in preventing the spread of COVID-19. Our idea is to spray disinfectants using mini helicopters that can be used indoors or outdoors. This mini helicopter is equipped with a camera so that it can be controlled remotely. Spraying disinfectant not only by land but also through the air, this is done so that prevention of the spread of COVID-19 is more effective (Nanda 2020).

2. Method

The method used in this study was a quantitative method based on questionnaires. This questionnaire was designed in such a way and distributed to Indonesian territory through social media so that data and information from the Indonesian people would be obtained. Questionnaires are data collection techniques that contain written questions to get responses from respondents. The data collected used as a reference in developing our ideas.

Our idea making a mini helicopter to spray disinfectant which is presented in Figure 1. This mini helicopter is small (mini), so it can be used indoors or outdoors. In the mini helicopter, there is a camera to see the surroundings, so it can be seen whether the situation is safe or not for spraying (Figure 2(a)). The mini helicopter is also driven by a remote control where the remote is controlled (Figure 2(b)). This helicopter also has a disinfectant liquid container and a tool for spraying the disinfectant. Spraying disinfectant could be easier especially at tall buildings using this mini helicopter.

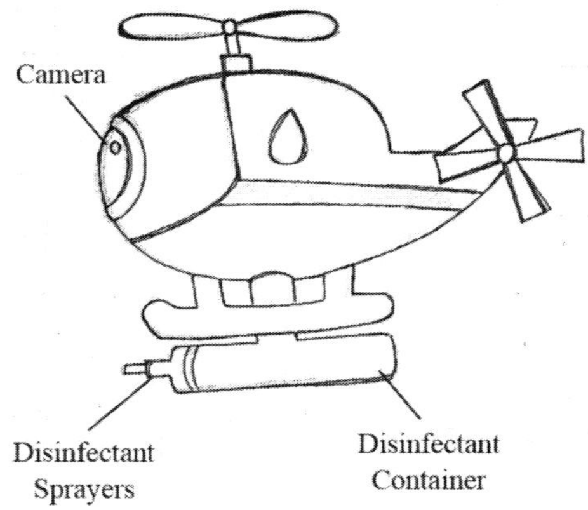

Figure 1. Mini helicopter as disinfectant sprayer.

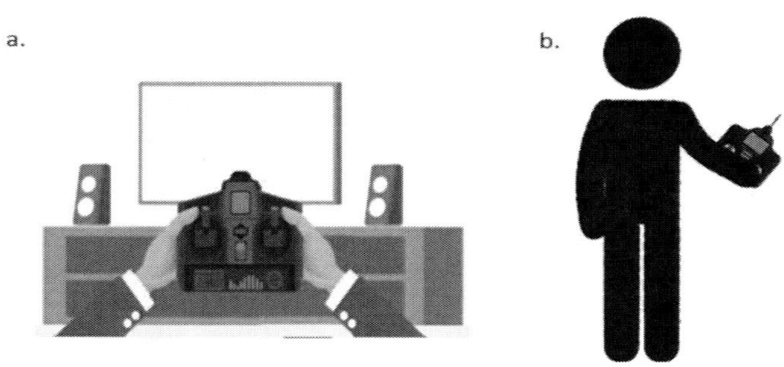

Figure 2. The situation around the helicopter can be seen through a monitor (a), the mini helicopter is also driven by a remote control (b).

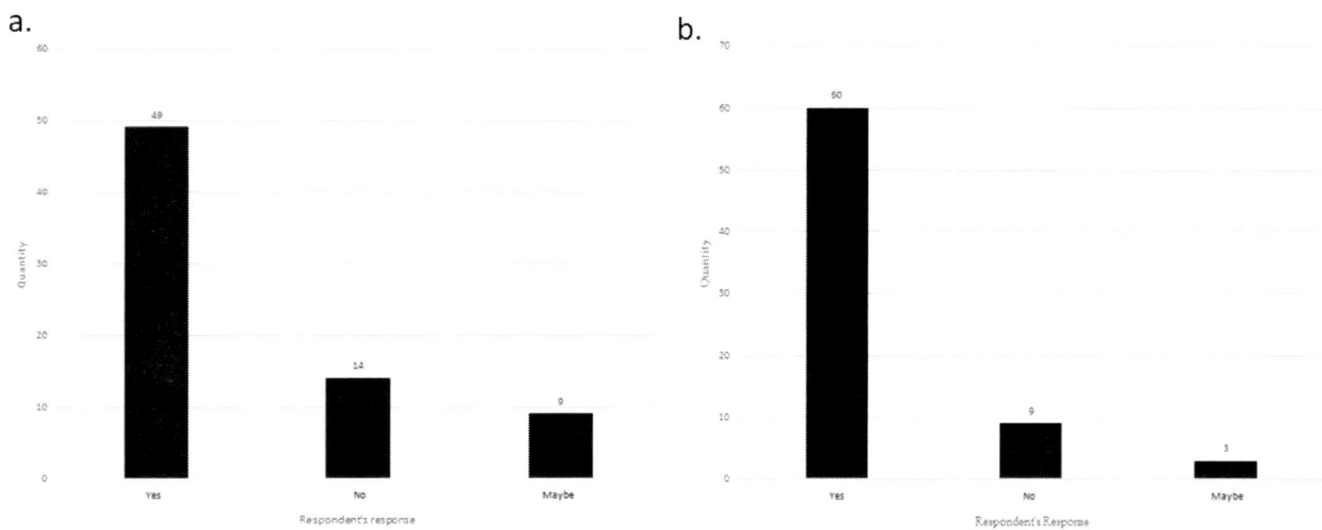

Figure 3. Spraying disinfectant is effective to prevent the spread of COVID-19 (a), it is necessary to spray in each area (b).

3. Results and Discussion

Based on data from 72 respondents on the questionnaire form that distributes, this idea is possible to be implemented. However, this idea has not been completely perfect. From this idea, we still have to consider other things. Most people believed that spraying disinfectants effectively reduces COVID-19 (Figure 3(a)). Spraying disinfectant was considered effective to prevent the spread of this virus because according to Juan Leon, a health scientist from Emory University, coronavirus is a virus that is covered with a protective fat layer which when exposed to disinfectants, the fat layer of the virus can be torn apart and make the virus weakened. Therefore, the use of disinfectants is recommended by a lot of scientists, especially to clean the surface of objects that are often touched by humans.

Spraying disinfectant in each area is needed to reduce the spread of COVID-19 (Figure 3(b)). Spraying of disinfectants is also done in places that have been visited by people with COVID-19. Spraying is conducted in an area where there is an indication that the patients exposed to COVID-19.

Meanwhile, spraying is also important in areas that have not been indicated by patients exposed to COVID-19 to reduce the spread of COVID-19.

The liquid used in spraying disinfectant is indeed safe and can reduce the spread of COVID-19 (Figure 4(a)). The disinfectant liquid is pulverizer at the right target, like at home, and the objects. It is not to be sprayed directly on a person's body because it can risk a person's health. Spraying disinfectant is done around the house (Figure 2(b)). The main priority in spraying this disinfectant is the object around the house. The part that needs to be sterilized is every surface of objects such as on door handles, toilets, and sinks. WHO does not recommend spraying disinfectants directly into the human body because it is dangerous. Alcohol or chlorine that is sprayer on the human body will not kill the virus that has entered the body but can be harmful if the alcohol and chlorine that is sprayed, are exposed to clothing or mucous membranes such as the mouth and eyes.

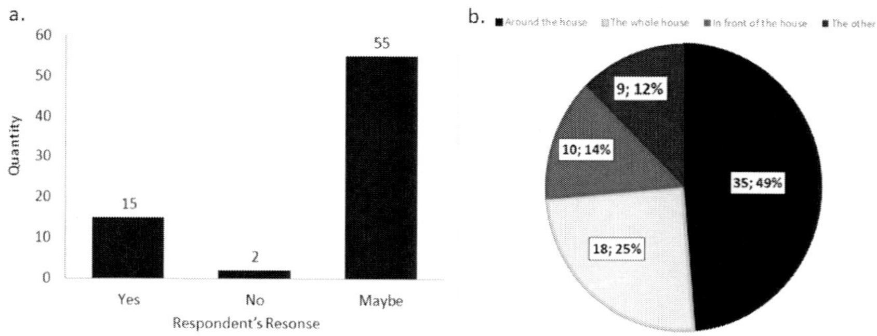

Figure 4. Disinfectant liquid is safe (a), and the part of the house that should be sprayed (b).

In the midst of this pandemic, a lot of Indonesian people have tried to anticipate the spread of COVID-19. Their efforts are like finding out or increasing knowledge about COVID-19 and ways to protect themselves from being infected by the virus. Many Indonesians already know how to make their own disinfectant liquid (Figure 5(a)). General knowledge about making disinfectants is certainly very useful for dealing with the current situation. Society can make their own forms of prevention without having to wait for government service. Therefore, this kind of knowledge is very important for our own good.

However, many people are still unsure about the safety of self-made disinfectants (Figure 5(b)). The public is also not entirely convinced that self-made disinfectants are effective in preventing the spread of COVID-19. This is because they do not know the ingredients that can be used to make disinfectants.

Regarding our idea of making a mini helicopter to help spray disinfectants in various regions, the results said that our idea could be implemented (Figure 6(a)). As if we implemented our idea in making this mini helicopter for spraying the disinfectant, around 56.90% of the survey results were willing to use it, while 31.90% of them still did not know whether they would use it, and the rest said they would not use it Figure 6(b)).

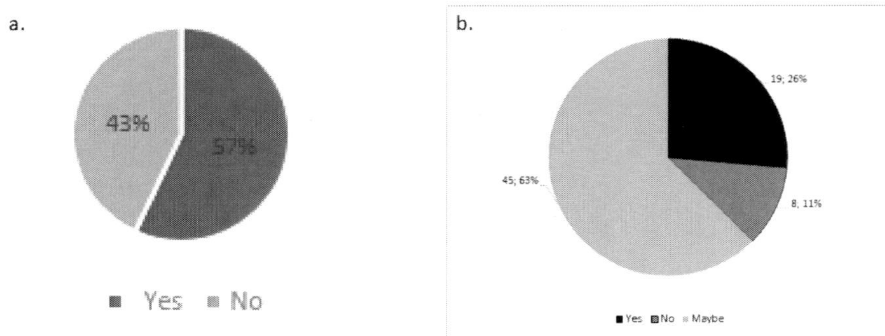

Figure 5. Lot of people can already make their own disinfectant (a), but there are still many who are not sure of the safety and effectiveness of the disinfectant that is made by themselves (b).

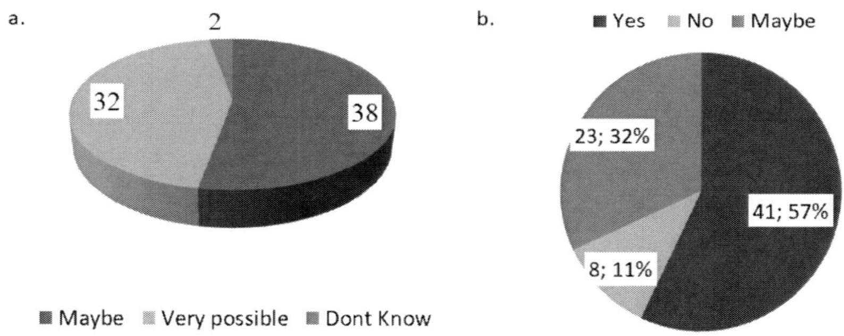

Figure 6. It is possible to develop mini helicopters for spraying disinfectants (a), and many people are willing to use mini helicopters to spray disinfectants (b).

Policies emerge due to the coronavirus outbreak can be seen with the closure of several access roads in a certain time, limitation on the amount of transportation, limitation on operating hours of transportation, which of course the policy is intended to be able to restrain the rate of society out of the house (Yunus and Rezki 2020). There are limitations to leave the house, therefore, the use of mini helicopters made unmanned to spray disinfectant on buildings and roads to reduce the spread of the COVID-19. This mini helicopter could be controlled from inside the building so that it still adheres to the government's recommendations to stay at home and reduce activities outside the home.

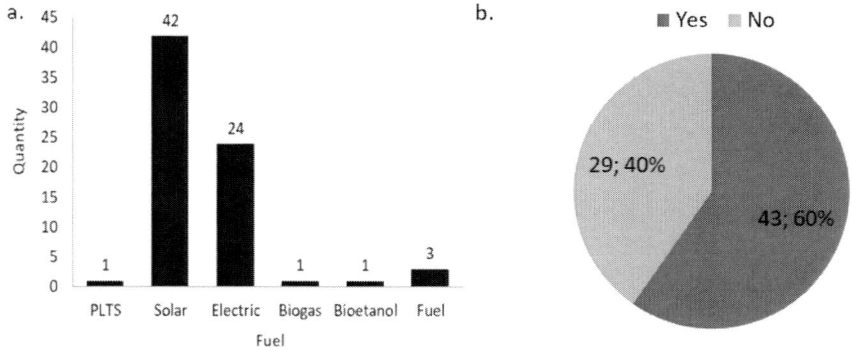

Figure 7. fuel that should be used for mini helicopters (a). effective hypochlorous acid (b).

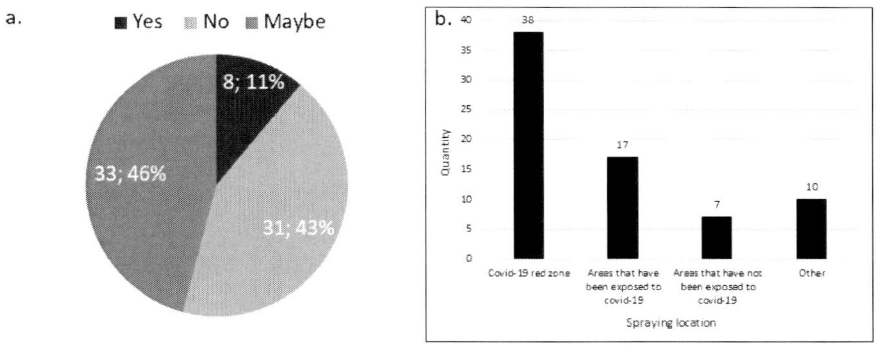

Figure 8. Effective or not spraying disinfectant through the air (a). effective parts for spraying disinfectant (b).

Based on the survey, around 42 people (58.30%) said that the fuel that should be used for this mini helicopter is solar power (Figure 7(a)), while others stated it would be better to use electricity. Another opinion said that we could use bioethanol or biogas fuel. It was suggested in order to maintain the environment and not adding a problem to the existing pollution. Hypochlorous acid can oxidize bacteria and other microorganisms in seconds and one of them is the coronavirus. Hypochlorous acid has anti-microbial, anti-inflammatory, and can also kill E. coli bacteria in just 12 seconds. So, 59.70% of them said that spraying disinfectants using hypochlorous acid was an effective step in reducing the spread of COVID-19 (Figure 7(b)). But there are still people who do not know the benefits and functions of these fluids. There are still some people who consider that the liquid is not effective in preventing the spread of the COVID-19. In fact, by spraying the liquid, it could prevent the spread of COVID-19.

Most people assume that spraying disinfectant through the air is still ineffective, also they still doubt whether spraying disinfectant would be effective (Figure 8(a)). The reasons are misconduct during the process which can endanger public safety. Therefore, when someone is spraying disinfectant through the air, it means that person must know the procedures. Spraying disinfectants is one step in preventing the spread of COVID-19, therefore, it is necessary to spray it in all areas. Especially areas marked by the COVID-19 red zone (Figure 8(b)) because these areas have a significant chance of COVID-19 transmission compared with areas that have been exposed to COVID-19 and areas that have not been affected by COVID-19.

CONCLUSION

This study concluded that this idea for applying mini helicopters is still very possible to be implemented. Most people think that spraying disinfectants using mini helicopters is possible and can reduce the spread of COVID-19. In addition, hypochlorous acid that does not contain alcohol can also be used as a disinfectant that can reduce COVID-19.

ACKNOWLEDGMENTS

We acknowledged Program Bangdos, Universitas Pendidikan Indonesia for supporting this study.

REFERENCES

Achmad. 2020. "Bahaya, jangan semprotkan langsung disinfektan ketubuh manusia WHO berikan penjelasan" ["Dangerous, do not spray disinfectant to human body directly. WHO provides an explanation"] *Madura Tribunews.com*, March 24, 2020. https://madura.tribunnews.com/2020/ 03/30/bahaya-jangan-semprotkan-disinfektan-langsung-ke-tubuh-manusia-who-berikan-penjelasan.

Anggraeni, S., Maulidina, A., Dewi, M. W., Rahmadianti, S., Rizky, Y. P. C., Arinalhaq, Z. F., Usdiyana, D., Nandiyanto, A. B. D., and Al-Obaidi, A. S. M. 2020. "The Deployment of Drones in Sending Drugs and Patient Blood Samples COVID-19." *Indonesian Journal of Science and Technology* 5, no. 2: 193-200.

Aris. 2020. "Pakar: penyemprotan disinfektan langsung ke tubuh berbahaya" ["Expert: spraying disinfectants directly on the body is dangerous"] *Antaranews.com*, March 30, 2020. https://www.antaranews.com/berita/1401630/pakar-penyemprotan-disinfektan-langsung-pada-tubuh-berbahaya.

BBC News. 2020. "Virus corona: Jokowi umumkan langkah pengendalian COVID-19, tapi tanpa 'komando nasional.'" ["Corona virus: Jokowi announced measures to control COVID-19, but without a 'national command'"] *BBCNews.com*, March 16, 2020. https://www.bbc.com/indonesia/indonesia-51897307.

Fathiyah. 2020. "Penyemprotan Disinfektan Dinilai Efektif Cegah Meluasnya Virus Corona." ["Spraying of Disinfectants is considered to be effective in preventing the spread of the Corona Virus"]. *Voaindonesia.com*, March 24, 2020 https://www.voaindonesia.com/a/penyemprotan-disinfektan-dinilai-efektif-cegah-meluasnya-virus-corona/5342058.html.

Hashim, S., Masek, A., Abdullah, N. S., Paimin, A. N., and Muda, W. H. N. W. "Students' Intention to Share Information via Social Media: A Case Study of COVID-19 Pandemic." *Indonesian Journal of Science and Technology* 5, no. 2: 246-245.

Kevin. 2020. "5 cara efektif mencegah corona." ["5 effective ways to prevent corona"]. *Alodokter.com*, March 16, 2020. http://www.alodokter.com/ketahui-cara-untuk-mencegah-penularan-virus-corona.

Maryanti, R., Hufad, A., Sunardi., Nandiyanto, A. B. D., and Al-Obaidi, S. M. 2020. "Understanding COVID-19 particle contagion through aerosol droplets for students with special needs." *Journal of Engineering Science and Technology* vol. 15, no. 3:1909-1920.

Merry. 2020. *Virus corona (COVID-19)*. KEMENKES RI: Indonesia.

Nanda. 2020. "Cara China Semprotkan Disinfektan ke Berbagai Penjuru Kota." ["The Chinese Way Spraying Disinfectant All Over the City"]. *Merdeka.com*, February 11, 2020. https://www.merdeka.com/foto/dunia/1146698/20200211122057-intip-cara-china-semprotkan-disinfektan-ke-berbagai-penjuru-kota-004-nfi.html.

Vembi, M. 2020. "Mengenal cairan disinfektan dan antiseptic" ["Recognize disinfectant and antiseptic fluids"] *Rancah.com*, March 27, 2020. https://www.rancah.com/kesehatan/46832/mengenal-cairan-desinfektan-dan-antiseptik/.

Verizarie, R. 2020. "Virus Corona: definisi, gejala, pengobatan, pencegahan." ["Corona virus: definition, symptoms, treatment, prevention"]. *The Time*, March 3, 2020. https:// doktersehat.com/virus-corona/.

Yunus, N. R., and Rezki, A. 2020. Yunus, Nur Rohim, and Annissa Rezki. "Kebijakan Pemberlakuan Lock Down Sebagai Antisipasi Penyebaran Corona Virus Covid-19" ["Lock Down Enforcement Policy in Anticipation of Corona Virus Covid-19 Spread"]. *Salam: Jurnal Sosial dan Budaya Syar-i 7*, no. 3: 227-238.

In: COVID-19 ISBN: 978-1-53618-903-2
Editors: A. B. D. Nandiyanto et al.

Chapter 26

MODIFICATION OF PUBLIC TRANSPORTATION TO PREVENT THE SPREAD OF COVID-19 IN WEST JAVA, INDONESIA

Putri Sakinah Hanafi[1], Asita Puji Astuti[1], Fajar Miraz Fauzi[1], Gabriela Chelvina Santiuly Girsang[1], Sri Anggraeni[1,*] and Asnul Dahar Minghat[2]

[1]Fakultas Pendidikan Matematika dan Ilmu Pengetahuan Alam, Universitas Pendidikan Indonesia, Bandung, Jawa Barat, Indonesia

[2]Razak Faculty of Technology and Informatics, Universiti Teknologi Malaysia, Skudai, Malaysia

* Corresponding Author's Email: anggraeni_said@upi.edu.

Abstract

Coronavirus disease 2019 (COVID-19) pandemic has influenced several areas, one of which is transportation, specifically public transportation. This affected captive groups or public transport users, especially public transportation cars, as city transportation. The purpose of this study is to investigate public transportation problems during the pandemic and find out community responses in West Java regarding the idea of modifying urban transport. The method used is a quantitative method based on the questionnaire. The results showed how the transportation system of urban transport was not yet effective enough to prevent COVID-19 exposure at the moment. Respondents support the idea of the modification of urban transport as a solution with affordable fees and minimal modification costs. Respondents also approved the use of electricity as a fuel for urban transport and encouraged the government to execute the idea of a modification of city transportation.

Keywords: public transportation, modification, COVID-19

1. Introduction

Corona or COVID-19 virus pandemic has caused problems in various parts of the world, including Indonesia. COVID-19 is a new type of virus that attacks the respiratory system (Maryanti et al., 2020). The COVID-19 case in Indonesia has been announced since 2 March 2020 and has become increasingly epidemic. Indonesian government adopts a policy to issue health protocols implemented in all regions in Indonesia led by the Ministry of Health of the Republic of Indonesia (Kementrian Kesehatan Indosesia (Indonesia Health Ministry), 2020). Nonetheless, COVID-19 continues to expand and the number of infected people continues to increase every day. The speaker of the Indonesian House of Representatives repeatedly reminded the government to create a national team that would deal with the COVID-19 outbreak (CNN Indonesia 2020). Limited information causes the community worried and confused because they do not get safe and convincing services when they feel there are indications of exposure to COVID-19. Another problem that arises is the authority to determine public health emergencies by the central government or regional governments. The President of the Republic of Indonesia stressed that lockdowns should not be carried out, however, if the municipal leaders felt the need to carry out a lockdown in the area is allowed. The slow response of the central government and weak regulation have been seen as something obvious (Telaumbalua 2018).

The community demands that the government immediately handle the threat of COVID-19. The solution has been written in Law Number 6 Year 2018 on Health Quarantine about health quarantine and the determination of public health emergencies by the government. The rules are also laid down in the law as a follow-up to the provisions on health quarantine. Efforts are made to limit activities outside the home, stop school activities at school, encourage people to work from home and conduct religious activities at home. This has been a standard government strategy and has been optimally evaluated (Rezki and Yunus, 2020). These efforts have had an impact on various sectors in Indonesia, one of which is transport. Existing transport is not yet in a position to support the COVID-19 prevention protocol. As a result, people have difficulty traveling without worrying about being exposed to COVID-19. Therefore, we have the idea of modifying one of the public transport services in West Java, namely *minicab* by following the COVID-19 prevention protocol.

The general public group is divided into two groups, based on users of transport services, namely choice and captives. The choice group is a private vehicle user group, while the captive group is a public transport user group (Siswoyo 2008). Although some stay and work at home, the community (captive group) still needs public transport to work or purchase daily needs. As a developing country, most people in Indonesia are from the lower middle class (Siswoyo 2008). Lower middle-class people commonly use public transport. Public transport, which promotes the use of the COVID-19 prevention program, is therefore needed to facilitate the public's need for public transport.

Public transport cars, commonly referred to as *minicab* or *angkot (in Indonesian languange)*, are chosen by the community to travel long and short distances. The distribution is fairly even and reaches different regions at a relatively affordable cost compared to other public transport services. *Minicab* has a flexible pick-up point for passengers and can carry around 10-12 people. These advantages make *minicab* dominates West Java transportation and can be accessed by all groups (Sutandi 2015). It is also the type of public transport mode that can be used as an alternative to public transport on the shortest, fastest and cheapest route. (Hobbs 1995; Hasyim et al., 2020). On the basis of these criteria, *minicab* is appropriate as a solution to the problems of public transport during this pandemic.

However, *minicab* modification is needed to prevent the spread of COVID-19. Illustration of changes in urban transport is shown in Figure 1. The modifications and background of the *minicab* selected are as follows.

1. Access to and from public transport is fairly simple, so that a body temperature thermometer can be installed before entering public transport (Figure 1a).
2. *Minicab* has a strategic area that can be modified to provide facilities/access to personal protective equipment. Automatic hand sanitizers can be supplied outside the *minicab* (Figure 1a) while masks are provided inside the *minicab* (Figure 1b).
3. Payment can be both digital and physical money. Money is one of the media which can spread COVID-19. *Minicab* can be equipped with digital wallet to prevent the spread of the virus through money. Payment can be made by scanning the QR code found on the *minicab* door (Figure 1b). However, *minicab* also accepts payment physical money, so that it is flexible in terms of payment.
4. The structure of the *minicab* is fairly simple compared to other four-wheeled public transportation modes. This facilitates surface sterilization of objects in public transportation (Figure 1b and 1c)
5. *Minicab* has good double-sided window air circulation (Figure 1c), to minimize the COVID-19 virus spread.
6. The distance between passengers can be easily adjusted by separating the position of the passenger seat and making it simple (Figure 1c).

7. In order to support physical-distancing efforts, the capacity of passengers is limited to 8 people by placing an X sign on the seats that cannot be occupied (Figure 1c).
8. The *minicab* pick-up points are flexible so that they can reach different regions.
9. Affordable price.
10. In addition to transporting passengers, *minicab* can carry a large quantity of food, such as sacks and boxes.
11. Modification of *minicab* requires only a small level of money and is prolonged.
12. The modification of *minicab* provides for public transport by preventing the spread of COVID-19. This solution uses active transport in West Java, so it does not cost money to create a new type of transport.

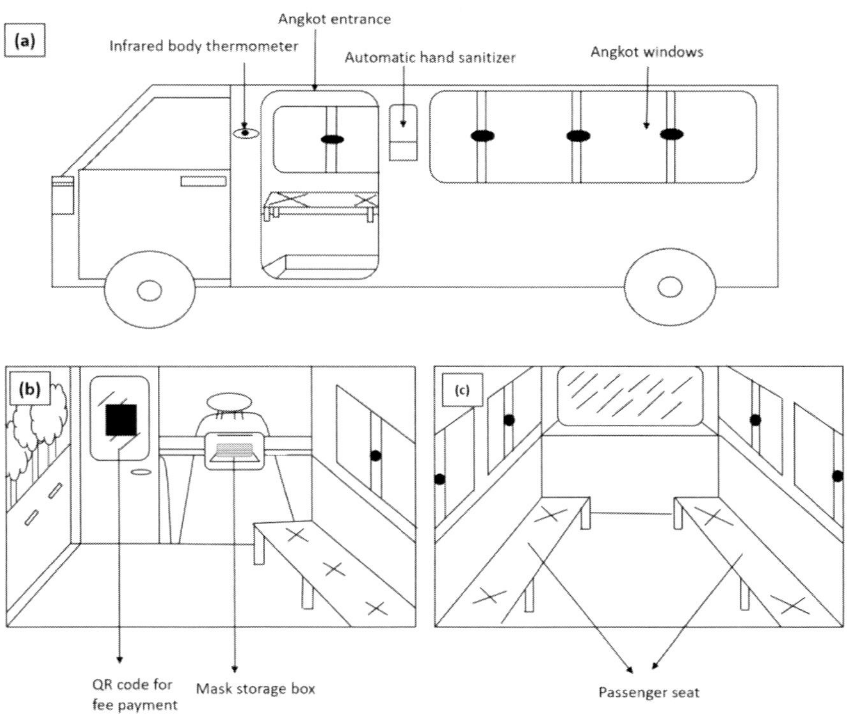

Figure 1. Illustration of exterior appearance (a), inside-front display (b), and inside-rear display on the modification of city transportation (c).

2. METHOD

A study was conducted in April 2020 with the implementation of the COVID-19 Distribution Prevention Protocol. The method used in this study was therefore a quantitative method based on a questionnaire. Questionnaire is a technique of collecting data through forms containing questions submitted in writing to a person or group of people to get the answers, responses, suggestions, or criticisms needed by researchers. Google form used to collect questionnaires. In addition, the literature review was also used to enhance references. Distribution of the questionnaire to all regions of West Java.

3. RESULTS AND DISCUSSION

The respondents were 54 people with the distribution of residential areas shown by Figure 2. The questionnaire was distributed with most of the respondents living in Cimahi, Bandung, and West Bandung Regency. The rest of the respondents lived in Depok, Cilegon, Purwakarta Regency, Sukabumi, Bogor, Garut Regency, Kuningan Regency, Sumedang Regency and Cirebon.

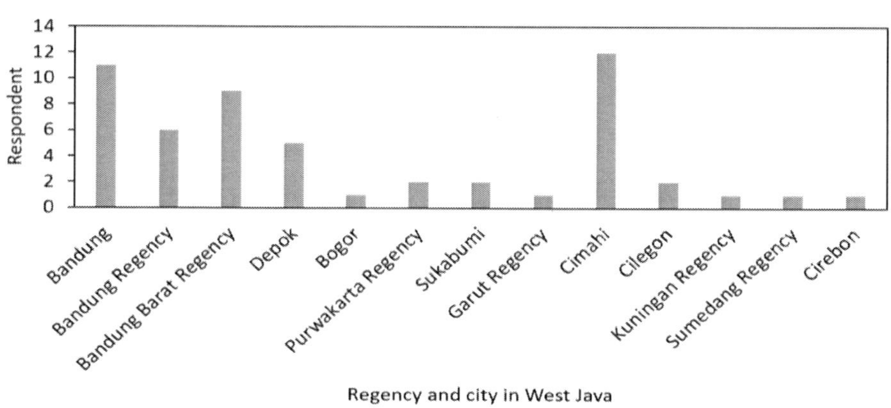

Figure 2. Distribution of respondent's residence in West Java.

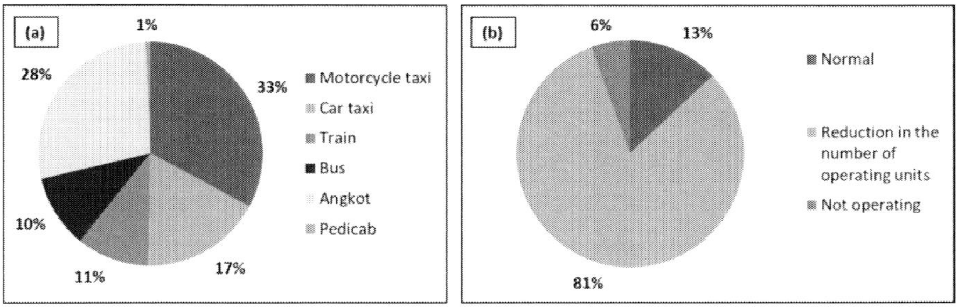

Figure 3. Public transportation in West Java, Indonesia: (a) active and (b) operation.

Each region has a different policy for public transport operations during this pandemic. Public transport was restricted as an effort to prevent the spread of COVID-19. Large numbers of public transportation have the potential to increase COVID-19 transmission (Kompas 2020a). Based on the results of the study, there were six modes of transportation chosen by the community during this pandemic, namely motorcycle taxi, taxi, train, bus, *minicab*, and pedicab (Figure 3a). The three modes of public transport most commonly used by the community are motorcycle taxi, taxi and *minicab*. All three of these transports underwent a dramatic change during this pandemic.

Motorcycle taxi still operates even though the operation is restricted by Pembatasan Sosial Berskala Besar (Large-Scale Social Restriction) rules in West Java. The Large-Scale Social Restriction (LSSR) rules state that a two-wheeled vehicle carries a maximum of two people living in the same house, as proven by their identity cards. In the meantime, both *minicab* and a car taxi could only carry 50% of their passenger capacity and are required to limit the distance between passengers (Kompas 2020b). The use of masks is mandatory when traveling during the LSSR. This is certainly a challenge for public transport operations.

A balance between the quantity of supply or unit and demand is needed in public transport operations (Juanita and Pinandita 2016). The call to stay at home and work from home (WFH) has an impact on current demand, resulting in a decrease in the number of passengers (Anggraeni et al., 2020). The decrease in passenger numbers has resulted in a decrease in public transport units (Figure 3b). In addition, several regions have issued policies so that public transport does not operate.

Efforts to protect passengers from exposure to COVID-19 in public transport may be made by passengers themselves or by an authorized institution to change the transport system. Passengers can use masks and apply hand sanitizers. These things are very simple, but in fact, there are still some people who are negligent in their implementation. Such negligence can increase the chance of being exposed to COVID-19 while on public transportation. However, the possibility of the negligence of users of public transportation can be anticipated by providing access to masks and hand sanitizers on public transportation.

The Indonesian Transportation Agency has changed the transportation system to support the prevention of the COVID-19 spread. Broadly speaking, public transport policies are limiting distance between passengers (physical distances), reducing the number of passengers to support distance restrictions, periodic sterilization of public transport surfaces, and reducing operating time due to reduced passenger volume. Body temperature measurements before entering public transport are also carried out to minimize contact with symptomatic people with COVID-19. Although these efforts have started to be socialized, not all public transport implement them. Based on the results of the questionnaire, *minicab* has not yet implemented overall preventive measures (Figure 4). This shows that *minicab* is vulnerable to COVID-19 exposure. Although such efforts have been done, respondents felt normal with the changes in the current public transportation system (Figure 5a). On a scale of 1-5, the majority of respondents are satisfied on a scale of 3. This is caused by prevention efforts that are not carried out in an optimal and thorough manner. On the other hand, the respondents assessed that efforts to prevent *minicab* from COVID-19 are still not effective in their implementation. (Figure 5b). Therefore, *minicab* modification to support efforts to prevent the spread of COVID-19 is needed to minimize the chance of COVID-19 exposure.

Based on Figure 6, the public welcomed the idea of modifying public transport. Respondents indicated that the modified *minicab* could reduce the spread of COVID-19. In addition, modified public transportation routes need special attention in order to be able to reach areas effectively, especially the PSBB zone and the red zone of COVID-19. The cost is expected to be affordable and modifications can be mass-produced. The community also supports the idea of using electricity as a modified public transport fuel. The idea emerged from public awareness of the impact of fuel transport on comfort, health and the environment. In addition, the use of electricity as fuel in public transport, in particular public transport, is a step towards a sustainable transport system (Sutandi 2015). The use of electrical energy will minimize air pollution caused by gasoline-fueled public transport. The community also supports this idea to be executed by the government.

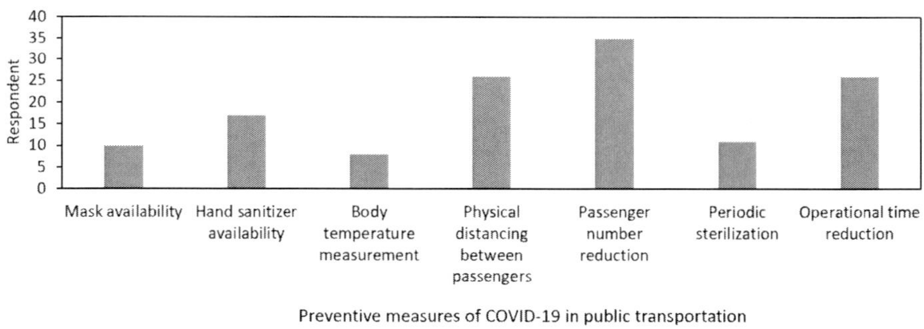

Figure 4. Changes in the city transportation system in West Java during the COVID-19 pandemic.

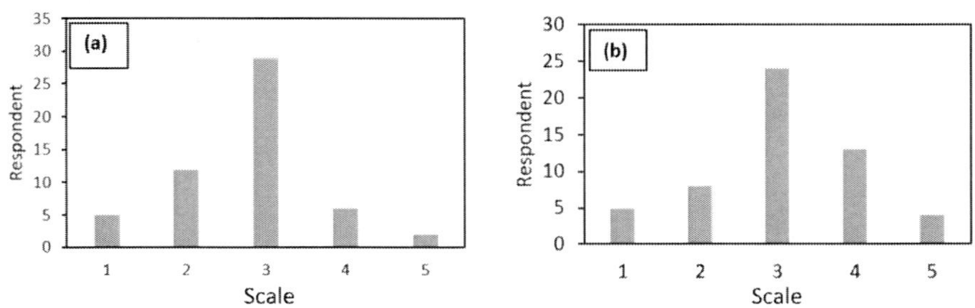

Figure 5. Satisfaction (a) and effectiveness (b) of the changes in the transportation system. Scales 1 to 5 are for dissatisfied to very satisfied, respectively.

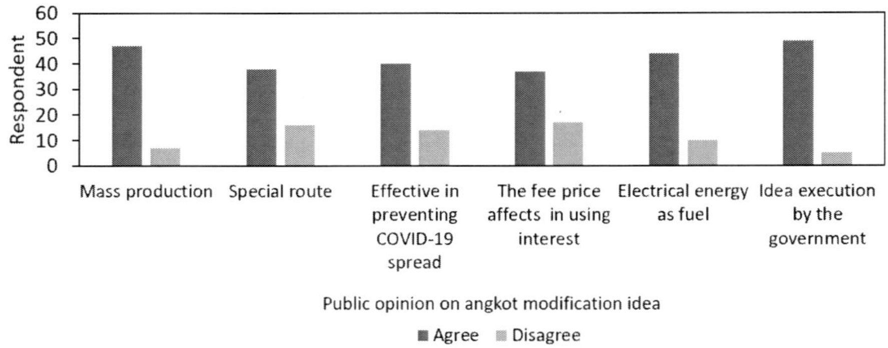

Figure 6. The idea in modifying public transportation.

CONCLUSION

Public transportation modification is needed as an effort to reduce the spread of COVID-19 in West Java, Indonesia. The modification maximizes self-protection from COVID-19 exposure by providing access to self-protective equipment and implementing physical distances, thereby reducing public concerns about travel by public transport. The community welcomes this idea with a condition that it has an affordable price and the modification is done as efficiently as possible. The public will also welcome the use of electricity as the *minicab* fuel and encourage the government to execute the idea of the *minicab* modification.

ACKNOWLEDGMENT

Program Bangdos, Universitas Pendidikan Indonesia is acknowledged.

REFERENCES

Anggraeni, S., Maulidina, A., Dewi, M. W, Rahmadianti, S., Rizky, Y. P. C., Arinalhaq, Z. F., Usdiyana, D., Nandiyanto, A. B. D., and Al-Obaidi,

A. S. M. 2020. "The Deployment of Drones in Sending Drugs and Patient Blood Samples COVID-19." *Indonesian Journal of Science and Technology* vol. 5, no. 2: 193-200.

Ansori, M. H. 2020. "Wabah COVID-19 dan Kelas Sosial di Indonesia" ["The COVID-19 Outbreak and Social Class in Indonesia"] *THC Insight*, no. 14 (April):1-5http://habibiecenter.or.id/img/publication/09da4f0fd333100e97d2b2bc1aec3163.pdf.

CNN Indonesia. 2020. "DPR Desak Pemerintah Bentuk Satgas Penanganan Virus Corona." ["Parliament Urges Government Forms Management Task Force Coronavirus"]. *CNNIndonesia.com*, March 29, 2020. [House of Representatives Urge the Government to Form a Task Force for Handling Corona Virus]. *CNNIndonesia.com,* March 29, 2020. www.cnnindonesia.com/nasional/20200312020329-20-482683/dpr-desak-pemerintah-bentuk-satgas-penanganan-virus-corona.

Hashim, S., Masek, A., Abdullah, N. S., Paimin, A. N., and Muda, W. H. N. W. "Students' Intention to Share Information via Social Media: A Case Study of COVID-19 Pandemic." *Indonesian Journal of Science and Technology* vol. 5, no. 2: 236-245.

Hobbs, F. D. 1995. *Perencanaan dan Teknik Lalu Lintas* [*Traffic Planning and Engineering*]. Penerbit Gadjah Mada University Press, Yogyakarta. Publisher: Gadjah Mada University Press, Yogyakarta. http://library.um.ac.id/free-contents/index.php/buku/detail/perencanaan-dan-teknik-lalu-lintas-f-d-hobbs-penerjemah-suprapto-t-m-waldijono-penyunting-achmad-djunaedi-24940.html.

Juanita, J., and Pinandita, T. 2016. "Studi Kelayakan Transportasi Umum Perkotaan" ["Urban Public Transportation Feasibility Study"] In *Prosiding Forum Studi Transportasi antar Perguruan Tinggi,* October 11-13, 2020. https://ojs.fstpt.info/index.php?journal=ProsFSTPT&page=article&op=view&path%5B%5D=178.

Kementerian Kesehatan Indonesia. 2020. "Lakukan Protokol Kesehatan Ini jika Mengalami Gejala Covid-19 Sehat Negeriku" ["Do this Health Protocol if you experience Covid-19 symptoms Sehat Negeriku"]. Kementerian kesehatan [Indonesia Health Ministry] *Indonesia.com,* March 16, 2020. http://sehatnegeriku.kemkes.go.id/baca/rilismedia/20200316/4033408/lakukanprotokol-kesehatan-jika-mengalami-gejala-covid-19.

Kompas. 2020a. "Memahami potensi Risiko Penularan Virus Corona di Transportasi Umum" ["Understanding the potential Risk of Corona Virus Transmission in Public Transportation"] *Kompas.com*, March 29, 2020. https://www.kompas.com/tren/read/2020/03/29/202100965/memahami-potensi-risiko-penularan-virus-corona-di-transportasi-umum?page=all.

Kompas. 2020b. "Aturan Berkendara Selama Penerapan PSBB di Jawa Barat" ["Driving Rules during the Implementation of large-scale social restrictions in West Java"]. *Kompas.com*, March 15, 2020. https://otomotif.kompas.com/read/2020/03/15/094200015/aturan-berkendara-selama-penerapan-psbb-di-jawa-barat.

Maryanti, R., Hufad, A., Sunardi, Nandiyanto, A. B. D., and Al-Obaidi, S. M. 2020. "Understanding COVID-19 particle contagion through aerosol droplets for students with special needs." *Journal of Engineering Science and Technology* vol. 15, no. 3: 1909-1920.

Rezki, A., and Yunus, N. R. 2020. "Kebijakan Pemberlakuan Lock Down Sebagai Antisipasi Penyebaran Corona Virus Covid-19" ["Lock Down Enforcement Policy in Anticipation of Corona Virus Covid-19 Spread"]. *Salam: Jurnal Sosial dan Budaya Syar-i* 7, no. 3 (2020): 227-238.

Siswoyo, M. P. 2008. "Kebijakan dan Tantangan Pelayanan Angkutan Umum" ["Public Transport Policy and Service Challenges"]. *Jurnal Teknik Sipil dan Perencanaan* 10, no. 2: 171-180.

Sutandi, A. C. 2015. "Pentingnya Transportasi Umum untuk Kepentingan Publik" ["The Importance of Public Transportation for Public Interest]. *Jurnal Administrasi Publik* 12, no. 1:19-34.

Telaumbanua, D. 2018. "Pembentukan Peraturan Daerah Kabupaten/Kota" ["Establishment of Regency/City Regulations"] *Jurnal Education and Development* 4, no. 1: 96-96.

In: COVID-19 ISBN: 978-1-53618-903-2
Editors: A. B. D. Nandiyanto et al.

Chapter 27

MICROFLUIDIC DEVICES IN PCR SYSTEM FOR THE APPLICATION OF COVID-19 RAPID DETECTION

Budi Mulyanti* and Roer Eka Pawinanto
Department of Electrical Engineering Education,
Universitas Pendidikan Indonesia, Bandung, Jawa Barat, Indonesia

ABSTRACT

The aim of this study was to review the development of microfluidic devices in the Polymerase Chain Reaction system for the application of corona virus disease 2019 (COVID-19) rapid detection. Materials used for microfluidic devices are briefly reviewed as well. Clear descriptions for every microfluidic device, namely micropump, microvalve, and micromixer used to develop the whole Polymerase Chain Reaction system are discussed in detail, including their advantages and disadvantages. It is concluded that much progress has been achieved in the microfluidic-based on the Polymerase Chain Reaction system. The future benefits of this review are to encourage the microfluidic involvement within the

* Corresponding Author's Email: bmulyanti@upi.edu.

Polymerase Chain Reaction system, especially for the application of COVID-19 rapid detection.

Keywords: COVID-19, microfluidic, micropump, microvalve, micromixer, PCR

1. Introduction

Since World Health Organization (WHO) on 11 March 11, officially stated that the corona virus disease 2019 (COVID-19) had become a global pandemic (Anjorin 2020; Anggraeni et al. 2020)), numerous countries all over the world have declared emergency state and shutdown public areas. Public areas have enormous potential for transmission of COVID-19 (Hasim et al. 2020). COVID-19 is a disease that is dangerous and can infect the human body. This disease is caused by a corona virus. This virus is transmitted through droplets (Maryanti et al. 2020a). The mouth or nose is a bridge for the virus to enter the human body. The very small size of the virus makes it easier for the virus to enter the human body (Maryanti et al. 2020b). Diagnostic tools can play a significant role to decrease the spreading rate of the virus. Polymerase Chain reaction (PCR) is one method that can be used as COVID-19 rapid detection. Since many microfluidic devices can be used for PCR application and rapidly identify the virus then make the microfluidic has the potential to offer an affordable point of care (POC) diagnostic.

In the recent decade, microfluidic has been particularly attractive for medical applications such as drug transportation, polymerase chain reactions (PCR), and chemical detection. Many devices in microfluidics can be integrated with one another such as on a single chip that can speed up biological analysis, reduce samples and reagents, and thus provide solutions for the medical field. PCR becomes a key process and a powerful tool in genetic investigations, clinical diagnostics, and the forensic field. Besides, currently, the PCR method is one of the techniques used for COVID-19 detection. Therefore, the role of microfluidic becomes more important and urgent because of its benefits such as rapid detection, few samples, short analysis time, good sensitivity, and disposable.

The advantages of micro-sized PCR devices have been widely studied by many researchers. Initially, the room-based PCR chip was introduced by Kopp (Kopp et al. 1998). The PCR chip model provided the basis for further development, and to date, they have been duplicated by many other researchers. The PCR chip transition from simple microfluidic components to advance integrated systems is still ongoing. Some microfluidic parts for several purposes such as sample preparation, DNA/RNA amplification, and sample detection can be integrated on a single chip (Cady et al. 2005). Micropump, microvalve, and micromixer successfully provide a higher level of integration and allow more than one sample to be run in parallel, which can reduce the analysis time.

Various progresses on the development of magnetic nanomaterials for micromixer has been reported. One of the reports presented a classification of micromixer divided into four types according to drive modes, such as external permanent magnet, electromagnet, micro stirrer, and the integrated electrode (Chen et al. 2017). Jeong et al. presented a report on micromixer based on its applications (Jeong et al. 2010). They classified the applications of micromixers into three categorized such as chemical applications, biological applications, and detection. Meanwhile, Au et al. presented a report on microvalves and micropumps for Bio-MEMS (Au et al. 2011). However, all previous reports were still too general in studying the detection process using the PCR system based on microfluidic devices.

Therefore, in this study, we reviewed the development of microfluidic devices in the PCR system for the application of COVID-19 rapid detection. Materials used for microfluidic devices are briefly explained as well. Furthermore, here explains the advantages and disadvantages of these functional components which indicate that micropump, microvalves, and micromixer technologies have played an important role in the development of integrated microfluidic chips.

2. Micropump for PCR Application

Several types of micropumps have been designed and fabricated with various structures and operating mechanisms. In general, micropumps for fluid pumping in PCR chips can be divided into two categories, namely: mechanical micropumps with moving parts and non-mechanical micropumps without mechanical components (Au et al. 2011).

In 2017, one group of researchers has succeeded in developing a peristaltic pump integrated into the PCR chip (Alam et al. 2017). 3D printing using VEROTM photopolymer materials was used to fabricate the micropump. Utilization of 3D printing technology allowed for relatively short fabrication time. The minipump design is based on the concept of a planetary gear and worked in the same way as a typical benchtop peristaltic pump. The micropump was able to pump fluids between 40 mL/min and 200 mL/min and continue to work well at a back pressure of 25 kPa. Therefore, this performance showed successful interfacing between chip and device where the conceptual polymerase chain reaction (PCR) chip is fabricated well without leakage or flow disturbance in the microchannels (Alam et al. 2017).

In the same year, another group of researchers developed diafiltration-on-chip microfluidics integrated with magnetic peristaltic micropumps (Liu et al., 2017). The integration of magnetically driven peristaltic micropumps has the role of achieving a continuous flow of recirculation as shown in Figure 1(a). This pump is operated using a three-dimensional microfluidic architecture, where magnetic material (iron filing) is joined into the layer above the flow channel which is divided from the flow channel by PDMS thin layer (Figure 1(b)). The filings of the iron are pulled down because the magnetic field deflecting the PDMS membrane and compressing the flow channel when a fixed magnet located below the flow channel separated from the sample by glass slide (Figure 1(b)). When an external magnet is moved in a plane along a flow channel, the place of this pressure in the channel moves with the magnet and forces the fluid to move in the direction of the magnet's movement, which is similar to a peristaltic pump. The on-chip magnetic pump promotes steady flow through permeable membranes and high-resistance microfluidic pinch channels. Flux across the membrane is controlled by the relative resistance of the pinched channel and the membrane (Figure 1(c)).

Furthermore, Li et al. developed passive micropump which can produce and transmit microdroplets inside a microchannel with several millimeters' length in a much longer periode (Li et al. 2018). Passive micropumps can consistently carry large volume (more than 2000 μL) of fluid/oil microdroplets inside 3D spiral microchannel (4 m long and 2 cm high) in 8 hours of the period. The droplet flow rate can be easily adjusted by changing the quartz capillary parameters connected to the microchannel ends. This passive micropump was successfully applied to the home-made setup of droplet-based surfactant-free quantitative PCRs using only two syringes for droplet generation, a Teflon tube for PCR amplification and single thermostatic heater for a thermal cycle with the amplification efficiency of the virus reaching 91% of commercial PCR thermocycler (Li et al. 2018).

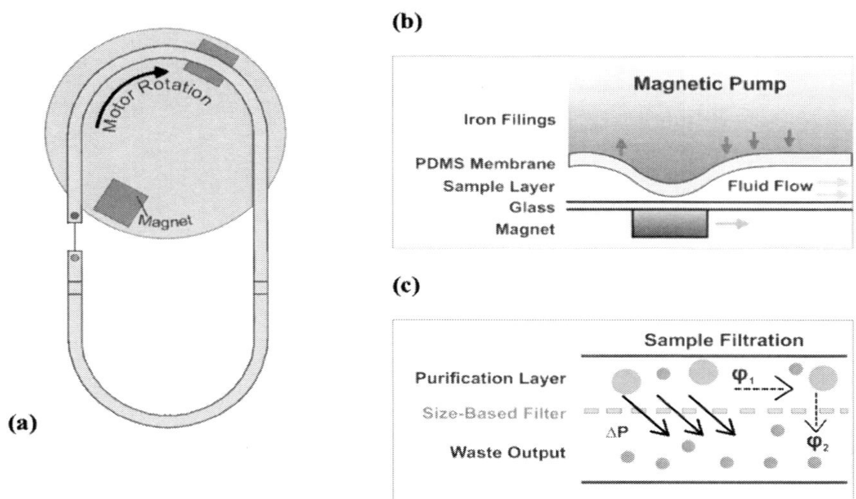

Figure 1. Magnetically-driven fluid flow. (a) As the motor rotates, (b) The cyclic magnetic pump comprises. (c) Sample filtration is driven by a pressure drop across the size-based filter (Liu et al., 2017).

3. Microvalve for PCR Application

The completely integrated microfluidic system such as lab-on-a-chip (LOC) or a micro total analysis system (μTAS) cannot be realized without microvalve development (Vilkner et al. 2004; Dittrich et al. 2006). Therefore, microvalve becomes one of the most important components to be successfully applied to the compact integrated on-chip PCR microfluidics. In general, microvalve can be classified into two main types: active microvalve and passive microvalve depending on mechanical or non-mechanical moving parts.

Generally, the deflection of the PDMS membrane is utilized to interrupt the flow in pneumatic microvalve. This easily integrated with standard soft lithography process caused pneumatic microvalve to become one of the common valve architectures. Liao et al. developed a miniaturized RT-PCR system for the diagnosis of RNA-based viruses, in which the reagent and sample flow were controlled automatically by utilizing two micropumps and one microvalve, as shown in Figure 2. The fluid flow could be effectively interrupted when the pneumatic microvalve was closed, and the pressure of 69 kPa could cause the microvalve to close the flow of a fluid moving at ~30 μL/min (Liao et al. 2005).

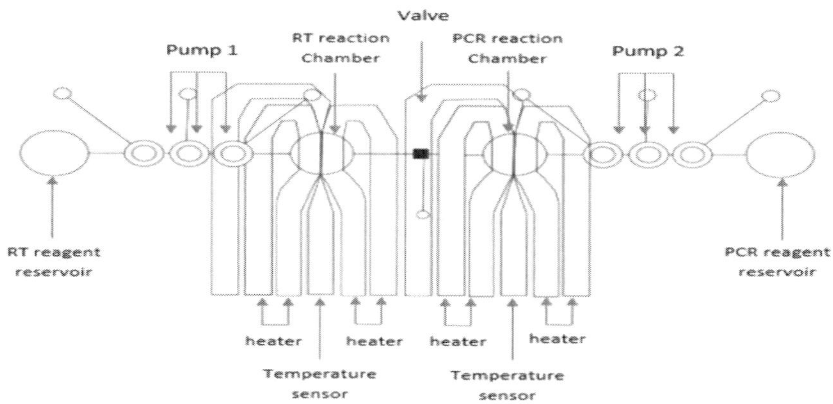

Figure 2. Schematic diagram of two-step micro RT-PCR chip integrated with two micropumps and one microvalve for controlling biosample transportation (Liao et al. 2005).

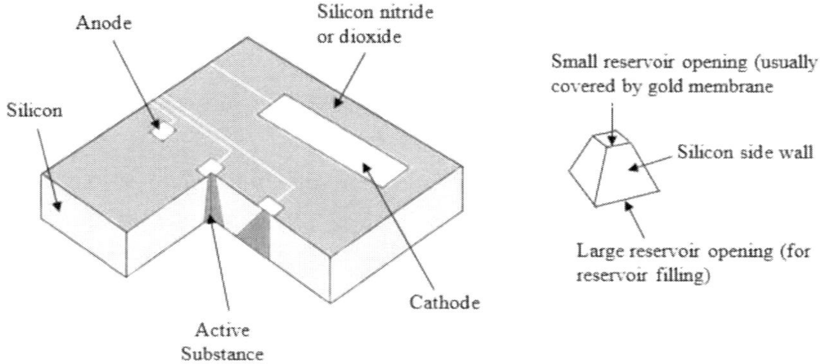

Figure 3. 3D schematics of a controlled-release microchip and a single anisotropically etched sacrificial membrane burst microvalves (Santini et al., 1999).

Manual microvalves system with 8 integrated channels for controlling up to 8 different flows of agents was developed by Lee et al. (2020). The working principle of the valve is based on flexible materials (PDMS) and mechanical structure. The plasma etching technique was used to bond 100 μm thickness of PDMS film fabricated on top microchannel. The mechanical structure for closing and opening the flow valve was integrated with two components. Firstly, the second slab of Plexiglass is fixed by a screw with 3 mm of diameter and width 0.5 mm of the thread pitch. Secondly, the screw hole is bigger than the PDMS piece (2.5 mm) make the PDMS piece move freely in this hole. The microreactor (~5 L of volume) and multi-liquid mixing component is successfully connected by the valve system. The function of controlling liquid flows to the microchamber was effectively succeeded in using this valve system (Lee et al. 2020).

The other microvalve principle utilizes a sacrificial membrane. This concept introduced by Robert Langer which designs a silicone-based "drug-release" microchip containing etched cavities capped with the sacrificial" gold membrane (Figure 3) (Santini et al. 1999). The drug-containing solutions are filling the cavities prior to being sealed with the membrane. The electrical supply of 1volt was used to electrochemically dissolve the membrane. Therefore, the release of one dose (25 nL) of "drug" for every cavity is controlled by a voltage pulse. Meanwhile, Moreno et al. (2010) and Allain et al. (2010) reported the sacrificial membrane composed of silicon nitride and SU-8. When electrical current or the heat is applied to the sacrificial membrane, the microvalves are open. The debris from the disintegration of the sacrificial membrane can be released into the fluid (Moreno et al. 2010; Allain et al. 2010).

Baek and Min investigated microvalves for selectively extracting nucleic acid from bacteria and viruses by physical adsorption and beat beating (Baek and Min 2015). The principle work of microvalves in the chambers is to switch between the packed bed for the pathogen concentration and beat beater. Meanwhile, Zahra et al. presented the microfluidic system integrated with temperature actuated microvalves. The "open" and "close" position of the valve is depending on the electrical supply to the heater. The atmospheric pressure obtained inside the chamber (microvalves) when there is no electrical supply. On the contrary, the temperature inside the chamber increases when the electrical supply is given and the generated pressure pushes up the valve membranes, which close the channel. The temperature of 92°C with an applied voltage of 4 V is given when the complete closure of the channel happened without liquid leakage. Furthermore, the time constant of the valve during the opening is 1.40 s (Zahra et al. 2015).

Tang et al. (2019) presented the multi-way microvalves with a rotor. The principle operation is based on a rotary mechanism. The five-degree rotational symmetry was obtained with a compressible rotor and a complementary stator seat valve. The Viton elastomer is used for a rotor to provide a seal and switch between outlets. The microvalves can be operated in two ways, including manually or automatically. The switching torque of below 0.03 Nm and the pressure of 370 kPa with no leakage is obtained by the microvalves (Tang et al. 2019).

Meanwhile, a high flow rate control under an ultra-low threshold pressure was realized through microfluidic passive valve comprising of a fluid chamber, a flexible membrane, and an ellipsoidal control chamber by Zhang et al. (2019). The UV laser-cutting and 3D printing technologies were used to fabricate the microvalves. The constant flow rate of 4.03 mL/min, with a variation of ~4.22% under the inlet liquid pressures varied from 6 to 12 kPa was achieved by the passive microvalves. Furthermore, the microvalves could stabilize the flow rate of liquid under the time-varying sinusoidal pressures or the square wave pressures (Zhang et al. 2019).

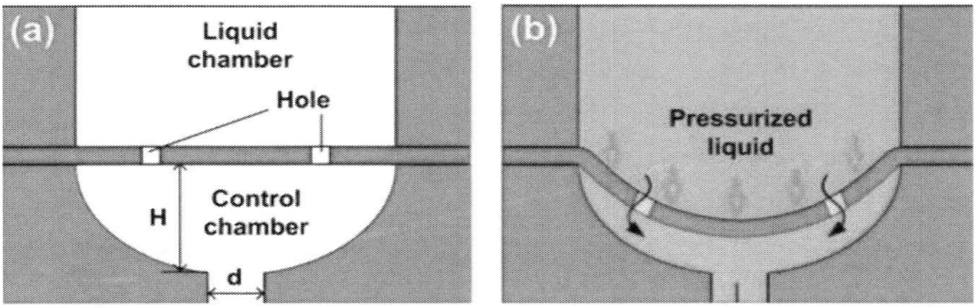

Figure 4. Working principle of the microfluidic passive valve. (a) Concept structure of the valve.(b) Schematic valve actuation under pressurized liquid (Zhang et al., 2019).

4. MICROMIXER FOR PCR APPLICATION

Besides the microvalves and micropump, the micromixer is often another important and necessary component in an integrated PCR microfluidic system. In general, two basic principles are followed to generate mixing at the microscale: passive micromixing and active micromixing. Passive micromixers do not require external energy, and the mixing process relies only on diffusion or chaotic advection. For this micromixing means, the flow energy due to pumping action or hydrostatic potential is used to rebuild a flow in a way that causes faster mixing. Active micromixers use energy input from the exterior for the mixing process. These external energy sources include electrokinetics, acoustics, magnetohydrodynamics, integrated microvalves/micropumps, and others.

The simplest micromixer structure is Y/T-type configurations that have been well applied for fluid mixing in the PCR chips (Hashimoto et al., 2006; Münchow et al. 2005). Hashimoto et al. presented Y-shaped passive micromixer to mix the continuous-flow PCR product and ligation detection reaction (LDR) cocktail for the detection of low-abundant DNA point mutations (Hashimoto et al. 2006). Meanwhile, the passive Y-type microchannel was developed to induce the reproducible metering and merging of two or more fluid volumes (0.1–10 μL) without any active valve components or external sensors in PCR chips (Münchow et al. 2005).

Chen and Zhao (2017) designed and optimized the obstacles of a three-dimensional T-type micromixer. The mixing index of above 0.9 is achieved for a wide range of Peclet numbers. The obstacles in T-type micromixers can improve the mixing performance than the conventional T-type micromixer (Chen and Zhao 2017). Another T-type micromixer with obstacles was presented also by Rasouli et al. (2018). The curve micromixer designed to create normal advection and curved microchannels to generate Dean vortices. The mixing index used in the range of 0.48-0.89 with a pressure drop of 195.6 Pa to 10,891.6 Pa for Reynolds number = 27 and mixing index range of 0.73–0.98 with a pressure drop of 1695.9 Pa to 35,543.8 Pa for Reynolds number = 81 is achieved (Rasouli et al. 2018).

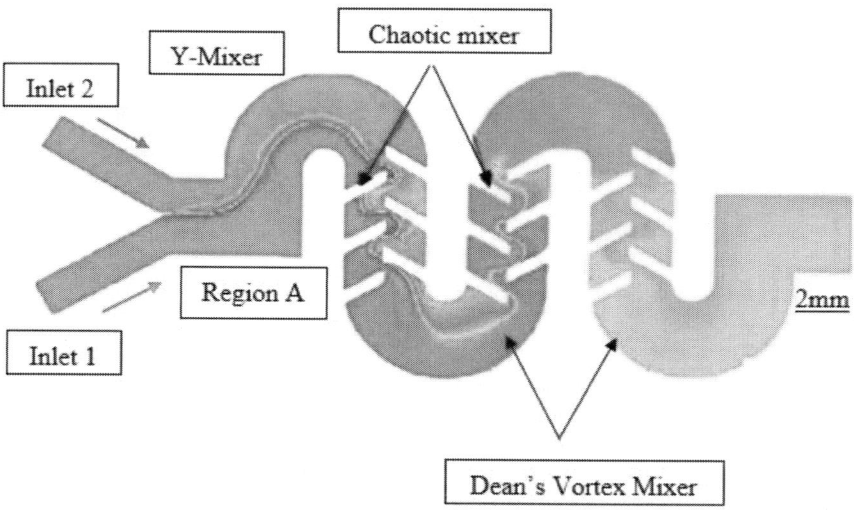

Figure 5. Schematic illustration of microfluidic mixer that simulates instant cross-contamination and sanitization scenarios (Zhang et al., 2015).

The micromixer integrated three different mixing designs including Y-junction, Dean vortex, and chaotic was presented by Zhang et al. (2015). The micromixer is used to determine precisely the reaction time and control the chlorine concentration as shown in Figure 5 (Zhang et al. 2015). Lee et al. (2009) presented an integrated microfluidic system consist of two micropumps, a pneumatic four-membrane-type micromixer, a micro coil array, and a sample purification chamber. The simultaneous detection of IgG and IgM in two different detection chambers can be done during the detection time of just 30 min. Also, the detection limit was found to be 2.1× 10^{-11}g (Lee et al. 2009).

Kastania et al., (2016) developed a passive polymeric micromixer integrated to the microfluidic chip for DNA purification. The micromixer design is zig-zag shaped PMMA microcolumn. For the DNA purification test, fluorescein (MW-332.21) which have a diffusion coefficient of 4.9 x 10-10 m2/s is used. The mixing index of 0.95 is reached for 5 μL/min per inlet and 0.88 for 10 μL/min per inlet (Kastani et al., 2016). Kefala et al. (2015). developed a planar split and merge passive micromixer with labyrinthine microchannels. The micromixer consists of concentric rings where flow split and merges. The mixing index above 0.85 was achieved with the 11 concentric rings and a flow rate of 2.7 μL/min (Kefala et al. 2015). Cai et al. (2019) developed a split-recombine passive micromixer integrated into the microfluidic chip for PCR application. The spit-recombine micromixer with multiple asymmetric rings has a function to mix the sample with H_2O_2. The mixing index of 0.85 is reached at the flow rate of 0.05 mL/min with 7 asymmetric rings applied and does not improve significantly when more asymmetric rings are added (Cai et al. 2019).

To accelerate the DNA hybridization process or to expand the immunomagnetic cell capture process efficiency, Liu et al. developed micromixer based on acoustic microstreaming (Liu et al. 2004). The micromixer was integrated with pump, valve, storage for PCR application as shown in Figure 6. The PZT actuator generates the field that induced Acoustic microstreaming. The complete mixing process in the 50 μL chamber was decreased from hours to only 6s. Furthermore, acoustic microstreaming resulted in up to 5-fold hybridization reaction kinetics acceleration with significantly improved signal uniformity. Acoustic microstreaming has many advantages over most existing chamber micromixing techniques, including simple apparatus, ease of implementation, low power consumption (~2 mW) (Liu et al. 2004b).

Another micromixer based on acoustics driven to increase antibodies-antigen binding which is forms the immunoassays such as enzyme-linked immunosorbent assay ELISA is presented by Gao et al. 2015). The external sound waves in the frequency range of 125 Hz to 150 Hz was used for micromixer. The acoustic micromixer is successfully increasing the initial binding rate of over 80% (Gao et al. 2015).

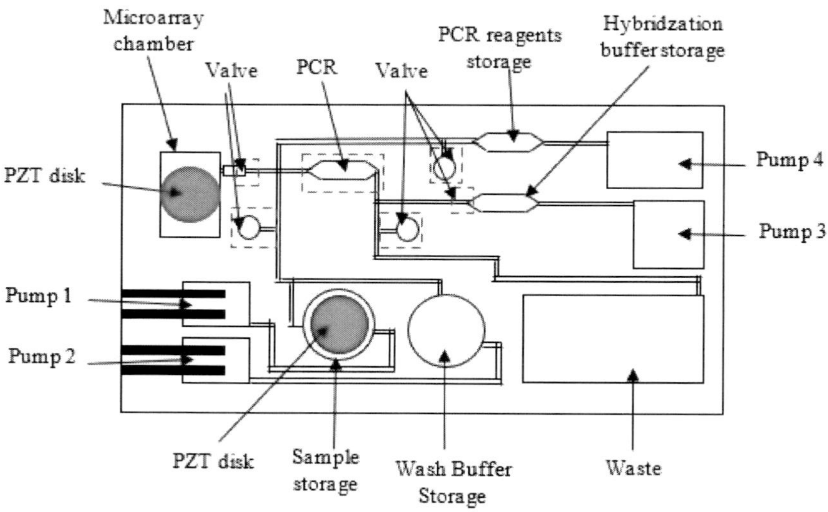

Figure 6. Schematic of the fully integrated PCR chip with a thermopneumatic air micropump and three electrochemical pumps (Liu et al., 2004b).

The bubble-based micromixer module fabricated with a combination of low-cost rapid prototyping techniques was presented by Coned et al. (Conde et al. 2020). The individual control of multiple micromixers embedded within the same monolithic chip can be integrated with any substrate. The static and continuous flow conditions can enhance mixing capabilities. The system is capable of performing cell-free DNA extractions from small volumes of blood plasma (≤500 μL) with up to a ten-fold increase. The convection mix method is used to mix the species and capillarity regulation to achieve sample transport on a single platform without the pump required is presented by Kim et al. as shown in Figure 7. The mixing rate as high as a few tens of seconds per microliter is achieved even at a low fluidic temperature of ~ 37°C (Kim et al. 2009).

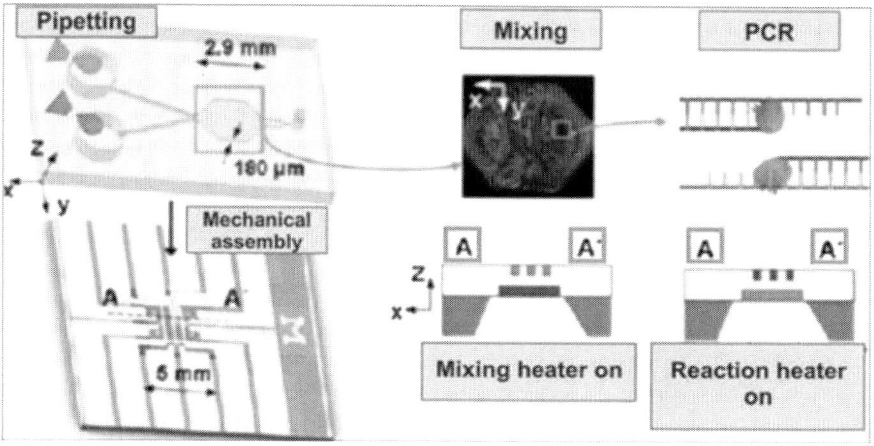

Figure 7. Schematic illustrations of single-chamber micromixing and PCR (Kim et al. 2009).

5. Research Challenges

One of these research challenges is materials limitations. Most of the microfluidic devices are fabricated using polyurethane methacrylate which is showing elastomeric behaviors such as polydimethylsiloxane (PDMS) (Kim et al. 2009; Conde et al. 2020; Kastani et al. 2016). In the late of 1990s, the utilization of PDMS is growth to fabricate much microfluidic research because of its compatibility with the soft lithography process (Kefala et al. 2015; Cai et al. 2019). However, PDMS has many limitations and is not suitable for mass production (Chiu et al. 2017). Also, PDMS also suffers from swelling with chemicals (Lee et al. 2003). On the other hand, glass or silicon substrates are robust but require advanced fabrication processes whose cost. Interestingly, the silicon and glass are emerging as important materials for microfluidic devices with integrated electrodes, high aspect ratio channels, and able to patterned by e-beam. However, the glass materials become one of constraint when the fabrication processes required to create a deep channel in glass (Toan et al. 2016). Furthermore, the other issue is the fragility of the material.

The issues of PDMS in all microfluidic devices also should be considered. Several issues using PDMS which are as follows:

1) Hydrophobic small molecular absorption: Due to the PDMS has hydrophobic property from polymer network structure, the utilization of fluorescent molecules to diffuse and absorb into PDMS walls can allow some hydrophobic pharmaceutical drugs. This absorption and diffusion of small molecules can affect the accuracy and reliability of the experiments conducted in PDMS based devices (Toepke et al. 2006; Ren et al. 2010).
2) The leaching of uncrosslinked oligomers from PDMS: The residual uncrosslinked polymer chains by cured PDMS can freely diffuse the bulk material (Regehr et al. 2009).
3) The unstable surface property caused by oxygen plasma treatment: to facilitate chip bonding, oxygen plasma commonly used to convert the hydrophobic surface of PDMS to hydrophilic surfaces. Unfortunately, the hydrophobic properties return because the polymer chain can replace the hydroxyl groups by diffusing from the bulk to the surface (Eddington et al. 2006).
4) It works only in moderate temperatures
5) Surface roughness: It depends to the fabrication of the master molding process. When the roughness increase, a larger area for adsorption and air bubble production occurs.

In terms of the fabrication method, the microfluidic device is limited to quasi-3D planar formats. Several research groups have used 3D printing involving to print 3D microfluidic reactors and reagents in situ, and to print the master mold of microfluidic (Ho et al. 2015; Chan et al. 2016; Bohr et al. 2015). Both the resolution and cost of consumer-grade 3D printers have been plunging in recent years and are currently at a point where they are starting to be applied to microfluidic device fabrication. Direct printing will not only greatly accelerate device prototyping but also give scientists an easily accessible and empowering tool to express their creativity in the way that the introduction of PDMS soft lithography (Waheed et al. 2016; Zips et al. 2018; Cuarte et al. 2017).

The potential breakthroughs in the designs and development of these microfluidic elements within PCR chips are included as follows. First, inexpensive materials which are developed with the compatibility of MEMS fabrication techniques expanded should encourage the micropump, microvalves/micromixer to be integrated. Second, the concept of active "self-supplied" in the microfluidic becomes important within PCR chips where no external bulky pneumatic supply, valve connection tubing, and even power supply required. Third, the single-chip contains microvalves/micropumps/micromixers integrated will get larger to perform the high-throughput PCR amplification and subsequent analysis.

6. FUTURE: SMART MICROFLUIDIC PLATFORMS

The automation design of microfluidic has the potential to provide many of the above interesting issues. For example, Thakur et al. developed the programmable microfluidic platform for spatiotemporal over nanoliter droplets (Thakur et al. 2015). To control the micropump such as the number of pump cycles and rate of valve actuation, a programmable microvalves controller is used. Yu et al. presented a microfluidic chip for PCR application that can automatically analyze the result detection within one hour (Yu et al. 2018). Meanwhile, Yehezkiel et al. designed a digital microfluidic with programmable order polymerization (Yehezkiel et al. 2015). The digital microfluidic can clone of assembled synthetic DNA by the PCR method. At present, the realization of functional digital microfluidic systems is still inception. Also, the digital microfluidic still equipped with many complex device apparatuses. However, the digital microfluidic performance will improve in a few years.

Many integrated circuit designers are rarely deal with semiconductor wafer or probe station. Therefore, the requirement for software experts that able to design and optimized the structure and then combine them with the fabrication experts and programmer experts so they can realize the smart microfluidic devices. Furthermore, the digital microfluidic will continue to have a significant potential application, especially in virus detection.

Future developments will relate also to bringing this technology into commercial devices worked on by non-specialists. Additionally, the requirement of standardization in microfluidic components is needed to be operated by unskilled end users. Commercialization of systems using microfluidic devices will become more frequent with many multinational companies investing heavily in microfluidic research. Devices for basic research will also remain very important, especially in the biological field due to researchers are trying to produce 'human-on-chips'. Future intelligent microfluidic platforms will also have a large impact on artificial intelligence and biological computations. This is ideal for applications, e.g., COVID-19 detection using the PCR method.

CONCLUSION

Much progress has been achieved in the microfluidic-based PCR system. Clear descriptions for every microfluidic device, namely micropump, microvalve, and micromixer used to develop the whole Polymerase Chain Reaction system are discussed in detail, including their advantages and disadvantages. It is concluded that much progress has been achieved in the microfluidic-based on the Polymerase Chain Reaction system. The future benefits of this review are to encourage the microfluidic involvement within the Polymerase Chain Reaction system, especially for the application of COVID-19 rapid detection.

REFERENCES

Alam, M. N. H. Z., Hossain, F., Vale. A., and Kouzani, A. 2017. "Design and Fabrication of a 3D Printed Miniature Pump for Integrated Microfluidic Applications." *Int. J. Precis. Eng* 18, no. 9: 1287-1296.

Allain, M., Berthier, J., Basrour, S., and Pouteau, P. 2010. "Electrically actuated sacrificial membranes for valving in microsystems." *Journal of Micromech. Microeng 20*, no.3: 035006.

Anggraeni, S., Maulidina, A., Dewi, M. W., Rahmadianti, S., Rizky, Y. P. C., Arinalhaq, Z. F., Usdiyana, D., Nandiyanto, A. B. D., and Al-Obaidi, A. S. M. 2020. The Deployment of Drones in Sending Drugs and Patient Blood Samples COVID-19. *Indonesian Journal of Science and Technology*, 5(2), 193–200.

Anjorin, A. A. 2020. "The coronavirus disease 2019 (COVID-19) pandemic: A review and an update on cases in Africa." *Asian Pac. J. Trop. Med* 13, no. 19: 199-203.

Au, A. K., Lai, H., Utela, B. R., and Folch, A. 2011. "Microvalves and micropumps for bioMEMS." *Micromachines* 2, no.2011: 179-220.

Baek, C., and Min, J. 2015. "Microvalves-assisted bead-beating system for selective nucleic acid preparation from bacteria and viruses." *Bio Chip Journal* 9, no.4: 332-338.

Bohr, A., Boetker, J., Wang, Y., Jensen, H., Rantanen, J., and Beck-Broichsitter, M. 2017. "High-throughput fabrication of nanocomplexes using 3D-printed micromixers." *Journal of pharmaceutical sciences* 106, no. 3: 835-842.

Cady, N. C., Stelick, S., Kunnavakkam, M. V., and Batt, C. A. 2005. "Real-time PCR detection of Listeria monocytogenes using an integrated microfluidics platform." *Sens Actuators B Chem* 107, no. 2005: 332–341.

Cai, G., Zheng, L., Liao, M., Li, Y., Wang, M., Liu, N., and Lin, J. 2019. "A microfluidic immunosensor for visual detection of foodborne bacteria using immunomagnetic separation, enzymatic catalysis and distance indication." *Microchim Acta.* 186, no.757: 1-9.

Chan, H. N., Shu, Y., Xiong, B., Chen, Y., Tian, Q., Michael, S. A., Shen, B., and Wu, H. 2016. "Simple, cost-effective 3D printed microfluidic components for disposable, point-of-care colorimetric analysis." *ACS Sens* 1, no.2016: 227–234.

Chen, X., and Zhao, Z. 2017. "Numerical investigation on layout optimization of obstacles in a threedimensional passive micromixer." *Analytica chimica acta* 964, no: 2017: 142-149.

Chen, X., and Zhang, L. 2017. "A review on micromixers actuated with magnetic nanomaterials." *Microchimica Acta* 184, no. 10: 3639-3649.

Chiu, D. T., deMello, A. J., Carlo, D. D., Doyle, P. S., Hansen, C., Maceiczyk, R. M., and Wootton, R. C. R. 2017. "Small but Perfectly Formed? Successes, Challenges, and Opportunities for Microfluidics in the Chemical and Biological Sciences." *Chem* 2, no.2: 201-223.

Conde, A. J., Keraite, A. I., Ongaro, A. E., and Kersaudy-Kerhoas, M. 2020. "Versatile hybrid acoustic micromixer with demonstration of circulating cell-free DNA extraction from sub-ml plasma samples." *Lab Chip* 20, no.4: 741-748.

Dittrich, P., S., Tachikawa, K., and Manz, A. 2006. "Micro total analysis systems. Latest advancements and trends." *Anal Chem* 78, no.12: 3887–3908.

Duarte, L. C., Chagas, C. L. S., Ribeiro, L. E. B., and Coltro, W. K. T. 2017. "3D printing of microfluidic devices with embedded sensing electrodes for generating and measuring the size of microdroplets based on contactless conductivity detection." *Sens Act Actuator B Chem.* 251, no.2017: 427-432.

Eddington, D. T., Puccinelli, J. P., and Beebe, D. J. 2006. "Thermal aging and reduced hydrophobic recovery of polydimethylsiloxane." *Sensors and Actuators B: Chemical* 114, no. 1: 170-172.

Gao, Y., Tran, P., Duran, K. P., Swalloe, T., and Zhu, Y. 2015. "Acoustic micromixing increases antibody-antigen binding in immunoassays." *Biomed Microdevices*, 17, no.79: 1-5.

Hashim, S., Masek, A., Abdullah, N. S., Paimin, A. N., & Muda, W. H. N. W. Students' Intention to Share "Information Via Social Media: A Case

Study of COVID-19 Pandemic." *Indonesian Journal of Science and Technology* vol.5, no.2:236-245.

Hashimoto, M., Barany, F., and Soper, S. A. 2006. "Polymerase chain reaction/ligase detection reaction/hybridization assays using flow-through microfluidic devices for the detection of low-abundant DNA point mutations." *Biosens Bioelectron* 21, no.10: 1915–1923.

Ho, C. M. B., Ng, S. H, Li, K. H. H., and Yoon, Y. J. 2015. "3D printed microfluidics for biological applications." *Lab Chip* 15, no.2015: 3627–3637.

Jeong, G. S., Chung, S., Kim, C. B., and Lee, S. H. 2010. "Applications of micromixing technology." *Analyst* 135, no.3: 460-473.

Kastania, A. S., Tsougeni, K., Papadakis, G., Gizeli, E., Kokkoris, G., Tserepi, A., and Gogolides, E. 2016. "Plasma micro-nanotextured polymeric micromixer for DNA purification with high efficiency and dynamic range." *Analytica chimica acta* 942, 2016: 58-67.

Kefala, I. N., Papadopoulos, V. E., Karpou, G., Kokkoris, G., Papadakis, G., and Tserepi, A. 2015. "A labyrinth split and merge micromixer for bioanalytical applications." *Microfluid Nanofluid* 19, no.2015: 1047-1059.

Kim, S. J., Wang, F., Burns, M. A., and Kurabayashi, K. 2009. "Temperature-programmednatural convection for micromixing and biochemical reaction in a singlemicrofluidic chamber." *Anal. Chem* 81. No.11: 4510–4516.

Kopp, M. U., and de Mello A. J., Manz, A. 1998. "Chemical amplification: continuous flow PCR on a chip." *Science* 280, no.1998: 1046–1054.

Le, T. N., Nguyen, V. A., Bach, G. L., Tran, L. D., and Cao, H. H. 2020. "Design and Fabrication of a PDMS-Based Manual Micro-Valve System for Microfluidic Applications." *Adv. Polym. Technol* 2020, no.2020: 1-7.

Lee, Y. F., Lien, K. Y., Lei, H. Y., and Lee, G. B. 2009. "An integrated microfluidic system forrapid diagnosis of dengue virus infection." *Biosens. Bioelectron* 25, no.2009: 745–752.

Lee, J. N., Park C., and Whitesides, G. M. 2003. "Solvent compatibility of poly (dimethylsiloxane)-based microfluidic devices." *Analytical chemistry* 75, no. 23: 6544-6554.

Li, Y., Jiang, Y., Wang, K., and Wu, W. 2018. "A passive micropump for highly-stable, long-termed and large volume of droplet generation/transport inside 3D microchannel capable of surfactant-free and droplet-based thermo-cycled RT-PCRs based on single thermostatic heater." *Anal. Chem* 90, no.20: 11925-11932.

Liao, C. S, Lee, G. B, Liu, H. S., Hsieh, T. M., and Luo, C. H. 2005. "Miniature RT–PCR system for diagnosis of RNA-based viruses." *Nucleic Acids Research* 33, no. 18: 156-166.

Liu, R. H., Yang, J., Lenigk, R., Bonanno, J., and Grodzinski, P. 2004. "Self-contained, fully integrated biochip for sample preparation, polymerase chain reaction amplification, and DNA microarray detection." *Anal Chem* 76, no:7: 1824–1831.

Liu, J. F., Yadavali, S., Tsourkas, A., and Issadore, D. 2017. "Microfluidic diafiltration-on-chip using an integrated magnetic peristaltic micropump." *Lab on a Chip* 17, no. 22 (2017): 3796-3803.

Maryanti, R., Hufad, A., Sunardi, Nandiyanto, A. B. D., and Al-Obaidi, S. M. 2020a. "Understanding COVID-19 particle contagion through aerosol droplets for students with special needs." *Journal of Engineering Science and Technology* vol.15, no.3:1909-1920

Maryanti, R, Hufad, A, Sunardi, Nandiyanto, A. B. D, Manullang, T. I. B. 2020b. "Understanding Coronavirus (COVID-19) as a Small Particle to Students with Special Needs." *Horizon* vol.2, no.1: 121-130.

Moreno, J. M., Quero, J. M. 2010. A novel single-use su-8 microvalves for pressure-driven microfluidic applications. *J. Micromech. Microeng*, *20*, 015005.

Münchow, G., Dadic, D., Doffing, F., Hardt, S., and Drese, K. S. 2005. "Automated chip-based device for simple and fast nucleic acid amplification." *Expert Rev Mol Diagn* 5, no.4: 613–620.

Rasouli, M., Mehrizi, A. A., Goharimanesh, M., Lashkaripour, A., and Bazaz, S. R. 2018. "Multi-criteria optimization of curved and baffle-embedded micromixers for bio-applications." *Chemical Engineering and Processing-Process Intensification*, *132*, no. 2018: 175-186.

Regehr, K. J., Domenech, M., Koepsel, J. T., Carver, K. C., Ellison-Zelski, S. J., Murphy, W. L., Schuler, L. A., Alarid, E. T., and Beebe, D. J. 2009. "Biological implications of polydimethylsiloxane-based microfluidic cell culture." *Lab on a Chip* 9, no. 15: 2132-2139.

Ren, K., Zhao, Y., Su, J., Ryan, D., and Wu, H. 2010. "Convenient method for modifying poly (dimethylsiloxane) to be airtight and resistive against absorption of small molecules." *Analytical chemistry* 82, no. 14: 5965-5971.

Santini, J. T., Cima, M. J., and Langer, R. A. 1999. "Controlled-release microchip." *Nature 397*, no.199: 335-338.

Tang, S. Q., Li, K. H. H., Lee, S. J., Zeng, J. J., and Ng, S. H. 2019. "Novel multi-way microvalves with ease of fabrication and integration for microfluidics application." *Sens Act Actuator B Chem* 286, no. 2019: 289-300.

Thakur, R., Zhang, Y., Amin, A., and Wereley, S. 2015. "Programmable microfluidic platform for spatiotemporal control over nanoliter droplets." *Microfluid Nanofluid* 18, no.5:1425-1431.

Toan, N. V., Toda, M., and Ono, T. 2016. An investigation of process for glass micromachining." *Micromachines* 7, no.51: 1-12.

Toepke, M. W., and Beebe, D. J. 2006. "PDMS absorption of small molecules and consequences in microfluidic applications." *Lab on a Chip* 6, no. 12: 1484-1486.

Vilkner, T., Janasek, D., and Manz, A. 2004. "Micro total analysis systems: recent developments." *Anal Chem* 76, no.12: 3373–86.

Waheed, S., Cabot, J. M., Macdonald, N. P., Lewis, T., Guijt, R. M., Paull, B., and Breadmore, M. C. 2016. 3D printed microfluidic devices: enablers and barriers. *Lab Chip* 16, no.2016: 1993-2013.

Yehezkel, T. B., Rival, A., Raz, O, Cohen, R., Marx, Z., Camara, M., Dubern, J. F., Koch, B., Heeb, S., Krasnogor, N., Delattre, C., and Shapiro, E. 2015. "Synthesis and cell-free cloning of DNA libraries using programmable microfluidics." *Nucleic Acids Res.* 44, no.4: 1–12

Yu, J. C., Hu, C. C., Chang, W. H., Chen, P. C., Lee, M. S., Peng, K. T., and Lee, G. B. 2018. "An integrated microfluidic system using mannose-binding lectin for bacteria isolation and biofilm-related gene detection." *Microfluid Nanofluid* 22, no.1: 13-23.

Zahra, A., Scipinotti, R., Caputo, D., Nascetti, A., and de Cesare, G. 2015. "Design and fabrication of microfluidics system integrated with temperature actuated microvalves." *Sens Act Actuator A Phys* 236, no.2015: 206-213.

Zhang, X., Oseyemi, A. E. 2019. Microfluidic Passive Valve with Ultra-Low Threshold Pressure for High-Throughput Liquid Delivery. *Micromachines*. 10, 1-12.

Zhang, B., Luo, Y., Zhou, B., Wang, Q., and Millner, P.D. 2015. "A novel microfluidicmixer-based approach for determining inactivation kinetics of Escherichia coli O157:H7 in chlorine solutions." *Food Microbiol* 49, no.2015: 152–160.

Zips, S., Wenzel, O. J., Rinklin, P., Grob, L., Terkan, K., Adly, N. Y., Weiß, L., and Wolfrum, B. 2018. "Direct Stereolithographic 3D Printing of Microfluidic Structures on Polymer Substrates for Printed Electronics." *In 9th International Nanomedicine Conference, Sydney, Australia 2018, no.*1800455: 1-5.

In: COVID-19 ISBN: 978-1-53618-903-2
Editors: A. B. D. Nandiyanto et al.

Chapter 28

COMMUNITY SERVICE DURING COVID-19 PANDEMIC AT UNIVERSITAS PENDIDIKAN INDONESIA

A. Ana[1], Asep Bayu Dani Nandiyanto[1,*], M. Syaom Barliana[1], Iwa Kuntadi[1], Dedi Suryadi[1], Vina Dwiyanti[1] and M. Muktiarni[1]

[1]Universitas Pendidikan Indonesia, Bandung, Jawa Barat, Indonesia

ABSTRACT

Coronavirus 2019 (COVID-19) epidemic has become an international concern and has posed challenges to psychological resilience in all areas. As one of the three pillars of higher education system in Indonesia, students and lecturers play a role in the community through community service program. In keeping with the present situation and circumstances, the community service program conducted this year related to the COVID-19 global pandemic. Universitas Pendidikan Indonesia lecturers and students invented and developed tools used to prevent the spread of COVID-19. The

* Corresponding Author's Email: bmulyanti@upi.edu.

invented and developed tools were disinfectant gate, portable sink, Nano Cabin Healing, SP-WASH-O Dual Chamber Automatic Disinfectant, masks and hand sanitizer. The innovation and development of these tools are part of partnership among lecturers, students, and the Anti-COVID-19 Brigade Team in Universitas Pendidikan Indonesia. Besides, it is also part of community service programs conducted by students who are members of the UPI Organization Movement Unit Team (SGO-UPI). The students shared foods, masks, and hand sanitizers to the locals live around the university. All the community service programs were conducted to break the COVID-19 spread chain as well as to overcome and reduce the negative impacts caused by the pandemic primarily from the community's public health, environment, and economic condition.

Keywords: COVID-19, community service, higher education, innovation

1. Introduction

At the beginning of 2020, a new history in Indonesia and in more than 200 countries in the world started as we experience the Corona Virus Disease pandemic outbreak (WHO 2020). On 11 February, 2020, the World Health Organization (WHO) named the disease from the corona virus as "COVID-19," an acronym of "coronavirus disease 2019" (Razon 2020). The WHO has officially declared the COVID-19 condition to be a global pandemic and the whole world should pay serious attention to it. Thus, all public activities, including educational institutions with a large number of masses, must be halted to reduce the amount of COVID-19 virus transmission and spread (Paules, Marston and Fauci 2020).

COVID-19 is a disease caused by acute coronavirus (known as SARS-CoV-2) respiratory syndrome (Darnell et al. 2004; Perlmans 2020). The deadly virus had infected the humankind after the consumption of some wild animals/birds which were being sold at the Chinese city of Wuhan (Anggraeni et al. 2020). Previous researches have shown that 54% of people in 194 cities in China encountered psychological impacts of the COVID-19 phenomena. Several factors can cause psychological impacts, one of which is the absence of human interaction due to lockdown and social isolation in different regions and countries around the world (WHO 2020). Women and students were the two most psychologically impacted groups (Wang et al. 2020).

In Indonesia, university students and lecturers as a part of the higher education components play three important roles in the implementation of the three pillars of Indonesian higher education system comprising education, research, and community service which is called *Tridharma Perguruan Tinggi*. These pillars motivate lecturers and students at Universitas Pendidikan Indonesia (UPI) to take an action as a part of its contribution and dedication to society and Indonesia amidst this COVID-19 pandemic. The students and lecturers collaborated to establish a range of resources that could support health workers and the community in the midst of COVID-19 pandemic.

2. Innovation and Device Development

The increasingly high spread of COVID-19 in the community encourages students and lecturers to develop devices that can be used by the community particularly the UPI community. The continuation of this device making is based on the issue that emerges amid the need of the community to address the COVID-19 high spread. The developed devices include the production of disinfectant gate to prevent the current spread the COVID-19 pandemic (Figure 1). It is made from a combination of iron with 2.1 meters high and 3.2 meters wide, and works by spraying the disinfectant liquid on vehicles (Medina 2020). The spraying chemicals are hydrogen peroxide (H_2O_2) and hypochlorite natrium (NaHOCl).

Furthermore, the disinfectant gate and disinfectant fluid innovation were made as a collaboration between UPI lecturers and students. Also, the UPI task force team created a portable sink tool (Figure 2) to support people who are still working outside the house and around UPI area, in an attempt to support the community and prevent COVID-19 (Humas UPI 2020).

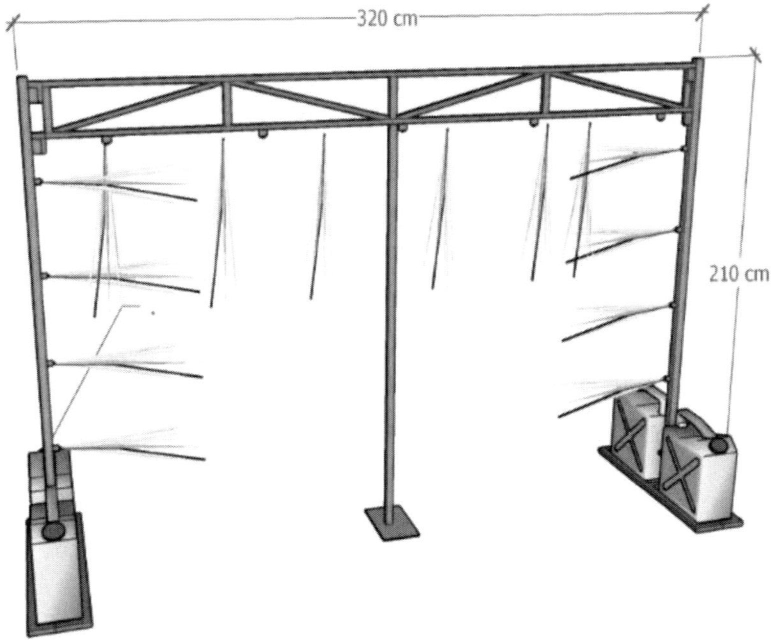

Figure 1. Disinfectant Gate.

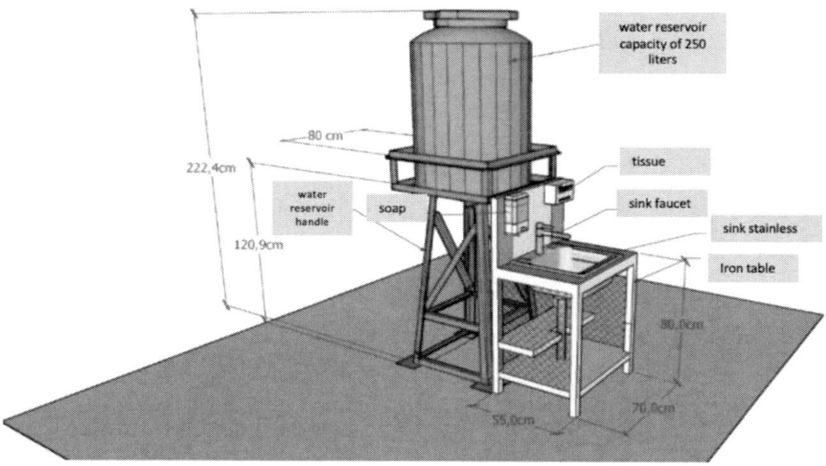

Figure 2. Portable sink.

Besides the aforementioned devices, lecturers and students also invented some other devices. Collaborating with the UPI Anti-COVID-19 Brigade Team, they created Nano Cabin Healing (Figure 3). The Nano Cabin Healing is a device used to overcome COVID-19 and other respiratory diseases, designed to improve the treatment of human immunity and the lung by means of a nano droplet injection technique. Nanoparticles are considered as the advanced materials that can perform excellently in terms of the electrical, chemical characteristics, and so on compared to the traditional ones (Digantari and Nandiyanto 2019). Nanotechnology is the branch of science and technology conducted at the nanoscale or a billionth of a meter and it first emerged in the modern era (Nandiyanto et al. 2018) and is capable of controlling nanometer-scale substances, materials, and systems, thus generating new functions. Additionally, 1 nanometer is equal to one-billionth of a meter and is 50,000 times smaller than a human hair's size. The system was created by referring to the breathing system or human respiration.

The interaction between artificial molecular assemblies or nanodevices and biomolecules can be used in extracellular media and human cells (Boisseau and Loubaton 2011). The use of nanotechnology in cabin healing is adapted to the human respiratory system, as has been done in previous studies in Europe and America, where nanotechnology has been used in healthcare technology (Khang et al. 2010). Therefore, this Nano Cabin Healing is used to increase human immunity and respiratory treatment through the nano droplet injection technology system. The system was formed by reference to the human respiratory system. It is easy and simple to use; the patient just sits on a chair with the head goes into the cabin and the smoke will be emitted.

UPI also collaborated with a ventilator expert. This collaboration aimed to create an active VENT-I device that can overcome the COVID-19 problems. Vent-I uses a Positive End-Expiratory Pressure (PEEP) ventilator for convenient operation by doctors and medical personnel.

In addition to producing nano-cabin healing, this collaboration between students and lecturers also produced Automatic Nano Sterilizer, which is a nano-technology sterilization chamber (Figure 4 on the left side).

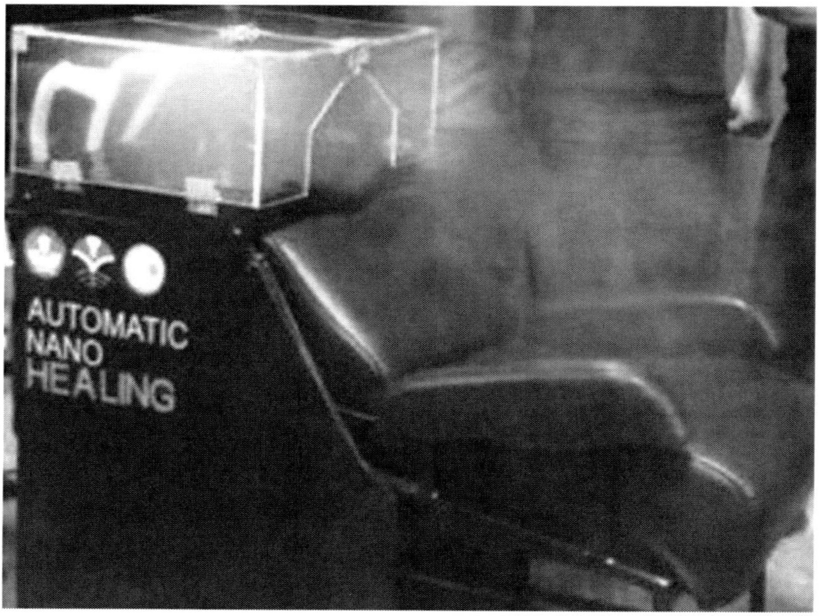

Figure 3. Automatic Nano Cabin Healing.

This chamber will address the issues of virus and bacteria. The chamber works simple and swiftly because the person enters the chamber only for 10 - 20 seconds. The sprayer will sterilize the water vapor. Since this sterilizer includes nanotechnology, the device allows the person to stay dry after sterilization. This Automatic Nano Sterilizer system could help reduce the bacteria or germs attached to the clothes or objects (Muharam 2020).

The innovation and productivity of students and lecturers as a community service process was carried out through the production of other devices. The team also created *Saung Paragi Wawasuh Awak diSemprot ku Halimun Otomatis* or SP-WASH-O (Figure 4 in the right side). It is a disinfectant chamber with two automatic disinfecting chambers with ultrasonic vibrator technology that can produce disinfectant steam with a size of 120-200 nanometers. The disinfection chamber has an entry point, an exit point, an enclosed area where disinfection takes place, a power supply, a solvent supply, a chemical room or mixer, an air supply, compressor (usually but not always), and a spray system (Darnell et al. 2004).

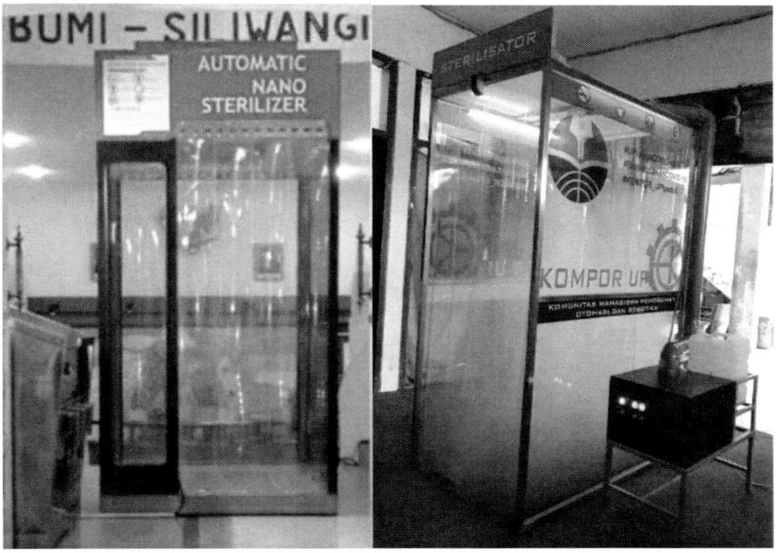

Figure 4. *Automatic Nano Sterilizer* (left) and SP-WASHO (right).

It also has optional features which include an electrical outlet for the room chamber, lighting features, audio or video options, temperature scanners, and chemical atomizers. This principle is used in the manufacture of SP-WASH-O and Automatic Nano Sterilizer tools in liquid or vapor form used for spraying disinfectants (Wickramatillake, and Kurukularatne 2020). This disinfectant chamber has been commonly used to provide medical personnel and the general public with protection and security, including many manufacturers from industries that produce and sell it.

3. Basic Personal Protective Equipment

The COVID-19 phenomenon has resulted in many changes and emerges panic in the society which has caused rising prices for PPE such as masks and hand sanitizer (Hendarto 2020). This condition motivates UPI students and lecturers to help develop resources which can be used as a community service by the local community, conducting experiments to make hand sanitizers (Figure 5 in the left side). Using hand sanitizer is also important because washing hand using soap and water is difficult to do while doing activities outside (Khosrowpour et al. 2019; Beiu et al. 2020). Being based on this, the hand sanitizers produced and distributed the local community around the university. During the COVID-19 pandemic outbreak, it also suggested that people put on masks to protect themselves as the discovery of an increase in human-to-human infection through droplets, contacts, and transmission (Pelman 2020) and people have to keep a distance and anticipate using the PPE as their personal protection especially for people with asymptomatic problem who are at high risk.

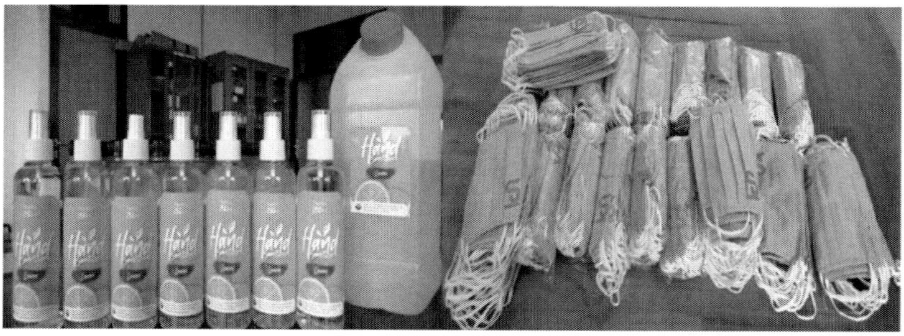

Figure 5. Hand sanitizer (left side) and face masks (right side).

Masks become one of the alternatives for protection from the COVID-19 spread as what massively happened in Wuhan, China (Cohen 2020) and the masks used have WHO standards and are adapted to the human respiratory system (Chan et al. 2020). In order to increase the awareness of using masks, the lecturers and students also produced masks (Figure 5 in the right side) and gave it to the local community along with the hand sanitizers and food. Generally, this community service is also part of the faculty to support the country in reducing and stopping the spread of the COVID-19 in the university and around its areas.

CONCLUSION

The limited conditions associated with the COVID-19 phenomenon require a great deal of creative and innovative work. Collaboration between lecturers and students in UPI established productive activities as evidence and contributions of UPI to Indonesia. Students and lecturers as a part of the elements in higher education have a role in community service activities. The community service activities carried out were collaboration between lecturers, students, UPI Anti-COVID 19 Brigade Team, and UPI Organizational Movement Unit Team (SGO-UPI) as contribution and participation for breaking the COVID-19 chain and the support to the economically affected communities around the university.

REFERENCES

Beiu, C., Mihai, M., Popa, L., Cima, L., Popescu, M. N. 2020. "Frequent Hand Washing for COVID-19 Prevention Can Cause Hand Dermatitis: Management Tips". *Cureus,* vol. 12, no. 4 (April): e7506. doi:10.7759/ cureus.7506.

Boisseau, P. and Loubaton, B. (2011). Nanomedicine, nanotechnology in medicine. *Comptes Rendus Physique,* vol. 12, no. 7:620 - 636. doi: 10.1016/j.crhy.2011.06.001.

Chan, J. F. W., Yuan, S., Kok, K. H., To, K. K. W., Chu, H., Yang, J., Yuen, K. Y. 2020. "A Familial Cluster of Pneumonia Associated with the 2019 Novel Coronavirus Indicating Person-to-Person Transmission: A Study of a Family Cluster". *The Lancet,* vol. 395, no. 10223 (February):514 - 523.

Cohen, E. 2020. "Disease detectives hunting down more information about 'super spreader' of Wuhan coronavirus". *CNN.com,* 23 January 2020. https://www.cnn.com/2020/01/23/health/wuhan-virus-super-spreader/index.html.

Darnell, M. E. R., Subbarao, K., Feinstone, S. M. and Taylor, D. R. 2004. Inactivation of the coronavirus that induces severe acute respiratory syndrome, SARS-CoV. *Journal of Virological Methods,* vol. 121, no. 1: 85 - 91.doi: 10.1016/j.jviromet.2004.06.006.

Dirgantari, P. D. and Nandiyanti, A. B. D. 2019. "Development Strategy of Earthworms Nanoparticle Products Using Ball Mill Methods in Indonesia". *Journal of Engineering Science and Technology,* vol. 14, no. 2 (April): 589 - 598.

Hendarto, Y. M. 2020. "Di Balik Melambungnya Harga" Hand Sanitizer" dan Masker Saat Wabah Covid-19" ["Behind the Soaring Prices of "Hand Sanitizers and Masks during the Covid-19 Outbreak"]. *Kompas.com*, 1 April 2020. https://kompas.id/ baca/riset/2020/04/01/di-balik-melambungnya-hand-sanitizer-dan-masker-saat-wabah-covid-19/.

Humas UPI. 2020. "Tim Satgas COVID-19 UPI Luncurkan Disinfectant Gate" ["UPI COVID-19 Task Force Team Launches Disinfectant Gate"] *Portal Berita UPI,* 25 March 2020. https://berita.upi.edu/tim-satgas-covid-19-upi-luncurkan-disinfectant-gate/.

Khang, D., Carpenter, J., Chun, Y. W., Pareta, R., Webster, T. J. 2010. "Nanotechnology for regenerative medicine". *Biomedical microdevices*, vol. 12, 4 (August): 575 - 87. doi:10.1007/s10544-008-9264-6.

Khosrowpour, Z., Ahmad Nasrollahi, S., Ayatollahi, A., Samadi, A., Firooz, A. 2019. "Effects of four soaps on skin trans-epidermal water loss and erythema index". *Journal of cosmetic dermatology*, vol. 18, 3 (June): 857 - 861. doi:10.1111/jocd.12758.

Medina, M. I. 2020. "UPI Develops Disinfectant Gate to Prevent Coronavirus". *Portal Berita UPI,* 13 April 2020. http://berita.upi.edu/ en/upi-develops-disinfectant-gate-to-prevent-coronavirus/.

Muharam, M. A. 2020. "Nano Technology Sterilization Chamber Made in Bandung". *Portal Berita UPI.* 24 March 2020. http://berita.upi.edu/en/ nano-technology-sterilization-chamber-made-in-bandung/.

Nandiyanto, A. B. D., Asyahidda, F. N., Danuwijaya, A. A., Abdullah, A. G., Amelia, N., Hudha, M. N. and Aziz, M. 2018. "Teaching "Nanotechnology" For Elementary Students with Deaf and Hard of Hearing". *Journal of Engineering Science and Technology,* vol. 13, no. 5 (May): 1352 - 1363.

Paules, C. I., Marston, H. D. and Fauci, A. S. 2020. "Coronavirus infections—more than just the common cold". *JAMA*, vol. 323 no. 8 (January):707 - 708. doi:10.1001/jama.2020.0757.

Perlman, S. 2020. "Another Decade, another Coronavirus". *The New England Journal of Medicine,* 382 (January): 760 - 762. doi: 10.1056/NEJMe2001126.

Razon, B. C. 2020. "COVID 19: Impetus for "Community Spirits" among Filipinos". *Indonesian Journal of Science and Technology,* vol. 5, no. 2 (March): 201 - 208.

Wang, C., Pan, R., Wan, X., Tan, Y., Xu, L., Ho, C. S. and Ho, R. C. 2020. "Immediate Psychological Responses and Associated Factors during the Initial Stage of the 2019 Coronavirus Disease (COVID-19) Epidemic among the General Population in China". *International Journal of Environmental Research and Public Health*, vol. 17, no. 5 (Mar):1729. doi:10.3390/ijerph17051729.

Wickramatillake, A. and Kurukularatne, C. 2020. "SARS-CoV-2 human disinfection chambers: a critical analysis". *Occupational Medicine*, Volume 70, no. 5, (May): 330 - 334, https://doi.org/10.1093/occmed/kqaa078.

World Health Organization (2020). "Coronavius Diseases (COVID-19) Pandemic". *WHO Worldwide.* https://www.who.int/emergencies/diseases/novel-coronavirus-2019.

In: COVID-19 ISBN: 978-1-53618-903-2
Editors: A. B. D. Nandiyanto et al.

Chapter 29

SIMULATION OF MULTI-HOP ROUTING WIRELESS SENSOR NETWORK TOPOLOGY PERFORMANCE AND ITS ADVANTAGES DURING COVID-19 PANDEMIC

Lilik Hasanah[1,*], Heru Yuwono[2], Ahmad Aminudin[1] and Budi Mulyanti[3]

[1]Department Pendidikan Fisika, FPMIPA,
Universitas Pendidikan Indonesia, Bandung, Jawa Barat, Indonesia
[2]PT Smartfren Telecom Tbk, Indonesia
[3]Department Pendidikan Teknik Elektro, FPTK,
Universitas Pendidikan Indonesia, Bandung, Jawa Barat, Indonesia

ABSTRACT

Wireless Sensor Network (WSN) application for remote monitoring and data acquisition especially during COVID-19 pandemic situation is performed. A simulation was conducted to determine the performance of

* Corresponding Author's Email: lilikhasanah@upi.edu.

WSN networks with different topologies and sizes using a Multi-hop routing. Analysis was also done in its energy usage. The WSN network in the simulation was made with Arduino-based hardware with a compatible radio transmitter module. The simulation was done in the MATLAB software environment. In the simulation, two network topologies were used, namely the Random and Grid topology and network sizes of 16 and 121 sensor nodes. It was found that the Grid topology has better performance compared to Random topology. The life time of a WSN network is not affected by the number of sensor nodes in the network, but by the amount of energy available at each sensor node.

Keywords: COVID-19, Random and Grid topology, Wireless Sensor Network

1. INTRODUCTION

On 11 February 2020, the World Health Organization (WHO) reported the disease, namely "COVID-19," an acronym of "coronavirus disease 2019" (Razon 2020). SARS-CoV-2 infection was first reported in Wuhan, China on 31 December, 2019 and the related literature henceforth published can help tracing the origin of the symptomatic individuals back to the early December 2019 (Anggraeni et al. 2020). During COVID-19 pandemic situation, remote monitoring and data acquisition facilitated by WSN is giving a way for application where limited human involvement and social distancing are required.

Many literatures published on the applications of wireless sensor networks (WSN) on daily life (Puccinelli and Haenggi 2005; Joshi, Nam and Kim 2003; Prathap et al. 2012; Alemdar and Ibnkahla 2007). Wireless Sensor Network (WSN) is a network of devices used to monitor the state of an environment, for example monitoring the condition of air pollution in an industrial complex, toxic gases exposure, water quality in fishponds, soil quality in agriculture, and so on. For environmental monitoring applications, WSN is characterized by the use of a large number of sensor nodes that continuously carry out measurements and send data to a number of base stations as data collectors.

Recently, the development of WSN hardware is increasingly matured supported by the development of intelligent hardware alternatives such as Xbee, Arduino and Raspberry Pi (Ferdoush and Li 2014; Kabir et al. 2014; Harikrishnan 2015; Kumbhar 2016). In this research, Arduino-based WSN nodes developed, considering its open hardware design and affordable price, although large-scale use still requires high costs. However, before the WSN hardware is developed, it is necessary to simulate the most optimal form of WSN network topology, the effect of the number of nodes, and routing schemes for transmitting data on power usage, and the efficient use of power from Arduino-based WSNs. Several studies conducted on WSN by simulation to examine the advantages of WSN (Korkalainen et al. 2009; Sobeih et al. 2006). For the application of specific hardware such as Arduino and its supporting modules, using the existing simulators is not suitable because it requires customizing the simulator software.

Thus, in this research, simulator software was made that was able to simulate the WSN in certain topologies and provide important data to researchers in analyzing WSN performance. This software made using Matlab from Mathworks, Inc. In this software, Arduino hardware is used as a reference since its ability in determining some parameters used in the simulation (Nandiyanto et al. 2018; Sukmafitri et al. 2019; Nandiyanto et al. 2019). The software created will be able to determine the most efficient topology in energy usage, fast data routing strategy, WSN network size, and maximum lifetime of a WSN network that will be implemented.

2. Research Methodology

2.1. Network Topology

A network with N nodes can be modelled as a curve diagram of G with N vertices so that $G = (V = \{1, \ldots N\})$, where the 2D/3D position of p of each vertex I point is expressed by the coordinates of $pi = (xi, yi, \text{and } zi)$. Since in this study the WSN network was simulated, the network was considered to be in a 2D plane so that the zi coordinates above could be eliminated.

The WSN network is considered to be fully connected to each sensor node, meaning that all nodes can be reached using the multi-hop communication method. In fact, connectivity between nodes is determined by the range of the radio signal so the parameters of the range of radio signals emitted by the node must be taken into account. Equation (1) can be used to calculate the estimated radio signal range from the sensor node (Simek and Moravek 2011).

$$R = \Phi\sqrt{\frac{\log N}{N}} \quad (1)$$

The parameter Φ is the 2D plane diameter that is proportional to the number of sensor nodes N. The range of the radio signal is expressed as R. By knowing the value of R, it can be determined how much energy is required by a node to send the signal to another node.

2.2. Multi-Hop Routing

In WSN applications for monitoring environmental condition, sensor nodes are generally powered by batteries, which can be replaced if their powers are depleted. The optimal routing strategy can reduce battery's power usage, so it can extend the operational life time of the WSN network.

Routing is the process of determining the route between the starting point and destination point in terms of data transmission. Several types of protocols have been proposed to extend the network life time and to determine the route of data delivery to the network data collector, including LEACH, HEED, PEGASIS, TEEN, and APTEEN (Joshi and Priya 2012). Multi-hop communication uses less energy than single-hop over long distances between nodes. Examples of multi-hop protocols are M-LEACH (Biradar et al. 2011) and MR-LEACH (Farooq, Dogar and Shah 2012).

In this research, multi-hop routing is applied using a simpler tree-diagram-based routing. In this routing strategy, no particular sensor node is selected to be the Head of the Group as there is possibility that the Head Group node is too far away, with distance of greater than *R* from the surrounding nodes. In tree-diagram-based routing, data from the initial sensor node is sent to the base station through a series of other nodes that form a tree structure. Thus, each node is responsible for resending data received from the node below it. Nodes with a significant number of neighbors below it can cause energy bottleneck, where these nodes can run out of battery power in a very short time. Furthermore, Dijkstra's algorithm for determining the closest distance between nodes in a curve structure can be used to determine tree-based multi-hop route. Using grTheory toolbox for Matlab, Dijkstra's algorithm is implemented (Sergi 2009).

2.3. Energy Consumption Model

The number of messages was processed by each node during the data collection process. For 4 sensor nodes, node *n1* starts sending data to the next node up until node *n4*. Node *n2* receives data, checks route information, and then sends the message again to the next node. Because the sensor node uses an omnidirectional type antenna, the same message is also received again by node *n1*. However, at this time, the message received *n1* is ignored because the recipient's identification in the message is not directed to node *n1*. Thus, node *n1* expends energy to send an initial message of ETX and ERX energy to receive a message back from *n2*. Thus, *n1* energy usage is:

$$E_{n1} = E_{TX} + E_{RX} \quad (2)$$

Then, node *n2* and node *n3* as a relay node used ERX energy to receive messages from the previous node, ETX to resend messages, and ERX to receive messages from the next node. Thus, the energy used by the relay node is:

$$E_{nr} = E_{TX} + 2E_{RX} \quad (3)$$

The last node *n4* as the base station node is only responsible for receiving messages so that the energy used is equal to ERX.

$$E_{SB} = E_{RX} \quad (4)$$

The hardware used was an Arduino Uno R3 system with the nRF24L01 radio transceiver module. Important parameters of the radio transceiver were the electrical current consumption when sending data which was 11.30 mA, receiving data of 11.80 mA, and when the stand-by was 22 uA, the transition time from the standby state to the ready to send and receive data state that is 130 us (micro seconds), and vice versa. Another parameter is the speed of data transfer of this radio which is equal to 1 Mbps.

The length of the message which contains sensor data sent by each node is assumed based on the results obtained by Milan (Simek and Moravek 2011). In the IEEE 802.15.4 protocol, the data payload length is 30 bytes. In addition, there are also other additional messages, namely Data Request messages as long as 12 bytes, ACK messages that are used as communication controls requires 5 bytes. Total length of data transmitted between sensor nodes is 47 bytes.

2.4. Simulation Scope

There are two types of network topologies to be simulated namely grid and random topology. In a grid topology, sensor nodes are arranged at similar distance from each other to form a square. In a random topology, sensor nodes are placed randomly where the distance between nodes is made to be smaller than the value of *R* as shown in equation (1). For each topology, different numbers of nodes are simulated, which are 16 and 121 nodes. All nodes are connected each other. The program determines a node that acts as the recipient of all data, called as the base station node.

Data transmission is done in a multi-hop strategy, where a sensor node sends its data to the base station node through several other nodes which serve as relay nodes. The relay node receives data and sends it again to the next relay node or directly to the base station node. It is assumed that the area where the sensor nodes installed is a rectangular area of 500 meters in length and 500 meters in width.

In the simulation, several assumptions were taken. The first assumption was that each node has energy of 1 Joule at the beginning, except the base station node which is considered to have unlimited energy so that the base station node never dies. Next assumption was that the power consumption of the Arduino base system is not taken into account as it will mask the effects of the sensor node power consumption. The last assumption was that the simulation does not considering the time for the sensor in the sleep/stand-by position.

The simulation was carried out in several rounds. One round means that all nodes, from node number 1 to number *N*, have sent data to the base station node. In the next round, the data transmission is repeated in similar manner. At each data transmission, the nodes use energy so that its total energy will be reduced. Nodes that do not have enough energy will be marked as a dead node and cannot participate in the next round. The simulation was stopped if the nodes located one hop before the base station node run out of energy or became a dead node, shown by the sending data to the base station node impossible.

3. Result and Analysis

The simulation was done with two types of network topologies: grid and random (as shown in Figures 1 and 2 with 16 nodes). For the random topology (Figure 1), if node 8 acts as the base station node, then nodes 1, 2, 4, 5, 6, and 13 are located 1 hop before the base station node. If all nodes die, the simulation is stopped. In the grid topology in Figure 2, if node 1 is a base station node, the node located 1 hop before is node 2, 5, and 6.

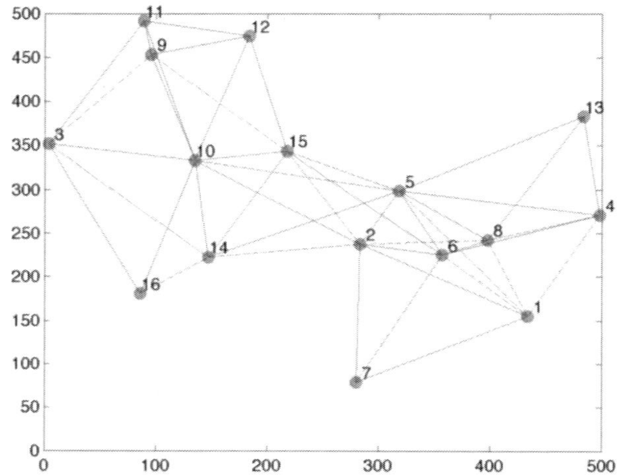

Figure 1. Random Network in Topology structure. Each node is numbered.

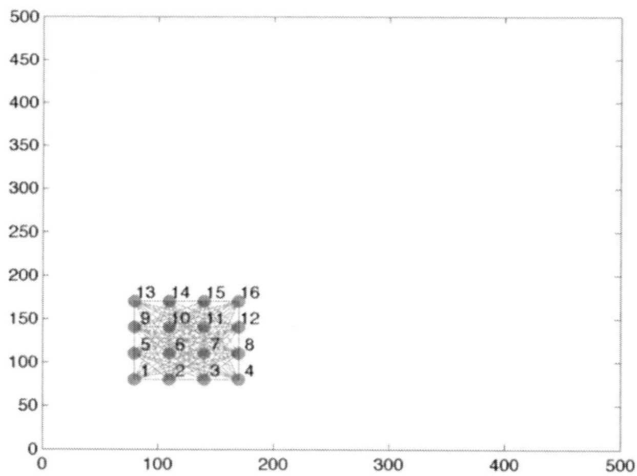

Figure 2. Random Network in Grid structure. Each node is numbered.

Figures 3, 4, 5, and 6 show the number of alive nodes at the end of each simulation round for random and grid topology with different numbers of nodes. From Figures 3 and 5, it can be seen that in the Random topology with the increasing number of sensor nodes. The dead nodes in random network happen earlier than that in grid network (see Figures 4 and 6). On the random network with 16 nodes, the first node dies at round 72, whereas at node number 121, it occurs at round 32. In the Grid topology, as shown in figures 4 and 6, for the number of nodes 16 the first node appears to die at round 143 while for the number of nodes 121 occurs at round 52. In both topology and number of nodes, all sensor nodes die at round 222.

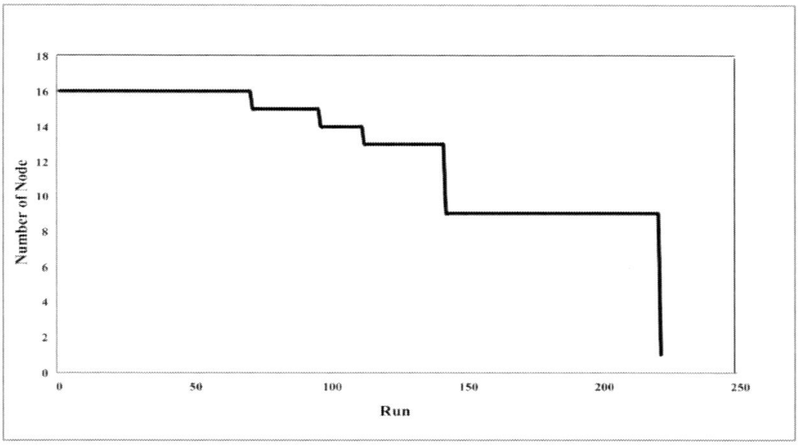

Figure 3. Number of alive nodes at the end of each round, for random topology with 16 nodes.

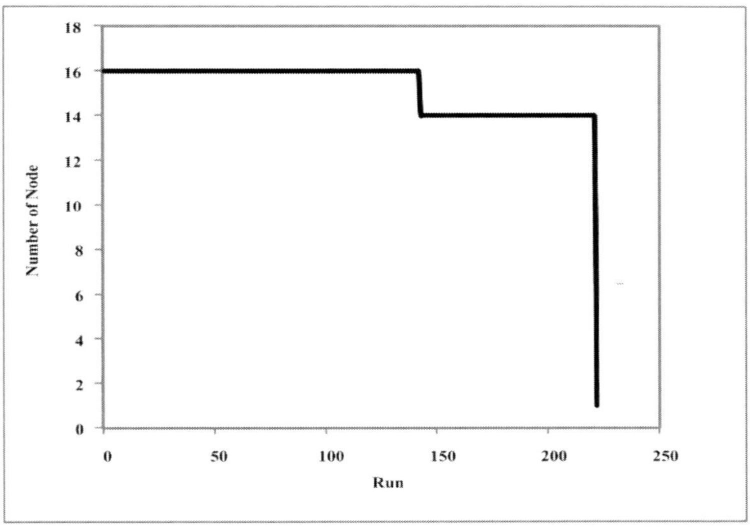

Figure 4. Number of alive nodes at the end of each round, for Grid topology with 16 nodes.

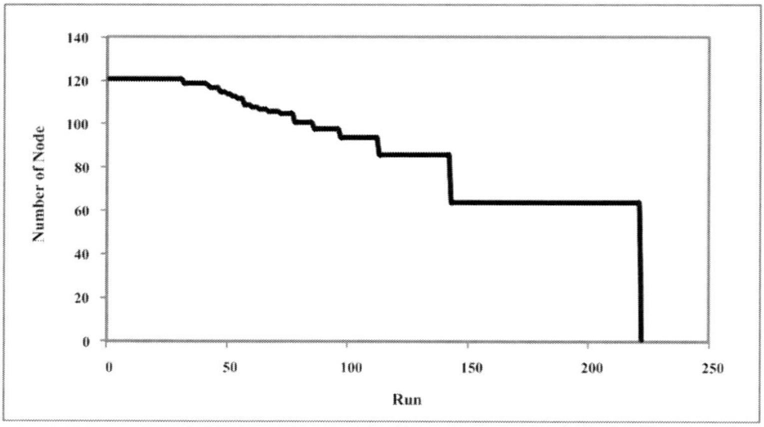

Figure 5. Number of alive nodes at the end of each round, for Random topology with 121 nodes.

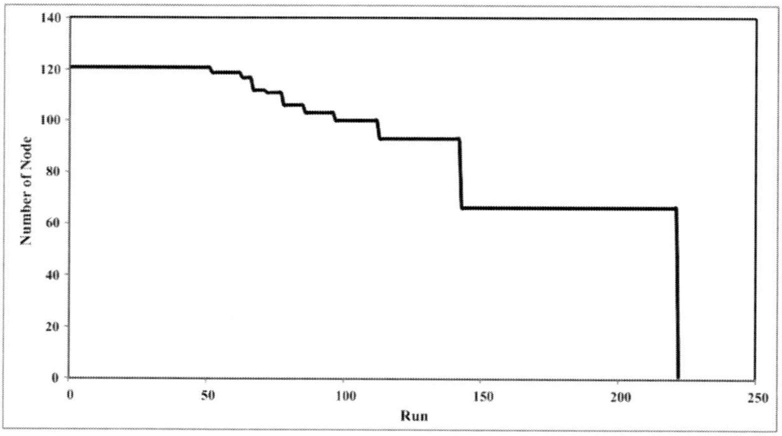

Figure 6. Number of alive nodes at the end of each round, for Grid topology with 121 nodes.

From above results, we can also analyze which topologies have better performance, whether random topologies or grid topologies. It has been mentioned before the criterion for the simulation to be considered as finished, there is no longer route for sending data from a sensor node to the base station node. This is because the node that located 1 hop before the base station node has run out of all energies. Thus, it can be counted how many data messages were successfully sent by the sensor nodes and received by the base station node. A topology with more data message received by the base station node is a better result. The number of messages received by the base station node is shown in Table 1 (Hasanah et al. 2018).

Table 1. Number of messages received by base station node for all network topologies

Number of Node	Topology					
	Random			Grid		
	Number of Messages	Round	Messages/ Node	Number of Messages	Round	Messages/ Node
16	2630	222	164.38	3172	222	198.25
121	19826	222	163.85	20658	222	170.73

Table 1 clearly shows that the increases in number of nodes in a network allow the more data messages received by the base station node. The number of data messages received is generally greater on the Grid topology than that on the Random topology. For the Random topology, the message/node value is almost the same in the range of 164 messages/node, while for the Grid topology is in the range of 179 messages/node.

With the increasing number of sensor nodes in a WSN network, the nodes (that are concurrently serving as relay nodes) get an additional workload to relay data transmission from other nodes before going to the base station node. With more data retransmission done by relay nodes, the more energy is used so that these relay nodes run out of energy faster and eventually die earlier.

Regarding the life time of a WSN network and its relationship to the number of nodes in the network, it appears that the number of nodes in a WSN network has no effect on the life time of the sensor network. Networks with the number of nodes 16 and 121 can both make 222 rounds before the network dies. It appears that the important factor is the amount of energy possessed by each node in the network. This can be seen from Figures 2-3, where there was a sharp decrease in the number of nodes that alive in the last round due to power run out.

CONCLUSION

WSN network performance simulation has been carried out successfully with different topologies and sizes. This WSN application can be used for remote monitoring and data acquisition especially during COVID-19 pandemic situation. With the increasing number of sensor nodes in the network, the correct placement of sensor nodes is very important to prevent important relay nodes from becoming a "bottleneck" in the communication path to the base station node and shortening the life time of the WSN network. Nodes that serve as relay nodes have a greater workload than other sensor nodes so that they require more energy to perform their duty and to prevent from dying earlier than other sensor nodes. Sensor network with Grid topology performs better than that network with random topology, as distance between nodes in Grid network can be controlled.

REFERENCES

Alemdar, A., and Ibnkahla, M. 2007. "Wireless sensor networks: Applications and challenges." In: *2007 9th International Symposium on Signal Processing and Its Applications* (February):1-6.

Anggraeni, S., Maulidina, A., Dewi, M. W., Rahmadianti, S., Rizky, Y. P. C., Arinalhaq, Z. F., Usdiyana, D., Nandiyanto, A. B. D., and Al-Obaidi, A. S. M. 2020. "The Deployment of Drones in Sending Drugs and Patient Blood Samples COVID-19." *Indonesian Journal of Science and Technology* vol. 5, no. 2 (March):193-200.

Biradar, R. V., Sawant, S. R., Mudholkar, R. R., and Patil, V. C. "Inter-Intra Cluster Multihop-LEACH Routing In Self-Organizing Wireless Sensor Networks." In: *International Journal of Research and Reviews in Computer Science (IJRRCS)* vol. 2, no. 1, March 2011, 88-95.

Farooq, M. O., Dogar, A. B. and Shah, G. A. "MR-LEACH: Multi-hop Routing with Low Energy Adaptive Clustering Hierarchy," *2010 Fourth*

International Conference on Sensor Technologies and Applications, Venice, 2010, 262-268. doi: 10.1109/SENSORCOMM. 2010.48.

Ferdoush, S., and Li, X. 2014. "Wireless sensor network system design using Raspberry Pi and Arduino for environmental monitoring applications." *Procedia Computer Science*, 34, 103-110. doi: 10.1016/ j.procs.2014.07.059.

Harikrishnan, R. 2015. "An integrated Xbee Arduino and Differential Evolution Approach for Localization in Wireless Sensor Networks." *Procedia Computer Science*, no. 48: 447-453.

Kumbhar, H. 2016. "Wireless sensor network using Xbee on Arduino Platform: An experimental study." In: *2016 International Conference on Computing Communication Control and automation (ICCUBEA)* August 2016, 1-5.

Hasanah, L., Yuwono, H., Aminudin, A., Suhendi, E., and Tayubi, Y. R. 2018. "Multi-Hop Wireless Sensor Network Performance and Energy Simulation." *Pertanika Journal of Science and Technology*, no. 26: 427-440.

Joshi, A and Muraleedharan, P. M. 2011. "A Survey of Hierarchical Routing Protocols in Wireless Sensor Network." In: *International Conference on Information Systems International Journal of Wireless & Mobile Networks (IJWMN)* vol. 4, no. 4, August 2012.

Joshi, G. P., Nam, S. Y., and Kim, S. W. 2013. "Cognitive radio wireless sensor networks: applications, challenges and research trends." *Sensors*, vol. 13, no. 9 (August): 11196-11228.

Kabir, A. S., Shorif, M. A., Li, H., and Yu, Q. 2014. "A study of secured wireless sensor networks with XBee and Arduino." In: *The 2nd International Conference on Systems and Informatics (ICSAI 2014), November 2014*: 492-496.

Korkalainen, M., Sallinen, M., Kärkkäinen, N., and Tukeva, P. 2009. "Survey of wireless sensor networks simulation tools for demanding applications." In: *2009 Fifth International Conference on Networking and Services*, April 2009, 102-106.

Nandiyanto, A. B. D., Zaen, R., Oktiani, R., Abdullah, A. G., and Riza, L. S. 2018. "A simple, rapid analysis, portable, low-cost, and Arduino-based spectrophotometer with white LED as a light source for analyzing solution concentration." *Telkomnika*, 16(2):580-585.

Nandiyanto, A. B. D., Ragadhita, R., Abdullah, A. G., Triawan, F., Ketut, G., and Sunnardianto, M. A. 2019. "Techno-economic feasibility study of low-cost and portable home-made spectrophotometer for analyzing solution concentration." *Journal of Engineering Science and Technology*, 14(2):599-609.

Prathap, U., Shenoy, P. D., Venugopal, K. R., and Patnaik, L. M. 2012. "Wireless sensor networks applications and routing protocols: survey and research challenges." In: *2012 international symposium on cloud and services computing* (December):49-56.

Puccinelli, D., and Haenggi, M. 2005. "Wireless sensor networks: applications and challenges of ubiquitous sensing." *IEEE Circuits and systems magazine*, vol. 5, no. 3: 19-31.

Razon, B. C. 2020. "COVID 19: Impetus for "Community Spirits" among Filipinos." *Indonesian Journal of Science and Technology* vol. 5, no. 2 (March): 201-208.

Sergii. I. 2009. "grTheory - Graph Theory Toolbox." *MATLAB Central File Exchange*. http://www.mathworks.com/matlabcentral/fileexchange /4266.

Simek, M., and Moravek, P. 2011. "Modeling of Energy Consumption of Zigbee Devices in Matlab Tool." *ElektroRevue* Vol. 2 No. 3 (September) 2011.

Sobeih, A., Hou, J. C., Kung, L. C., Li, N., Zhang, H., Chen, W. P., and Lim, H. 2006. "J-Sim: A Simulation and Emulation Environment for Wireless Sensor Networks." *Wireless Communications*, vol. 13, no. 4, (September):104-119.

Sukmafitri, A., Nandiyanto, A. B. D., Oktiani, R., Ragadhita, R., and Abdullah, A. G. 2019. "Temperature on the effectiveness of Arduino-based portable spectrophotometer with white light-emitting diode (led) as a light source for analyzing solution concentration." *Journal of Engineering Science and Technology*, 14(3):1653-1661.

About the Editors

Asep Bayu Dani Nandiyanto
Associate Professor
Universitas Pendidikan Indonesia, Bandung, Jawa Barat, Indonesia
Corresponding Editor's Email: nandiyanto@upi.edu

Asep Bayu Dani Nandiyanto is an Associate Professor in Chemistry at Universitas Pendidikan Indonesia, Indonesia. He received B.Eng. (2005) in Chemical Engineering at Institut Teknologi Bandung. He received M. Eng. (2008) and Dr. Eng. (2011) in Chemical Engineering at Hiroshima University. He was selected as a prestigious JSPS fellow (2011-2013). He was also a Visiting Professor at King Fahd University of Petroleum and Minerals in Saudi Arabia (2011) and an Assistant Professor at Hiroshima University in Japan (2013-2014). He was a visiting Assistant Professor at Tokyo Institute of Technology (2018) and a visiting scholar at Virginia Commonwealth University (2018) under RISTEK DIKTI Fulbright fellowship. Nandiyanto's research is in the area of particle technology, specifically the production of fine particles and their applications. He also works in science education. He has published eight patents and 35 copyright, 11 books, three book chapters, three review papers, 56 peer-reviewed

Scopus-indexed articles, and 105 refereed Scopus-indexed journal articles. He has received numerous awards (more than 13 awards), such as the Society of Chemical Engineers Japan Award for Outstanding Young Researcher (2013) and the George Klinzing Award from American Institute of Chemical Engineer (2014).

Tryastuti Irawati Belliny Manullang
PhD Candidate
Universitas Pendidikan Indonesia, Bandung, Jawa Barat, Indonesia

Tryastuti Irawati Belliny Manullang is a PhD candidate in Special Needs Education Program at Universitas Pendidikan Indonesia. She has experiences in teaching preschool students, special needs students. She is actively involved in Continuous Professional Development through Lesson Study in West Java and the Innovation Lab at Universitas Pendidikan Indonesia. Her research focuses on inclusive education and special education implementation in Indonesia.

Rina Maryanti
PhD Candidate
Universitas Pendidikan Indonesia, Bandung, Jawa Barat, Indonesia

Rina Maryanti is a PhD candidate in Special Need Education Program at Universitas Pendidikan Indonesia. She studied Special Education program for her undergraduate and postgraduate in Universitas Pendidikan Indonesia. She has an experience as a teacher and principal at Special School in Kuningan, Indonesia. She is also actively involved in the organization, carrying out social activities, fostering teachers and the community, and making the assessment program for children with special needs in West Java Province.

Her research focuses on increasing the life skills of students with special needs through science learning at school. She has also published several international journals indexed by Scopus through the research she is working on.

Amir Machmud

Associate Professor
Universitas Pendidikan Indonesia, Bandung, Jawa Barat, Indonesia

Amir Machmud is an Associate Professor at Faculty of Business and Economics Universitas Pendidikan Indonesia. He completed his studies in Human Resources Management from IKOPIN Sumedang (1993), then graduated from Economics and Development Studies from Universitas Padjajaran Bandung (1996) and completed his PhD in Economics. His research is in the fields of economics and business. He has had wide-ranging research experience and has published several articles both in national and international journals.

A. Ana

Associate Professor
Universitas Pendidikan Indonesia, Bandung, Jawa Barat, Indonesia

A. Ana is an Associate Professor and Vice Dean in Faculty of Technology and Vocational Education Universitas Pendidikan Indonesia. She completed her education from the culinary art from IKIP Bandung. She graduated from Technology and Vocational Education Universitas Negeri Yogyakarta in 2004 and completed her doctoral degree from the same university. She has served as the Head of the Child and Elderly Services Laboratory of Culinary Art Department Faculty of Technology and Vocational Education Universitas Pendidikan Indonesia (2011-2016). She is also a research counselor in RMUTT Thailand. She was chosen as the best lecturer in Faculty of Technology and Vocational Education Universitas Pendidikan Indonesia in 2013. She has published two books, five patents, and around 54 research articles. She has also been a keynote speaker at several national and international conferences.

Asnul Dahar Minghad
Professor
Razak Faculty of Technology and Informatics,
Universiti Teknologi Malaysia;
University College of Islam Melaka, Malaysia

Asnul Dahar Bin Minghat is an Associate Professor in Universiti Teknologi Malaysia. He completed his studies in Mechanical Engineering from Universiti Teknologi Malaysia in 1997, then completed his master from the Vocational Education program in Universiti Putra Malaysia (2000) and his PhD from Universiti Kebangsaan Malaysia in 2012. He had served as a teacher in a vocational school before becoming a lecturer. His research is in the field of Technical and Vocational Education. He has published eleven research articles that have been indexed by Scopus, eight non-indexed journals, two book chapters, and his articles have been cited twenty times. He is also actively involved in national and international conferences and has been a keynote speaker on conferences and general lectures for several times.

INDEX

#

A

B

C

H

I

K

L

M

N

O

P

R

S

U

V

W